Springer
Tokyo
Berlin
Heidelberg
New York
Barcelona
Hong Kong
London
Milan
Paris

H. Kikuchi (Ed.)

Strategic Medical Science Against Brain Attack

With 115 Figures, Including 28 in Color

Springer

Haruhiko Kikuchi
President Emeritus
NATIONAL CARDIO-VASCULAR CENTER
5-7-1 Fujishiro-dai, Suita
Osaka 565-8565, Japan

ISBN-13: 978-4-431-68432-9 e-ISBN-13: 978-4-431-68430-5
DOI: 10.1007/978-4-431-68430-5

Library of Congress Cataloging-in-Publication Data
Strategic medical science against brain attack / H. Kikuchi, ed.
p. cm.
Includes bibliographical references and index.

1. Cerebrovascular disease. 2. Cerebral ischemia. I. Kikuchi, Haruhiko.

RC388.5 .S826 2002
616.8'1—dc21

2002021805

Printed on acid-free paper

Softcover reprint of the hardcover 1st edition 2002

Typesetting: Authors

SPIN: 10868599

Foreword

The importance of the therapeutic time window for ischemic stroke has been widely accepted for a long time. Consequently, I have been thinking about the past, when the term "brain attack," which was reimported from the United States, began to spread by repetition.

In the 1980s, I had made an enthusiastic study of acute-phase cerebral revascularization for ischemic stroke. At that time, we could cure only a quite limited number of patients, such as those who already were hospitalized or who, fortunately, were brought to the hospital within a few hours from the onset of the stroke.

RM Crowell, in his 1977 report[1] on cases of failure, had identified the considerable problems in acute-phase cerebral revascularization as diagnosis of tissue reversibility, brain-protective reagents or methods, and effective techniques for revascularization. I remember that we strongly endorsed his opinion.

Recently, the basic study of stroke has advanced significantly, resulting in newly developed materials and new experimental techniques, which are introduced in this book. I hope that new basic knowledge will be clinically applied.

Strategic Medical Science Against Brain Attack will serve as a source book bridging basic studies and clinical application. This edited volume is one in which the contributors share their expertise and specialized knowledge in their field of work. They introduce the possibility of neuritic reconstruction and neurogeneration, by cells or tissue transplantation to the damaged organ. They also demonstrate the role of the MEK/ERK pathway, for instance, as a biological pathway, and cortical spreading depression as a biophysiological pathway of the mechanism for ischemic neuronal cell damage. In considering the process of neuronal cell death, there is a focus on signal transduction and gene expression in neuronal cells, which are significant factors in cell death. In a molecular approach to subarachnoid hemorrhage, the process from aneurysm formation to the mechanism of cerebral vasospasm is discussed in detail. In addition, the effects of hypothermia and the usefulness of MR imaging in ischemic stroke are summarized for clinical application.

---

[1]Crowell RM (1977) STA-MCA bypass for acute focal cerebral ischemia, In: Schmiedek P et al (eds) Microsurgery for stroke. Springer, Berlin Heidelberg New York, pp 244–250.

It is hoped that these strategies one day in the future will make us entirely free from brain attack, which now is of such great clinical concern.

Takashi Yoshimoto

Dean, Tohoku University Graduate School of Medicine
Professor and Chairman, Department of Neurosurgery
Tohoku University Graduate School of Medicine
Sendai

February 2002

Preface

There are two kinds of strategies in the world: one, which should remain secret, is to protect society from attacks by enemies; the other, which should be actively propagated, is to protect anyone and everyone from catastrophes, including diseases. Based on the belief that a human being is an invaluable entity that should survive on the earth as long as possible, this book is one of the most advanced records of scientists and clinicians who have tried to fight numerous etiologic factors that cause "stroke" and who also have tried to make progress against cerebral disorders that appear in the battle against brain attack.

Up to now, we have lost tremendous numbers of battles to protect the brain because of the lack of effective weapons, resulting in the loss of very important persons or their cerebral functions. However, recent progress in medical science that focuses on the central nervous system is on the way to creating new weapons with which it may be possible to fight life- and brain-threatening attacks effectively.

There are several approaches to joining the battle: protecting the brain from slowly and latently progressing cerebrovascular injuries; assessing the strength of brain attacks and diagnosing the depth of injury in deciding how best to treat disease; protecting the brain from the rapid progression of cerebrovascular disorders following the onset of stroke; and promoting brain recovery or re-establishing brain functions after initial stroke damage, using techniques of neuroregeneration. All the approaches described in this book may not be enough yet to construct the best defense system against brain attack because modern medical science is advancing rapidly, which may make another new approach possible soon. I hope, however, that the new information provided here, composed of data from researchers and clinicians who are fighting a real and ongoing battle, will open a door for many readers and will give them insight into a world where humans will be able to avoid any possible discomfort caused by brain attacks.

On the timescale of human history, these advances in medical science have reached the point when we are going to receive the first group of photons on a light-beam directly from the rising sun.

Haruhiko Kikuchi
President Emeritus
NATIONAL CARDIO-VASCULAR CENTER
Osaka

Acknowledgments

This book includes the results of the research project entitled "Protection of the Brain Against Brain Attacks" (1997–2002), supported by Special Coordination Funds for the Promotion of Science and Technology from the Ministry of Education, Culture, Sports, Science and Technology (MEXT) of Japan. The contributions from the authors and the secretarial assistance by Ms. Tomoko Yasuda are gratefully acknowledged. We thank Springer-Verlag Tokyo for accepting our proposal for this publication.

Contents

3. Strategies using survival or death signals in neurons

4. Strategies for and from cortical spreading depression

5. Strategies using hypothermia

6. Strategies for cerebral aneurysm and vasospasm

7. Developments in brain-imaging technology

List of Contributors

1. Strategies using neuritic reconstruction and neuroregeneration

Neural stem cells as a tool for cell transplantation

Jun Takahashi, Hiroki Toda, and Nobuo Hashimoto

Department of Neurosurgery, Clinical Neuroscience, Kyoto University Graduate School of Medicine, Kyoto 606-8507, Japan

Summary: Basic fibroblast growth factor responsive neural stem cells (NSCs) derived from adult rat hippocampus were earlier demonstrated to generate neurons and glia. These stem cell-derived neurons express GABA, acetylcholinesterase, tyrosine hydroxylase, or calbindin.
We cultured these adult NSCs on a glial feeder layer to test the competence of adult NSCs. We observed that the differentiated adult NSCs possessed membrane excitability and demonstrated glutamatergic and GABAergic synaptic transmission. These results suggested that NSCs from adult rat hippocampus differentiated into functional neurons which were able to form functional synapses in vitro.
Next, to determine the therapeutic effects of NSCs in the ischemic brain, we grafted these NSCs derived from adult rat hippocampus into the hippocampus of rats with transient global ischemia. In this study, grafted NSCs survived and differentiated into neurons in the hippocampus. Furthermore, the rats with more than 120 neurons showed recovery from the impairment of spatial recognition in the water maze test.
These results support the concept that NSCs in the adult brain have a potential to differentiate into functional neurons that can be integrated into the neuronal circuitry.

Key words: Neural stem cells, Differentiation, Transplantation, Ischemia

Introduction

Much previous evidence from animal studies has shown that cell transplantation is an effective strategy for functional regeneration in central nervous system (CNS) disorders [1]. Furthermore, transplantation of embryonic neural cells has been justified for patients with Parkinson's disease [2]. In a double-blinded study, human embryonic dopamine-neuron transplants survived in patients with Parkinson's disease and resulted in some clinical benefit in younger patients. However the supply of embryonic tissue is limited, and ethical issues also remain to be solved.

Under these circumstances, neural stem cells (NSCs) are expected to be another source of cell transplantation therapy for various neurological disorders, including cerebral infarction. In this article, we would like to discuss about the therapeutic potentials of NSCs against "Brain Attack".

NSCs differentiate into neurons which express neurotransmitters

Neural stem cells (NSCs) are immature cells with the ability of self-renewal, and they give rise to neurons, astrocytes, and oligodendrocytes (Fig. 1). These cells persist in the subventricular zone, hippocampus, and spinal cord, even in adult CNS [3].

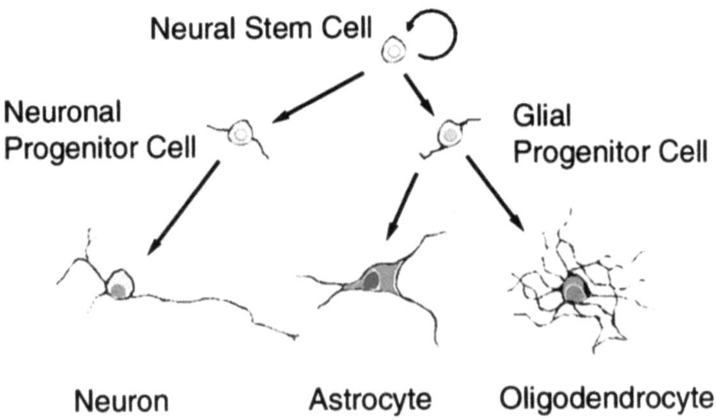

Fig. 1. The ontogeny of neural stem cells. Neural stem cells proliferate in response to fibroblast growth fractor-2 (FGF-2) and/or epidermal growth factor (EGF). Without mitogen, these cells commit to a neuoral or glial lineage, and become neurons, astrocytes and oligodendrocytes.

We have reported that FGF-2-responsive progenitor cells can be isolated from the hippocampus of embryonic [4] and adult rats [5,6]. Furthermore, detailed analyses of clonal populations derived from these cultures revealed that FGF-2-responsive cells from adult rat hippocampus have characteristics of stem cells: the ability to self-renew and to generate both neurons and glia *in vitro* [7]. To better understand the molecular signaling that regulates adult stem cell differentiation, a genetically marked normal diploid clone of multipotent stem cells isolated from the adult rat hippocampus [7] were used to examine the role of retinoic acid (RA) and neurotrophins in neuronal differentiation.

For proliferating conditions, clonal stem cells (AP14) were cultured in Dulbecco's Modified Eagles Medium/Ham's F12 (DMEM/F12, 1:1) containing N2 supplement (Gibco BRL, Gaithersburg, MD) and 20 ng/ml rhFGF-2 (provided by A. Baird, Prizm Pharmaceuticals Inc., La Jolla, CA). For differentiation experiments, cells were plated into polyornithine/laminin coated glass chamber slides (Nunc, Naperville, IL) at a density of 2.5 x 10^3 per cm^2. The cells were incubated for 24 hrs in normal N2 medium containing 20 ng/ml FGF-2, and then the medium was replaced by N2 medium containing 0.5% fetal bovine serum (FBS) and 0.01% DMSO (control solvent) or 0.5 mM all-trans retinoic acid (Sigma, St. Louis, MO). For further differentiation, the medium was replaced by N2 medium containing 0.5% FBS and one of the following; sterile water (control solvent), mouse 2.5S NGF (50 ng/ml, Boehringer Mannheim, Indianapolis, IN), rhBDNF (20 ng/ml, Alomone Labs, Jerusalem, Israel), rhNT-3 (40 ng/ml, Genentech, South San Francisco, CA).

RA treatment significantly increased the number of cells differentiating into microtubule-associated protein 2ab (MAP2ab)-immunoreactive neurons. RT-PCR analysis revealed that RA was stimulating an immediate upregulation of *NeuroD*, a more gradual upregulation of *p21* and a simultaneous reduction in cell proliferation. RA also induced the expression of *trk*A, B, C and *p75*NGFR, thus making the cells responsive to neurotrophins. To determine how the RA-induced responsiveness to neurotrophins affected neuronal differentiation and/or maturation, we first treated the multipotent stem cells with RA for 6 days, then withdrew RA and added either NGF, BDNF or NT-3 for another 6 or 12 days. The application of RA followed by neurotrophins led to a significant increase in the proportion of neurons displaying mature gamma-aminobutyric acid (GABA), acetylcholinesterase (AChE), tyrosine hydroxylase (TH), or calbindin phenotypes but had little effect on the total number of neurons generated in response to RA alone. These results suggest that RA and neurotrophins act sequentially to first trigger the early events of neuronal commitment and subsequently promote neuronal maturation. Together, these processes are sufficient to direct the differentiation of a single adult-derived neural stem cell into mature neurons displaying a variety of transmitter phenotypes (Fig. 2).

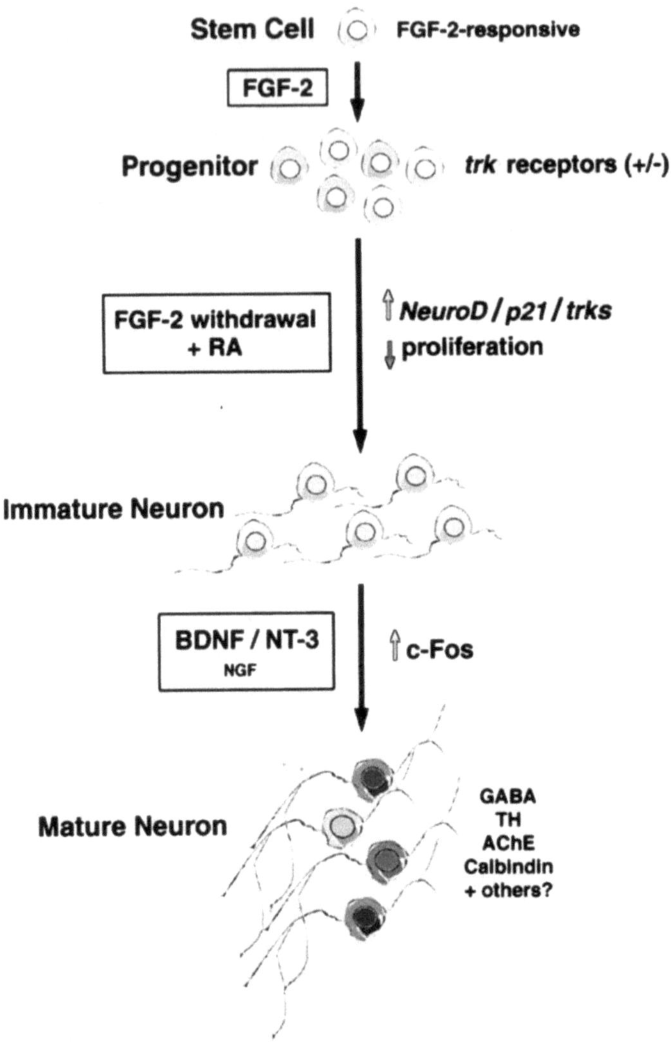

Fig. 2. Sequential regulatory events in adult hippocampus-derived stem cell neurogenesis. A single stem cell proliferates in the presence of FGF-2 to generate a clonal population of daughter cells that include new stem cells and progenitors committed to neuronal or glial lineages. In cells destined to become neurons, growth factor withdrawal and RA stimulation trigger the expression of NeuroD, elicit a gradual increase in the cell-cycle moderator, p21, and render the cells sensitive to neurotrophins by maintaining or up-regulating expression of the Trk receptors. RA treatment alone is sufficient to maximally stimulate the accumulation of MAP2ab-immunoreactive neurons; however, subsequent treatment with neurotrophins promotes the maturation of these immature cells into mature neurons that display one or more neurotransmitter phenotype. (Adapted with permission from Ref. 8)

NSCs form functional glutamatergic and GABAergic synapses in vitro

As mentioned above, we demonstrated that bFGF-responsive NSCs from adult rat hippocampus gave rise to neurons and glial cells after treatment with retinoic acid in the absence of bFGF [7]. Five to 10% of the differentiated adult NSCs expressed MAP2ab or other neuronal markers such as MAP5, NeuN, or neurofilament 200 (NF200). In a following study [8], the GABAergic, dopaminergic, or cholinergic phenotypes were identified in NSC neurons by immunofluorescence or histochemical staining methods.

As a cell source for transplantation, NSCs have to form synapses with host neurons. Other studies using differently isolated NSCs have demonstrated that neurons from NSCs generate action potentials [9,10]. However, there was no direct evidence that demonstrates the formation of functional synapses by NSCs *in vivo* or *in vitro*. So we decided to test the competence of adult NSCs to do so in order to evaluate their potential for cell therapy against various neurological diseases [11,12] and also to examine the concept of continual neuronal replacement in the adult CNS.

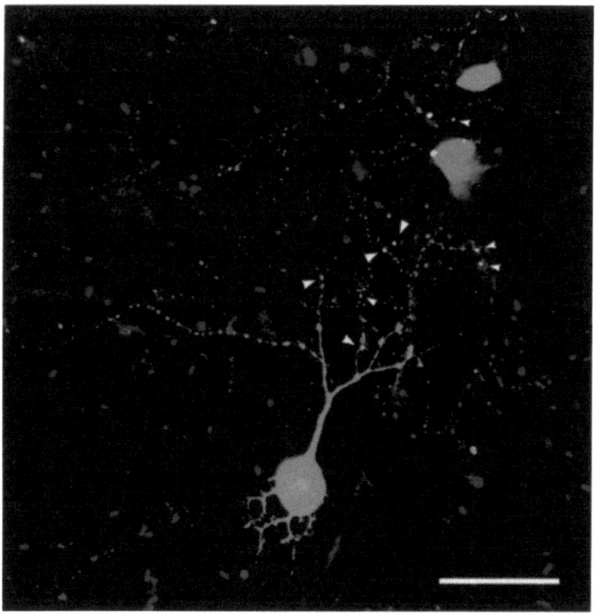

Fig. 3. Confocal micrographs of differentiated NSCs (GFP-labeled) and E18 hippocampal neurons. NSCs were GFP-positive (green), and synaptobrevin-immunoreactive cells were stained with Texas red (red). There were some contacts between the neurites that extended from E18 neurons and NSC neurons (appeared yellow, arrowheads). Scale bar, 50 μm. (Adapted with permission from Ref. 22)

In this experiment we used clonal NSCs previously isolated from adult rat hippocampus, PZ5 cells [7]. We marked PZ5 cells with green fluorescent protein (GFP) by use of a GFP-expressing retroviral vector, which also carried the hygromycin B resistance gene. GFP-positive PZ5 cells were selected in the presence of 50 μg / ml hygromycin B. The selected cells were plated on a glial feeder layer prepared from rat hippocampus of embryonic day 18 to postnatal day 1. NSCs were discriminated from other cells by their fluorescence. GFP fluorescence enabled us to recognize the morphological changes of differentiated NSCs. Some of the differentiated NSCs increased in their size and possessed neurite-like processes. Neuronal differentiation and synaptic specialization of differentiated NSCs were demonstrated by double staining of GFP-marked NSCs for synaptobrevin and MAP2ab on 18 DIV (Fig. 3). Synaptobrevin and MAP2ab were co-localized in GFP-positive PZ5 cells, and some of their neurites showed intense punctate immunoreactivity for synaptobrevin. After 18 DIV the proportions of MAP2ab-positive and synaptobrevin-positive cells were estimated. MAP2ab-positive cells were 5.0±1.4 percent of the GFP-positive cell population in glia-free cultures and 5.6±1.8% in cocultures. Cells both MAP2ab and synaptobrevin-positive were 3.3 ± 1.8% in glia-free cultures and 3.8±1.5% in cocultures. PZ5 cells were also immunoreactive for both NF200 and synaptophysin. NF200-positive cells were 2.2±1.3% of the GFP-positive cells in glia-free cultures and 2.4±1.5% in cocultures. Cells both NF200 and synaptophysin-positive were 2.2±1.2% in glia-free cultures and 2.1±1.2% in cocultures. GFAP-positive cells were 6.6±4.9% of the GFP-positive cells in glia-free cultures and 5.1±4.1% in cocultures. These results suggest that pre-synaptic specialization had occurred on the nerve terminals of NSC-derived neurons by 18 DIV. These neurons from NSCs made contact with each other or with primary hippocampal neurons that had been added to the cultures after 7 DIV.

Ultrastructural observation of these nerve terminals by immunoelectron microscopy utilizing immunogold particles to label GFP-positive cells with anti-GFP antibody showed cell-cell contacts with synapse-like ultrastructures, between a primary cultured neuron and a GFP-positive nerve terminal or between two GFP-positive nerve terminals. These cell-cell contacts consisted of closely apposed membranes of two neural components, and one of the components contained clusters of pleiomorphic vesicles characteristic of chemical synapses. These vesicle-like structures were noted in three samples of the eight examined cell-cell contact sites between NSCs or between NSCs and primary hippocampal cells on the glial feeder layer. There were no such contact regions with similar structures in 10 samples taken from glia-free cultures, though there were cell-cell contacts with slightly increased membrane density.

PZ5 cells were recognized under a fluorescence microscope by their GFP fluorescence (Fig. 5A). Cells on astroglial monolayers were tested for their membrane excitability. After 6 DIV, 33 % of the NSCs tested (four of 12 cells) on glial feeder layer showed TTX-sensitive fast inward currents, namely, sodium currents, under the voltage-clamp condition. These currents were shown in 83% of the tested cells (10 of 12 cells) after 12 DIV, and in 80% of the tested cells (eight of 10 cells) after 18 DIV. The amplitude of the sodium current was enhanced with days in culture: -0.55 ± 0.10 nA on 6 DIV and -2.07 ± 0.67 nA after 18 DIV (Table 2). The resting membrane potential was -32.7 ± 3.9 mV on 6 DIV and -46.2 ± 5.1 mV on 18 DIV. Some of these NSCs generated action potentials when stimulated with a depolarizing current. After 12 DIV, immature action potentials of low amplitude and long duration were recorded in 30 % of the cells (three of 10 cells) displaying a TTX-sensitive sodium current. The resting membrane potential of these cells was from -38.6 mV to -46 mV (N=3). After 18 DIV, in 37% of the cells (3 of 8 cells) having a TTX-sensitive sodium current, typical overshooting action potentials were elicited; and their amplitudes were up to 60 mV, and their duration was 3.2 to 3.5 msec (Fig. 5B). Their resting membrane potentials were from -52.2 to -57.1 mV. Sodium currents recorded from these cells were larger than those of cells at 6 DIV or 12 DIV: from -2.2 to -6.5 nA (N=3). A much prolonged time in culture up to 35 DIV did not result in any changes in the shape of the action potentials.

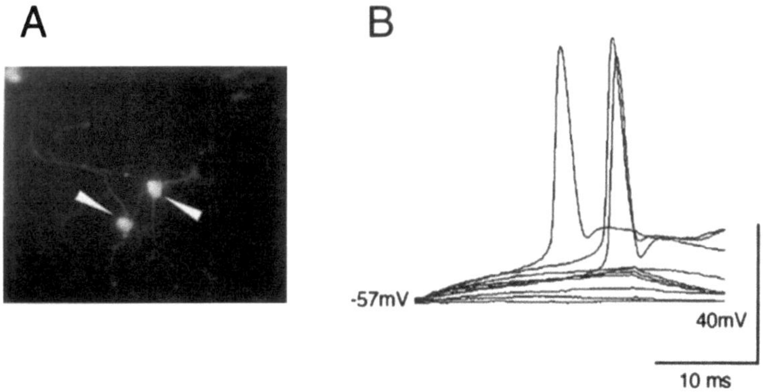

Fig. 4. Electrophysiological recordings from differentiated NSCs on 18-35 DIV in culture by the whole-cell patch clamp method. (**A**) Differentiated NSCs (arrowheads) on DIV18 with neurites, rather large cell bodies, and green fluorescence from GFP. (**B**) Action potentials from a NSC-derived neuron on 18 DIV. Superimposed responses elicited from resting membrane potential of –57mV by brief current pulses. The amplitudes of action potentials are up to 60 mV, and the durations are 3.2 to 3.5 msec. Small afterhyperpolarizations are observed (arrow). (Adapted with permission from Ref. 22)

Cells from glia-free culture (N=70) from 0-28 DIV did not show the expression of action potentials. After 18 DIV, 58.3% of NSCs tested (7 of 12 cells) from glia-free cultures showed TTX-sensitive fast inward currents with an amplitude of -0.74 ± 0.51 nA, namely, immature sodium currents.

During 0-35 days, 354 of 520 cells tested in coculture showed TTX-sensitive fast inward currents, and they were treated with TTX and Barium to record mPSCs. Among these tested cells, six cells from NSCs in coculture (DIV 28-35) showed spontaneous mPSCs, suggesting the presence of functional synaptic transmission. Using the voltage-clamp method at a holding potential of –69 mV, we elicited mPSCs with two different kinetics by exposing the cells to 10 m*M* barium in the presence of 1 *μM* TTX (Fig. 6 upper trace). The mPSCs with rapid kinetics (N=95) were blocked by 10 *μM* DNQX, but not by 20 *μM* bicuculline (excitatory mPSCs: mEPSCs) (Fig. 6B lower, left). The remaining mPSCs (N=114) had slower kinetics and were blocked by 20 *μ*M bicuculline, but not by 10 *μM* DNQX (inhibitory mPSCs: mIPSCs) (Fig. 6B lower, right). From an average of 18 mEPSCs with rapid kinetics, the decay time constant was calculated by a best fit of a single exponential function to be 6.3 msec. From the average of 20 mIPSCs, the decay time constant was similarly calculated to be 15.3 msec. An amplitude histogram of mEPSCs showed a distribution with a skew, and its mean value was 29.2 pA. Amplitudes of mIPSCs were distributed over a wide range, and the mean value was 54.1 pA. mPSCs were not observed up to 28 DIV when NSCs were in a glia-free culture.

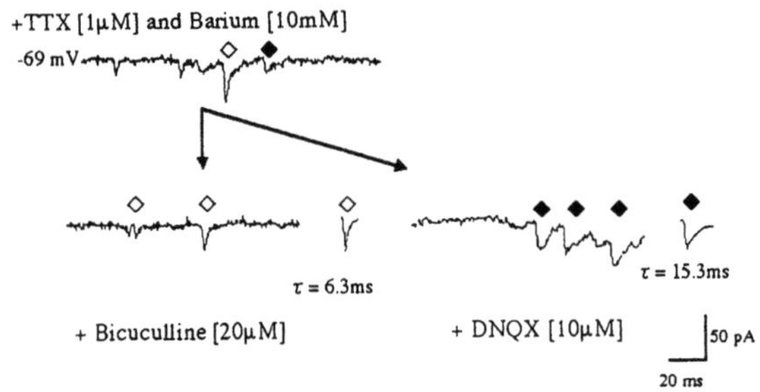

Fig. 5. Sample traces of spontaneous mPSCs with fast- (◇) and slow-decaying (◆) responses. mEPSCs (◇) elicited in the presence of bicuculline and blocked by DNQX. mIPSCs (◆) elicited in the presence of DNQX and blocked by bicuculline. The decay time constant of mEPSCs is 6.3 msec; and that of mIPSCs, 15.3 msec. CsCl and CsOH were used instead of KCl and KOH in the internal solution, when miniature post-synaptic currents were recorded. (Adapted with permission from Ref. 22)

Our morphological data suggest that neurons from adult NSCs seem to acquire presynaptic and postsynaptic specialization by 18 DIV. However, as was reported previously [13], morphological appearance is not always predictive of electrophysiological properties. Our physiological data showed that the differentiated NSCs with neuronal morphology underwent maturation of membrane excitability within 6 days after induction of differentiation and that this maturational process progressed until 18 DIV. The increase in amplitude of sodium channel current and the late appearance of the action potentials suggest that functional sodium channels developed gradually and that their density increased with time in culture. The increase in the resting membrane potentials also suggests the development of other components of membrane ionic channels such as potassium channels and some transporters, which also contribute to the generation of mature action potentials. From the electrophysiological recording of mouse multipotent stem cells [9], their resting membrane potentials or magnitude of the action potentials were similar to those found as our results, but a larger afterhyperpolarization with shorter duration of spikes was noted than that found as our results. In rat neural precursor cells from SVZ and spinal cord (SC), resting membrane potentials and amplitude of action potentials were similar to those we found, though SC cells showed relatively lower resting membrane potentials and smaller action potentials [10]. Human NSCs have TTX-sensitive sustained firing in their action potentials [14]. These variances between studies are considered to be partly due to the differences in species, region of CNS, methods of isolation, or age of cells in culture.

Formation of functional synapses occurred in 1.2 percent of the tested cells (six of 520 cells) during 28-35 DIV, suggesting that the synaptic maturation was delayed to match the maturation of membrane excitability (N=6). Approximately 55% of mPSCs with rapid kinetics (time constant of 6.3 msec) were glutamatergic through the activation of AMPA type-glutamatergic receptors (mEPSCs) because they were blocked by 10 μM DNQX, but not by 20 μM bicuculline (Fig. 4 lower, left). The remaining mPSCs with slower kinetics (time constant of 15.3 msec) were GABAergic mediated by $GABA_A$ receptors (mIPSCs), as they were blocked by 20 μM bicuculline, but not by 10 μM DNQX (Fig. 4 lower, right). The properties in the amplitude histogram of mEPSCs and mIPSCs are similar to those described for cultured hippocampal neurons [15,16]. These results demonstrate that adult NSCs differentiate into neurons that acquire functional and morphological specialization of both excitatory and inhibitory synapses and also that a single neuron derived from a NSC receives both excitatory and inhibitory synaptic inputs. The use of fluorescence and morphological chatacteristics for the detection of NSC-derived neurons might lead us to choose non-neuronal cell for the electrophysiological study. Therefore, the percentage of cells showing neuronal activities among the tested cells might actually be higher than that presented in this study.

In our present study, the glial feeder layer seems to play an important role for maturation of membrane excitability and synaptogenesis of NSCs, because no synaptic currents were recorded under glia-free conditions, though several exogenous trophic factors such as BDNF and NT3 were present. As depicted in the previous studies, several neurotrophic effects by glia may have occurred, such as trophic signals from glia for neuronal differentiation [17], metabolic coupling in glucose or glutamate uptake [18], induction of the sodium channel cluster by glia [19], or enhancement of synapse formation [20]. Moreover, interaction with astrocytes has been reported to stimulate neurogenesis by SVZ precursors [21]. Some soluble factors from glia or cell/cell contact between stem cells and glia could be essential for the differentiation and maturation of neurons derived from NSCs.

NSCs differentiate into neurons in the ischemic brain, and improve spatial recognition

As shown in our data mentioned above and also data from another laboratory, neurons derived from NSCs are able to form functional synapses in vitro[22,23] and in vivo [24]. These results suggest that NSCs have a potential to differentiate into appropriate neurons to form a functional neuronal circuitry around the graft site. Therefore, NSCs are expected to be an alternative source of cell transplantation therapy for various neurological disorders.

Transient global ischemia in rats causes relatively circumscribed and specific damage to the CA1 pyramidal neurons of the hippocampus [25], resulting in impairment of spatial learning and memory tasks [26]. So, as a next step, to determine the therapeutic effects of NSCs in the ischemic brain, we grafted NSCs derived from adult rat hippocampus into the hippocampus of rats with transient global ischemia.

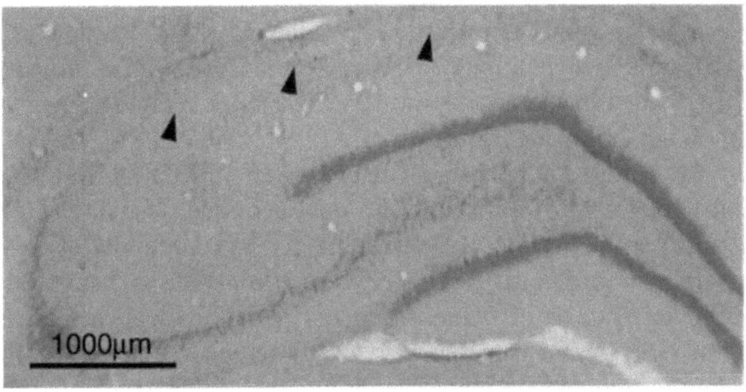

Fig. 6. Loss of CA1 pyramidal cells was shown in hematoxylin-eosin steining (arrows). Scale bar, 1000 μm.

First, the survival and differentiation of the grafted NSCs were analyzed. Male adult Fischer-344 rats weighing 260-300g (Charles River Japan, Yokohama, Japan) were used as both the source of the donor cells and as recipients. All the procedures were performed under anesthesia achieved with an intraperitoneal injection of sodium pentobarbital. Transient global ischemia was induced by the four-vessel occlusion method of Pulsinelli [25]. As Fischer rats are vulnerable to ischemic insult, some modifications were made as described below. Vertebral arteries were coagulated on the first day. Seven days later, silastic threads were inserted around the carotid arteries and brought to the surface. Then three days later, the threads were tightened for 15 minutes. Fourteen controls were subjected to an identical procedure, except the threads were not tightened. Two weeks after ischemia surgery, groups of rats were randomly selected to receive NSCs. For controls, 14 ischemic rats and 14 non-ischemic rats were injected with only the vehicle. NSCs used in this experiment, named as PZ5, were derived from the adult hippocampus and monoclonally isolated [7,22]. For nuclear labeling, NSCs were pretreated with 5μM of 5-bromo-2'-deoxyuridine (BrdU) for three days before grafting. A cell suspension was prepared at the density of 5×10^4 cells/μl, and 1.5 μl of the suspension was stereotaxically injected into the dorsal hippocampus bilaterally. The coordinates, anterior-posterior (AP) measured from bregma, lateral (ML) from the midline, and depth (DV) from dura, were as follow (in mm): AP –3.5; ML ±3.0; DV –2.8.

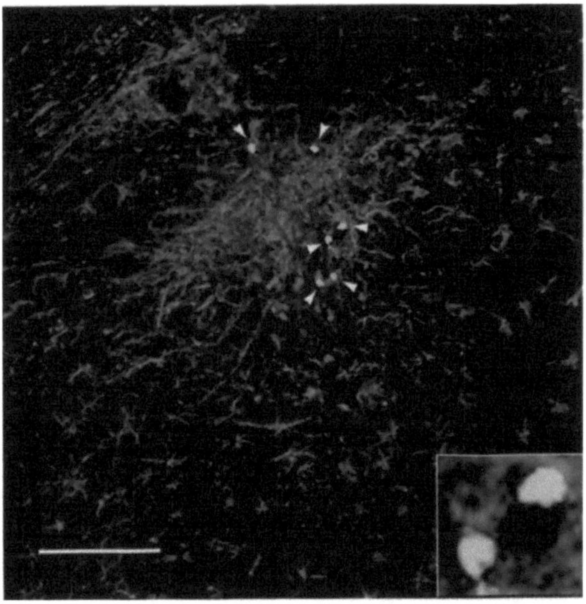

Fig. 7. Triple-labeled confocal imaging of the grafted cells. BrdU-labeled (green) and NeuN-positive (red) and GFAP-positive cells (blue) were observed in the grafted area in the hippocampus. Double-labeled cells for BrdU and NeuN appeared to be yellow (arrowheads and insets), which indicate NSC-derived neurons. Scale bar, 200 μm. (Adapted with permission from Ref. 35)

On day 10 of the behavioral test described below, the rats were perfused with 4% paraformaldehyde. Coronal sections stained with hematoxylin/eosin were examined for hippocampal pathology. Cell loss was graded bilaterally on a five-point scale [27]. Anti-BrdU staining was performed, and the number of BrdU-labeled cells was quantified in every sixth section through the hippocampus by using a stereological procedure as previously described [5]. Triple- and double-labeled immunofluorescence staining was performed to analyze the grafted NSCs. Transient global ischemia by the four-vessel occlusion yielded selective loss of pyramidal neurons in the hippocampal CA1 region (Fig. 6). Eleven out of 14 ischemic control rats and 10 out of 15 grafted rats showed 90 to 95% losses of the cells. Only these animals were included in the following analyses. Nuclear labeling of NSCs with BrdU made 90% of the cells positive for BrdU *in vitro*. Immunostaining for BrdU revealed that the grafted cells were localized in the hippocampal CA1, corpus callosum, and along the needle tract. The number of surviving cells in the CA1 region of each side was about 500 – 2000. These cells were dispersed throughout the graft area in CA1, but seemed to reconstitute the laminar organization of the normal CA1 field. The triple-labeling immunofluorescence study showed that 3-9% of the BrdU-positive cells was also positive for NeuN, indicating differentiation of the grafted NSCs into neurons (Fig. 7).

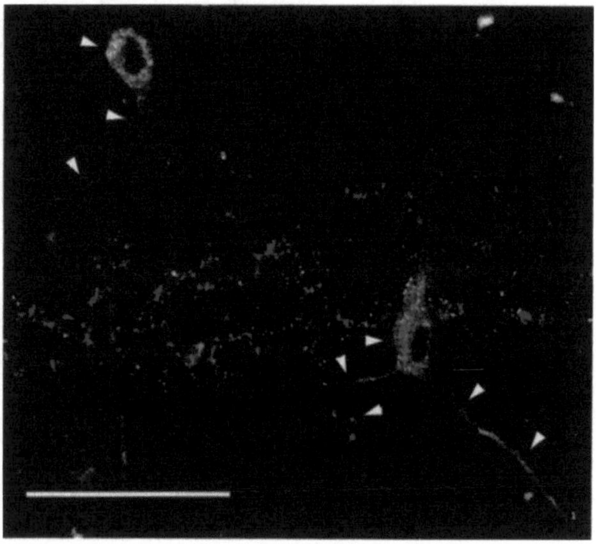

Fig. 8. Grafted NSCs stained with the mouse anti-β-gal antibody (green) and anti-synaptobrevin antibody (red). β-gal-positive cells (arrowheads) in the CA1 pyramidal cell layer exhibited neurite-like processes, and they were co-localized with synaptobrevin. Scale bar, 50 μm. (Adapted with permission from Ref. 35)

The hippocampus-derived NSCs, PZ5, used in this study also have a cytoplasmic b-galactosidase gene introduced by a retroviral vector [7]. Immunostaining with anti-ß-gal and anti-synaptobrevin antibodies showed that the grafted cells located in the pyramidal cell layer had neurite-like processes, and were co-localized with synaptobrevin (Fig. 8). Gliotic changes around the grafts were also noted in several rats. There was a tendency that the rats with more gliosis had fewer neurons. No tumor formation was observed.

Next, to determine if grafting NSCs into ischemic rats could alter spatial learning, the Morris water maze test [28] was performed. Rats were trained to find a platform submerged below the surface since three weeks after transplantation surgery. They were given two trials per day with a 10-minute inter-trial interval for 10 days. This sparse training regime has been shown to be more sensitive to detect lesion-induced deficits than multiple daily trials with short inter-trial interval [29].

In this test, the examiners were totally different from those who had cultured and transplanted the NSCs, and were not informed of the operation a given rat had undergone. After water maze test and immunofluorescence staining were completed, the treatments were disclosed. According to the number of survived grafted cells, the rats were divided into the following four groups: Group 1, rats with a sham operation (n=14); Group 2, rats with transient ischemia with no graft (n=11); Group 3, rats with transient ischemia with a high number of surviving grafted cells (n=5); and Group 4, rats with transient ischemia with a low number of surviving grafted cells (n=5). Group 3 was composed of the rats with more than 1500 BrdU-positive cells and more than 120 NeuN-positive grafted cells in the CA1 region. The average number of BrdU-positive cells was 1656, and 8.7% of them were NeuN-positive. Group 4 was composed of the rats with less than 60 NeuN-positive grafted cells. The average number of BrdU-positive cells was only 618, and 5.8% of them were NeuN-positive.

During the 10-day training period, the swimming time and path length to reach the platform declined day by day in all groups (repeated measures ANOVA, effect of days on latency, $F_{9,270} = 18.8$, $p < 0.001$; Fig.9). By the multiple comparison Scheffé's test, reliable deficits in spatial navigation and acquisition of a hidden platform navigation in the Morris water maze were found between Group 1 and 2 ($p < 0.001$). A Group effect and Group x Days effect (Group, $F_{3,9} = 13.049$, $p < 0.0001$; Group x Days, $F_{3,27} = 1.794$, $p < 0.011$) were also observed, suggesting that different groups learned the task at different rates. Multiple comparison of latency between groups on days 8-10 revealed a statistical difference between Group 2 and 3 ($p < 0.021$) or between Group 3 and 4 ($p < 0.0005$) with Posthoc Scheffé's test. Rats in Group 4 took more time than the ones in Group 2 during 5-10 days, but no significant difference was observed ($p < 0.2084$ at Days 8-10). Pearson's correlation coefficient test showed a significant negative correlation between the number of surviving NSCs and the latency on days 8-10 ($r = -0.755$, $p < 0.01$). The analysis with respect to path length gave the same results.

One possible mechanism of functional effect in the present study is the re-formation of neuronal networks, which were damaged by ischemic insult. In a previous *in vitro* study of ours, NSC-derived neurons exhibited action potentials 12 days after differentiation, and synapse formation by them was observed in 28-

35 days [22]. In the present study, we started water maze test three weeks after the transplantation, when the grafted NSCs were supposed to differentiate into functional neurons. The timing of significant improvement in water maze test was coincident with that of synapse formation in culture. Furthermore, grafted NSCs having neurite-like structure in the pyramidal layer were co-localized with synapse-related protein, synaptobrevin. Take these results into account; it is reasonable to expect that primary networks would have formed in the hippocampus by the end of water maze test although they might not be mature enough.

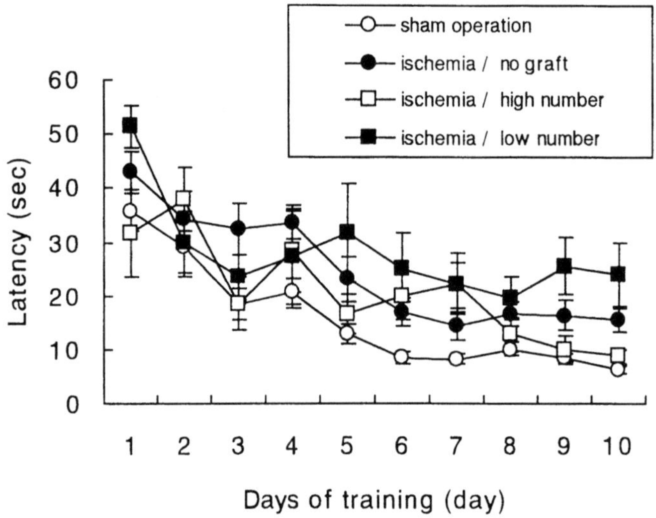

Fig. 9. Latency to find the platform in water maze test. The swim path was recorded with a CCD camera, and latency to reach the platform and swim path length were computed by an image analyzing system. These results were analyzed by one-way or two-way analysis of variance (ANOVA). On days 8-10, significant recovery was observed in the ischemia/ high number versus the ischemia/ no graft group. Values are means +/- SEM. (Adapted with permission from Ref. 35)

Functional recovery from spatial impairment in ischemic rats was previously observed by grafting CA1 fetal cells or cells of an immortalized hippocampal neuroepithelial cell line [30,31]. In those studies, cell suspensions (30,000 cells/site) were grafted into bilaterally into the hippocampus at two points on each side, and 80% of the cells survived. However, the precise number of the neurons located in the CA1 region was not mentioned. In our case, the minimum number of surviving NSC-derived neurons for the behavioral effect was approximately 120. In a rat model of Parkinson's disease, the survival of as few as 100-200 dopaminergic neurons could reverse Parkinson symptoms [32]. Although the mechanism of functional recovery might be different, it is thus quite possible that the small number of surviving cells that differentiated into neurons would have a behavioral effect in ischemic rats.

The number of surviving cells in the CA1 region was about 500 – 2000. This number was equivalent to 1-3% of the grafted cells. As some of the surviving cells were found outside of the CA1 region, the actual survival rate of all surviving cells was higher. But in comparison with the report that about one-half of the NSCs survived in the normal hippocampus [33], this rate is low. It is possible that ischemic insult has the effect of preventing cell survival. Especially in the rats with a large gliotic reaction, both survival rate and neuronal differentiation were lower. In these rats, the results of water maze test were worse than those from the high number group. Gliosis and cytokines from dying cells might have prevented neuronal differentiation and sprouting of the neurites, resulting in poor scores. To increase the number of surviving cells, the method of grafting should become more sophisticated. Also, the optimum timing of grafting NSCs after ischemia for adequate neuronal differentiation should be determined.

CA1 is not a native neurogenic region. In a study on grafting NSCs into the hippocampus of normal rats, no NSC-derived neurons were found in the CA1 region [33]. However, it is possible that cytokines and/or membrane-bound proteins are upregulated after ischemia to support the differentiation and migration of NSCs. Several neurotrophic factors are reported to be upregulated after ischemia in the hippocampus [34]. These factors may have contributed to the neuronal differentiation or maturation of the grafted NSCs. In view of our results, we speculate that some factors in the CA1 play a role in the neuronal differentiation of grafted NSCs, but the actual mechanism remains unknown.

Conclusion

As mentioned above, NSCs from adult rat hippocampus differentiated into neurons which expressed neurotransmitters, and they were able to form functional synapses in vitro. When these cells were grafted into the brain of ischemic rats, they survived and differentiated into neurons. Furthermore, the rats with more than 120 neurons showed recovery from the impairment of spatial recognition in the water maze test [35]. The timing of significant improvement in water maze test was coincident with that of synapse formation in culture.

These results support the concept that NSCs in the adult brain have a potential to differentiate into functional neurons that can be integrated into the neuronal circuitry. This means that grafting NSCs have a potential to reverse a impaired CNS dysfunction in brain damages such as neurodegenerative diseases, ischemia, and trauma. Because of this potential, NSCs could be a tool for us to fight against "Brain Attack".

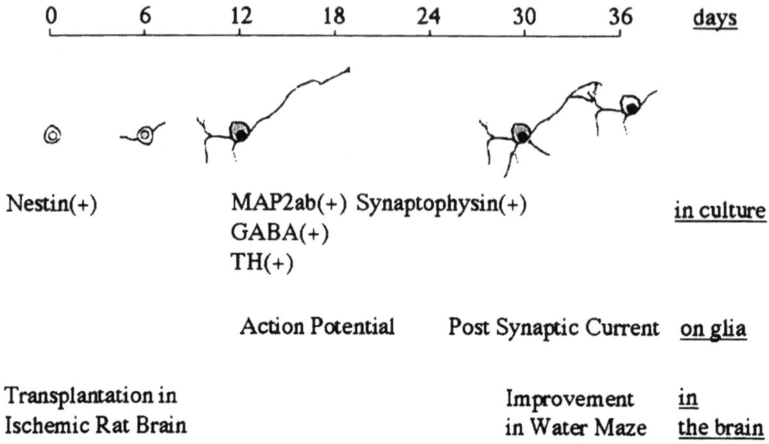

Fig. 10. Time-course of differentiation from neural stem cells into functional neurons. In 2 weeks, the cells express neurotransmitters and elicit action potentials. The timing of improvement in water maze test was coincident with that of synapse formation in culture.

Ackowledgement

The authors thank Fred H. Gage of Laboratory of Genetics at The Salk Institute for Biological Studies, and Theo D. Palmer of Department of Neurosurgery at Stanford University for collaborating to achieve the in vitro analyses of adult hippocampus-derived NSCs. We also thank Haruhiko Kikuchi, the Dean of Kobe City General Hospital, for giving a good opportunity to enter the stem cell world.

References

1. Björklund A and Lindvall O (2000) Cell replacement therapies for central nervous system disorders. Nat Neurosci 3:537-544
2. Freed CR, Greene PE, Breeze RE, et al (2001) Transplantation of embryonic dopamine neurons for severe Parkinson's disease. N Engl J Med 344:710-719
3. Temple S and Alvarez-Buylla A (1999) Stem cells in the adult mammalian central nervous system. Curr Opin Neurobiol 9:135-141
4. Ray J, Peterson DA, Schinstine M, et al (1993) Proliferation, differentiation and long-term culture of primary hippocampal neurons. Proc Natl Acad Sci USA 90:3602-3606
5. Gage FH, Coates PW, Palmer TD, et al (1995) Survival and differentiation of adult neuronal progenitor cells transplanted to the adult brain. Proc Natl Acad Sci USA 92:11879-11883
6. Palmer TD, Ray J, Gage FH (1995) FGF-2-responsive neuronal progenitors reside in proliferative and quiescent regions of the adult rodent brain. Mol Cell Neurosci 6:474-486
7. Palmer TD, Takahashi J and Gage FH (1997) The adult rat hippocampus contains

primordial neural stem cells. Mol Cell Neurosci 8:389-404
8. Takahashi J, Palmer TD and Gage FH (1999) Retinoic acid and neurotrophins collaborate to regulate neurogenesis in adult-derived neural stem cell cultures. J Neurobiol 38:65-81
9. Gritti A, Parati EA, Cova L, et al (1996) Multipotential stem cells from the adult mouse brain proliferate and self-renew in response to basic fibroblast growth factor. J Neurosci 16:1091-1100
10. Liu RH, Morassutti DJ, Whittemore SR, et al (1999) Electrophysiological properties of mitogen-expanded adult rat spinal cord and subventricular zone neural precursor cells. Exp Neurol 158:143-154
11. Gage FH (1998) Cell therapy. Nature 392:18-24
12. Svendsen CN, and Smith AG (1999) New prospects for human stem-cell therapy in the nervous system. Trends Neurosci 22:357-364
13. Ryder EF, Snyder EY and Cepko CL (1990) Establishment and characterization of multipotent neural cell lines using retrovirus vector-mediated oncogene transfer. J Neurobiol 21:356-375
14. Vescovi AL, Parati EA, Gritti A, et al (1999) Isolation and cloning of mutipotential stem cells from the embryonic human CNS and establishment of transplantable human neural stem cell lines by epigenetic stimulation. Exp Neurol 156:71-83
15. Liu G and Tsien R W (1995) Properties of synaptic transmission at single hippocampal synaptic buttons. Nature 375:400-404
16. Vicario-Abejön C, Collin C, McKay RDG, et al (1998) Neurotrophins induce formation of functional excitatory and inhibitory synapses between cultured hippocampal neurons. J Neurosci 18:7256-7271
17. Pfrieger FW and Barres BA (1995) What the fly's glia tell the fly's brain. Cell 83:671-674
18. Tsacopoulos M and Magistretti PJ (1996) Metabolic coupling between glia and neurons. J Neurosci 16:877-885
19. Kaplan MR, Meyer-Franke A, Lambert S, et al (1997) Induction of sodium channel clustering by oligodendrocytes. Nature 386:724-728
20. Pfrieger FW and Barres BA (1997) Synaptic efficacy enhanced by glial cells in vitro. Science 277:1684-1687
21. Lim DA and Alvarez-Buylla A (1999) Interaction between astrocytes and adult subventricular zone precursors stimulates neurogenesis. Proc Natl Acad Sci USA 96:7526-31
22. Toda H, Takahashi J, Mizoguchi A, et al (2000) Neurons generated from adult rat hippocampal stem cells form functional glutamatergic and GABAergic synapses in vitro. Exp Neurol 165:66-76
23. Vicario-Abejön C, Collin C, Tsoulfas P, et al (2000) Hippocampal stem cells differentiate into excitatory and inhibitory neurons. Eur J Neurosci 12:677-688
24. Auerbach JM, Eiden MV and McKay RDG (2000) Transplanted CNS stem cells form functional synapses in vivo. Eur J Neurosci 12:1696-1704
25. Pulsinelli WA and Brierley JB (1979) A new model of bilateral hemispheric ischemia in the unanesthetized rat. Stroke 10:267-272
26. Nunn JA and Hodges H (1994) Cognitive deficits induced by global cerebral ischaemia: relationship to brain damage and reversal by transplants. Behav Brain Res 65:1-31
27. Nunn JA, LePeillet E, Netto CA, et al (1994) Global ischaemia: hippocampal

pathology and spatial deficits in the water maze. Behav Brain Res 62:41-54
28. Morris RGM, Garrud P, Rawlins JNP, et al (1982) Place navigation is impaired in rats with hippocampal lesions. Nature 297:681-683
29. Mandel RJ, Gage FH and Thal LJ (1989) Enhanced detection of nucleus basalis magnocellularis lesion-induced spatial learning deficit in rats by modification of training regimen. Behav Brain Res 31:221-229
30. Hodges H, Sowinski P, Fleming P, et al (1996) Contrasting effects of fetal CA1 and CA3 hippocampal grafts on deficits in spatial learning and working memory induced by global cerebral ischaemia in rats. Neuroscience 72:959-988
31. Sinden JD, Rashid-Doubell F, Kershaw TR, et al (1997) Recovery of spatial learning by grafts of a conditionally immortalized hippocampal neuroepithelial cell line into the ischaemia-lesioned hippocampus. Neuroscience 81:599-608
32. Brundin P, Barbin G, Strecker RE, et al (1988) Survival and function of dissociated rat dopamine neurones grafted at different developmental stages or after being cultured in vitro. Dev Brain Res 39:233-243
33. Suhonen JO, Peterson DA, Ray J, et al (1996) Differentiation of adult hippocampus-derived progenitors into olfactory neurons in vivo. Nature 383:624-627
34. Lindvall O, Kokaia Z, Bengzon J, et al (1994) Neurotrophins and brain insults. TINS 17:490-496
35. Toda H, Takahashi J, Iwakami N, et al (2001) Grafting neural stem cells improved the impaired spatial recognition in ischemic rats. Neurosci Lett 316:9-12

Repair of mammalian central nervous pathways: attempts to reconstruct normal neural connections with marked functional recovery

Saburo Kawaguchi and Takeshi Nishio

Department of Integrative Brain Science, Graduate School of Medicine, Kyoto University, Yoshida-Konoe-cho, Kyoto 606-8501, Japan

Summary: In contrast to the widely-held view that regeneration of the mammalian CNS is limited because myelin, glial cells, and extracellular matrices make CNS environment non-permissive for regrowth of axons, here, we advocate that CNS environment is permissive and regeneration of mammalian CNS pathways is possible to the extent of almost normal projections with marked recovery of function. It is based on the findings of three kinds of experiments: 1) replacement of spinal cord segments in neonatal rats, 2) a sharp transection of the spinal cord or the brain stem in young rats, and 3) grafting embryonic spinal cord or glial cells into the injured spinal cord in adult rats. In these experiments, when regenerating fibers entered the normal path, they extended all the way correctly to terminate in the proper target areas. This indicates that the mammalian CNS possesses an adequately arranged guiding system that enables regenerating axons to find path and target correctly. Failure of regeneration or occurrence of erroneous reconnection appeared likely due to local conditions in the lesion site under which the axon guiding system is damaged. The present findings offer a new perspective for repair strategy after damage to the brain and spinal cord.

Key words: Spinal cord repair, Axonal regeneration, Embryonic CNS graft

Introduction

Studies over the past two decades have provided convincing evidence for the occurrence of axonal regeneration in the mammalian central nervous system (CNS) and opened up the possibility of neural repair after damage to the brain and spinal cord. There are two categories of CNS projections to be repaired. One is the global projections like the monoaminergic pathways in which a relatively small number of neurons project widely upon various CNS structures without showing somatotopic organization. The other is the point-to-point projections with precise somatotopic organization which constitute the majority of sensory and motor pathways. Here we state repair of the latter projections focusing on the spinal cord injuries.

Various attempts have been made on neural repair of spinal cord injuries: grafting embryonic spinal cord [1,2] or peripheral nerve segments [3], transplanting cultured cells including olfactory ensheathing cells [4,5] or embryonic stem cells [6,7], and neutralizing Nogo-A [8,9]. The achievements to date, however, are not great. The regenerated projections were mostly very restricted in amount and extension, and inevitably mostly aberrant. Consequently the recovery of function was poor. To achieve a marked recovery of function it would be necessary to break the restriction and restore the projections similar to normal. Is it possible to break the restriction and restore projections to nearly normal extent? We think it is possible because we know the occurrence of such restoration in the cerebellofugal projections in kittens [10]: the regenerated projections coursed in the normal path, terminated in the normal target areas, and elicited normal functional activity. The textbook [11] that described for the first time the occurrence of marked regeneration of the mammalian CNS pathways cited our report as convincing for that.

It appears likely that path and target finding of axons during ontogenesis is controlled by guidance cues [12,13]. It is also the case during regeneration because regeneration recapitulates ontogenesis [14]. Path and target finding is associated with extension of axons. Extension of axons is, therefore, likely regulated by guidance cues. An adequately arranged organization of guidance cues of axons is considered to exist along the presumptive pathway of a projection during ontogenesis [14] and persist stably after the projection is formed [10]. It is, therefore, assumable that robust regrowth of axons and reconstruction of a neural circuitry similar to normal are possible when such an organization of guidance cues is provided along the tract. On the basis of this assumption we hypothesized firstly that grafting embryonic homologous CNS structures into the host CNS in the correct place in the correct orientation would make it possible to provide such cues along the entire course of projections through the host-graft interface and thereby break the restriction of regeneration; Secondly that a sharp transection to minimize damage to the organization of such cues would permit severed axons to regrow robustly; Thirdly that regeneration would be possible provided that the local unfavorable conditions are ameliorated. The hypothesis was thus tested by the three kind of experiments: replacement of spinal cord segments in neonatal rats, a sharp transection of the spinal cord or the brain stem in young rats, and grafting embryonic spinal cord or cultured glial cells into the injured spinal cord in adult rats.

Replacement of spinal cord segments in neonatal rats

Spinal cord segments in neonatal rats were removed at the midthoracic level and embryonic spinal cord (ESC) segments were grafted into the vacancy [15-18]. Control animals were grafted with a peripheral nerve (PN) segment or left ungrafted. Neural connections across the graft were examined by the anterograde and retrograde tracing methods [16]. Anterogradely labeled pyramidal tract fibers enetered the PN segment meanderingly and were dispersed; most stopped at the caudal end of the graft. Although a small fraction of fibers reentered the host spinal cord, they terminated near the host-graft interface without further extension. Outcomes in anatomical regeneration in the animals with ESC segment grafts varied among the operated animals. When the graft was nicely fused with the host spinal cord without formation of scars and cysts, regeneration was excellent, whereas reconnection between the supraspinal structures and the lumbar enlargement was poor when the fusion was bad with formation of cysts [17]. In the excellent cases, the labeled pyramidal tract fibers entering the ESC segments crossed the graft and extended further to reach the lumbar segments. The fibers were fasciculated or defasciculated in the graft. Even when the fibers were defasciculated in the graft they became fasciculated and oriented dorsally near the caudal end of the graft, and descended in the normal path [16].

Consistent with these findings, the retrograde tracing study revealed that in the animals with ESC segment grafts but not in those with PN segment grafts, many neurons in the upper brain strucrures were labeled when Fast Blue was injected into the lumbar enlargement. In the animals with PN segment grafts, when the tracer was injected into the graft/host interface neurons in the upper brain structures were labeled as many as in the animals with ESC segment grafts. The difference between the two kinds of graft as a conduit for CNS axons is likely to be due to differences in matching growing axons and their guidance cues through the graft-host interface.

Locomotor performance in the rats with ESC segment grafts that had excellent regeneration was almost normal [15,17]. In the rats that had brainstem-spinal regeneration but not corticospinal connections showed hind-forelimb coordination consistently in some and occasionally in others. In addition to such a relationship between distribution of the regenerated projections and functional recovery, a positive correlation was observed between the number of regenerated connections in each of the supraspinal projection and locomotor performance of the animal [18]. Thus distribution and number of the regenerated supraspinal-lumbar projections were intimately related to the grade of functional recovery. These results suggest that accurate reconstruction of neural connections is essential for marked recovery of function after spinal cord repair [15-18].

Spontaneous regeneration of the pyramidal tract and dorsal column axons in young rats after transection

Spontaneous regeneration of spinal cord tracts occurred in rats younger than one month of age [19,20]. When transection was made so sharply as to produce edema-free lesions without subsequent formation of either scars or cysts, marked regeneration occurred in the pyramidal tract [19]and dorsal column axons [20]. When the tracts were less sharply transected, regenerated fibers crossed the lesion dispersedly and extended aberrantly for a relatively short distance, whereas after a blunt transection which produced edema and later glial scars at the lesion regenerative outgrowth could not cross the lesion. The pyramidal tract that was cut sharply at the pontomedullary junction crossed the lesion site, descended in the ventralmost part as a compact bundle forming the pyramid, decussated completely in the lower medulla to turn dorsally and distribute terminals into the dorsal column nuclei, and extended in the base of the contralateral dorsal funiculus to reach the sacral segments, giving off collaterals through the entire length which terminate in laminae 3-7 [19]. Pyramidal tract neurons as many as in the normal control animals were retrogradely labeled when tracer was injected into the lumbar enlargement.

The dorsal column axons cut sharply at a level of T12~13 regenerated to cross the lesion and ascended in the normal path as a compact bundle in the superficial part of the dorsal column and terminated correctly in the gracile nucleus [20]. The terminals were immature when observed at 9 days postlesion but became mature in two to three weeks. Many neurons in the dorsal root ganglia (DRG) in the lumbar segments were retrogradely labeled with tracer injected into the gracile nucleus. Nuclei of DRG neurons were swallen and displaced to the cell periphery to form cytoplasm a crescent shape. This morphologival change is characteristic of chromatolysis that is known to occur after injury and during regeneration of a peripheral branch of DRG neurons. In either the pyramidal tract and dorsal column axons restriction of regrowth was undetectable so far as the fibers traversed the normal path.

Spinal cord repair in adult paraplegic rats by amelioration of local unfavorable conditions

In adult rats regeneration of spinal cord tracts never occurred spontaneously, whereas a marked regeneration occurred after grafting embryonic spinal cord tissue [21]. In rats aged 2 to 3 months the spinal cord was overhemisected under ether anesthesia at the level of Th10-11 and homologous structures taken from E13-14 embryos were grafted in the lesion. Control animals were left ungrafted. Occurrence of regeneration of the corticospinal and rubrospinal tracts was examined by the anterograde and retrograde labeling methods. In the grafted rats but not in the controls both tracts were regenerated to cross the lesion, descended the normal path, and reached the caudalmost end of the sacral segments. The regenerated tracts were similar to normal projections in various aspects: amount, extension, path, formation of a compact bundle, and termination. With respect to the effectiveness of embryonic spinal cord tissue two possibilities can be envisaged: one is the possibility that diffusible substances contained in the embryonic tissue may suppress formation of glial scars and cysts at the lesion site and enhance regeneration, and the other is the possibility that cellular element in the graft, presumably gial cells may ameliorate the local unfavorable conditions and make environment pertinent for growth of axons. To test the latter possibility we cultured glial cells harvested from the spinal cord of neonatal Sprague-Dawley rats expressing enhanced green fluorescent protein (EGFP) transgene [22] and implanted them in the spinal cord of adult rats after a complete transection at a lower thoracic level [23]. Neural reconnection was examined by tracers and behavioral recovery was assessed by BBB scoring [24].

Rats were completely paraplegic for 3 to 5 postoperative days. They began to move hindlimbs in a week, and in the best cases walked with hind-forelimb coordination in 3 weeks after surgery. The BBB scores at the 4th postoperative week ranged from 8 (sweeping with no weight support) to 20 (consistent plantar stepping, coordinated gait and toe clearance). EGFP-positive glial cells migrated towards the lesion site to be aligned in parallel to axons. In the best cases regenerated projections were similar to normal in amount, extension, path, and termination [23].

Conclusion and comments

Findings described in the present paper dispute the widely-held view that regeneration of the mammalian CNS is limited because myelin, glial cells, and extracellular matrices make CNS environment non-permissive for regrowth of axons. The occurrence of marked regeneration coursing in the normal path and terminating in the normal targets indicates that the axonal environment is permissive. Failure of regeneration is due to the local unfavorable conditions rather than the global inhospitable axonal environment. The local unfavorable conditions in the lesion are ameliorable by grafting embryonic CNS structures or cultured glial cells. The mammalian CNS has an incredible potential of axonal regrowth and self-organization to lead the regrowing axons to make neural connections similar to normal, which makes it possible to achieve marked recovery of function. To let the spinal cord injured walk again is not an impossible dream but a realistic goal.

The results of our experiments indicate that there is an adequately arranged guiding system of axons not only during ontogenesis but also after establishment of neural connections, which provides permissive environment for regrowing axons along the correct path. Outside the normal path and targets the guiding system must exert inhibitory influences on regrowing axons not to extend and terminate aberrantly. The inhibitory influences might have been taken as non-permissive environment. Endeavours to make CNS environment permissive may perturb the inherent axon guiding system, which would account for why regenerated projections induced by such procedure are so restricted and aberrant.

Acknowledgements

The work from the author's laboratory was supported by grants: JSPS-RFTF96100203 from the Japan Society for the Promotion of Science, Special Coordination Funds for Promoting Science and Technology, STA, Health Sciences Research Grants for Research on Brain Science, and the Uehara Memorial Foundation.

References

1. Howland DR, Bregman BS, Tessler A, Goldberger ME (1995) Transplants enhance locomotion in neonatal kittens whose spinal cords transected: a behavioral and anatomical study. Exp Neurol 135:123-145
2. Miya D, Giszter S, Mori F, Adipudi V, Tessler A, Murray M (1997) Fetal transplants alter the development of function after spinal cord transection in new born rats. J Neurosci 17:4856-4872
3. Cheng H, Cao Y, Olson L (1996) Spinal cord repair in adult paraplegic rats: partial restoration of hind limb function. Science 273:510-513
4. Li Y, Field PM, Raisman G (1997) Repair of adult rat corticospinal tract by transplants of olfactory ensheathing cells. Science 277:2000-2002
5. Ramón-Cueto, A, Cordero MI, Santos-Benito FF, Avila J (2000) Functional recovery of paraplegic rats and motor axon regeneration in their spinal cord by olfactory ensheathing glia. Neuron 25:425-435
6. Liu S, Qu Y, Stewart TJ, Howard MJ, Chakrabortty S, Holekamp TF, McDonald JW (2000) Embryonic stem cells differentiate into oligodendrocytes and myelinate in culture and after spinal cord transplantation. Proc Natl Acad Sci USA 97:6126-6131
7. McDonald JW, Liu XZ, Qu Y, Liu S, Mickey SK, Turetsky D, Gottlieb DI, Choi DW (1999) Transplanted embryonic stem cells survive, differentiate and promote recovery in injured rat spinal cord. Nat Med 12:1410-1412
8. Brosamle C, Huber AB, Fiedler M, Skerra A, Schwab ME (2000) Regeneration of lesioned corticospinal tract fibers in the adult rat induced by a recombinant, humanized IN-1 antibody fragment. J Neurosci. 20: 8061-8068
9. Thallmair M, Metz GA, Z'graggen WJ, Raineteau O, Kartje GL, Schwab ME (1998) Neurite growth inhibitors restrict plasticity and functional recovery following corticospinal tract lesions. Nat Neurosci 1:124-131
10. Kawaguchi S, Miyata H, Kato N (1986) Regeneration of the cerebellofugal projection after transection of the superior cerebellar peduncle in kittens: morphorogical and electrophysiological studies. J Comp Neurol 245:258-273
11. McGeer PL, Eccles JC, McGeer EG (1987) Molecular neurobiology of the mammalian brain. 2nd Ed, Plenum Press, New York, pp 448-450

12. Silver J, Lorenz SE, Wahlsten D, Coughlin J (1982) Axonal guidance during development of the great commissures: descriptive and experimental studies in vivo, on the role of performed glial pathways. J Comp Neurol 210:10-29
13. Serafini T, Colamarino SA, Leonardo ED, Wang H, Beddington R, Skarnes WC, Tessier-Lavigne M (1996) Netrin-1 is required for commissural axon guidance in the developing vertebrate nervous system. Cell 87:1001-1014
14. Kawaguchi S, Murata M, Kurimoto Y (1991) Ontogenesis of the cerebellofugal projection in the rats. Dev Brain Res 61:285-289
15. Iwashita Y, Kawaguchi S, Murata M (1994) Restoration of function by replacement of spinal cord segments in the rat. Nature 367:167-170
16. Asada Y, Kawaguchi S, Hayashi H, Nakamura T (1998) Neural repair of the injured spinal cord by grafting: comparison between peripheral nerve segments and embryonic homologous structures as a conduit of CNS axons. Neurosci Res 31:241-249
17. Hase T, Kawaguchi S, Hayashi H, Nishio T, Asada Y, Nakamura T (2002) Locomotor performance of the rat after neonatal repairing of spinal cord injuries: Quantitative assessment and electromyographic study. J Neurotrauma 19:267-277
18. Hase T, Kawaguchi S, Hayashi H, Nishio T, Mizoguchi A, Nakamura T (2002) Spinal cord repair in neonatal rats: A correlation between axonal regeneration and functional recovery. Eur J Neurosci. (in press)
19. Inoue T, Kawaguchi S, Kurisu K (1998) Spontaneous regeneration of the pyramidal tract after transection in young rats. Neurosci Lett 247:151-154
20. Kikukawa S, Kawaguchi S, Mizoguchi A, Ide C, Koshinaga M (1998) Regeneration of dorsal column axons after spinal cord injury in young rats. Neurosci Lett 249:135-138
21. Kawaguchi S, Kojima K, Hasebe T, Kikukawa S, Murata M, Iwashita Y (1999) Spinal cord repair in adult rats: restoration of corticospinal and rubrospinal tracts to almost normal extent. In: Uemura K, Kawamura K, Yazaki T. (eds) Keio University Symposia for Life Science and Medicine 2 on Neural Development, Springer-Verlag Publications, Berlin, p. 506
22. Okabe M, Ikawa M, Kominami K, Nakanishi T, Nishimune Y (1997) 'Green mice' as a source of ubiquitous green cells. FEBS Lett 407:313-319
23. Nishio T, Kawaguchi S, Iseda T, Hase T, Kojima K, Kawasaki T (2001) Spinal cord repair in afult paraplegic rats by glial transplantation: recovery of walking with hind-forelimb coordination. 34th International Union of Physiological Sciences, Abstract.
24. Basso, D.M., Beattie, M.S. & Bresnahan, J.C. (1995) A sensitive and reliable locomotor rating scale for open field testing in rats. J Neurotrauma 12: 1-21

2. Strategies of neuroprotection

The MEK/ERK pathway as a target for stroke therapy

Shobu Namura[1], and Alessandro Alessandrini[2]

[1]Stroke and Brain Protection Laboratory, NATIONAL CARDIO-VASCULAR CENTER Research Institute, 5-7-1 Fujishirodai, Suita, Osaka 565-8565, Japan
[2]Renal Unit, Massachusetts General Hospital, Harvard Medical School, Charlestown, MA 02129, U.S.A.

Summary: Oxidative stress is implicated in aging or cell death. Accumulating evidence suggests that oxidative stress also plays a crucial role in brain tissue damage resulting from ischemic stroke. Several mechanisms of oxidative stress have been proposed. During the past several years, mitogen-activated protein kinases [MAPKs] have been shown to be key signaling components in oxidative stress from the cell surface into the nucleus. We recently demonstrated that re-perfusion following brain ischemia dramatically activates the MEK/ERK pathway within damaged brain regions. In addition, we have shown that MEK inhibitors protect brain against damage resulting from ischemia and reperfusion. We further demonstrated that MEK inhibitors protect neurons at the cellular level against hypoxia as well as oxidative stress induced by glutamate or nitric oxide toxicity. These data indicate that the MEK/ERK pathway is crucial in neuronal damage resulting from ischemia and reperfusion or other related oxidative stresses. It is suggested that the MEK/ERK pathway may be a novel target for stroke treatment. This article will review the evidence that implicates the MEK/ERK pathway in cerebral ischemia and reperfusion. In addition, we will discuss the potential thera-peutic relevance of MEK/ERK inhibition in ischemic stroke and other related neurological diseases.

Key words: Oxidative stress, MAP kinase, MEK/ERK, Cerebral ischemia, Re-perfusion, Stroke

Introduction

Stroke is the third leading cause of death in the U.S., the European Union, and Japan. A large part of stroke prevention has involved life style changes and treatment of related diseases (e.g., hypertension and heart disease). There is also a great need to develop brain protection therapy, which is effective even when initiated after an onset of stroke.

One of the most exciting occurrences in recent years in the stroke research field has been the approval of intravenous injection of tissue type plasminogen activator (t-PA) within 3 hours of onset [1, 2]. This treatment is primarily aimed to restore cerebral blood flow by removing blood clots that block arterial blood flow. On the other hand, great efforts have been made to develop neuroprotective drugs targeting molecular events that occur in the brain tissue after ischemia.

During the past two decades, evidence has been gained suggesting contribution of oxidative stress to brain tissue damage resulting from ischemia and reperfusion. In addition, intracellular mechanisms for oxidative stress have been elucidated. This chapter will review the evidence implicating oxidative stress in ischemic stroke, and to consider therapeutic approaches for brain ischemia, targeting signaling components activated during oxidative stress.

Oxidative stress and ischemic stroke

Oxidative stress has been implicated in ischemic brain injury. This mechanistic insight was derived from several pieces of evidence. First, brain subjected to ischemia/reperfusion produces reactive oxygen species (ROS) during reperfusion phase [3,4]. Since the microvasculature of the brain represents a huge surface area, the produced ROS could be generated by the brain microvasculature. The same group demonstrated that hydroxyl free radicals are produced during anoxia/reoxygenation in isolated brain microvessels, which are inhibited with catalase and superoxide dismutase [5]. Besides the microvasculature, neurons also generate ROS. Oxidized hydroethidine formation, an indicator of ROS generation, has been shown in neurons after ischemia/reperfusion [6, 7]. Damaged mitochondria in ischemic neurons are thought to be a major source of ROS. Polymorphic lymphocytes brought into damaged brain areas after reperfusion are also likely to be a source of ROS. Second, antioxidant enzymes or antioxidant such as free radical scavengers or vitamin E have been shown to protect brain against ischemia [8, 9]. Third, the use of transgenic mouse models has been quite useful in testing this hypothesis. For example, neuronal nitric oxide synthase knockout mice and iNOS knockout mice are less sensitive to brain ischemia [10, 11]. Overexpression of the human copper/zinc superoxide dismutase gene protects brain against ischemia in mice and rats [12, 13], whereas gene deletion of copper/zinc superoxide dismutase or manganese superoxide dismutase enhanced brain tissue injury in mice [6, 14]. Several clinical trial studies targeting oxidative stress have shown that antioxidant drugs are effective [8, 15]. Recent approval of MCI-186 (edaravone), a free radical scavenger, as a neuroprotectant against ischemic stroke by Japanese authorities indicates the important role of oxidative injury in human ischemic stroke.

Molecular mechanisms of oxidative stress

Prooxidant and antioxidant enzyme

Many oxidant-producing enzymes have been shown to be involved in ischemic brain injury. Based on their producing oxidant, these prooxidant enzymes are classified into three groups. The first group, nitric oxide synthases (NOSs), produces nitric oxide radical. NOSs have three isoforms: neuronal NOS (nNOS) and endothelial NOS (eNOS) are constitutively expressed in neurons and endothelium, respectively; whereas an inducible isoform (iNOS) is produced in microglia/macrophages, astrocytes, and endothelial cells in the brain. The second group including cyclooxygenases, xanthine dehydrogenase, xanthine oxidase, NADPH oxidase produces superoxide anion. Superoxide reacts with nitric oxide to form peroxynitrite, a strong oxidant. The last group includes myeloperoxidase and monoamine oxidase, which produces hydroxy anion and hydrogen peroxide, respectively.

There are enzymes that detoxify free radicals. Superoxide dismutases (SODs) are antioxidant enzymes that specifically convert superoxide anion to hydrogen peroxide. There are three SOD isoforms: copper/zinc SOD (CuSOD), manganese SOD (Mn-SOD), and extracellular SOD (ECSOD). Converted hydrogen peroxide is in turn detoxified by catalase and glutathione peroxidase (GSHPx) by consuming glutathione (GSH). GSHPx also scavenges lipid peroxides. Besides these enzymes, the thioredoxin system can exert an antioxidant property by reducing the disulfide bond in protein or GSH. Drs. Yodoi et al. will discuss the thioredoxin system in more detail in this book. In addition, Bcl-2 expression decreases the net cellular generation of reactive oxygen species production, contributing to inhibition of both apoptosis and necrosis [16].

Signal transduction of oxidative stress

Excessive formation of ROS results in macromolecular damage including lipid peroxidation, protein oxidation, DNA oxidation, all of which contribute to cell damage. In addition, ROS can regulate signaling by modifying the redox states of molecules. Many transcripton factors such as AP-1, HIF-1, SP-1, and Elk-1 are controlled by their redox states. Therefore, the functions of these molecules are likely to be affected by oxidative stress. One of the well-characterized redox-sensitive molecules is nuclear factor-κ B (NF-κB), a transcription factor. NF-κB is activated by ROS, typically in response to inflammatory stimuli. And importantly, down stream target genes regulated by NF-κB include iNOS, COX-2, matrix metalloproteinases, all of which have been implicated in ischemic brain tissue injury. Oxidative stress may exert cellular damage by affecting these redox-sensitive molecules.

Oxidization of sulfhydryl (thiol) groups on protein cysteine residues has also been shown to attribute to cell protection. For example, *N*-methyl-D-aspartate (NMDA) receptor activity and caspase enzymatic activity can be diminished by S-nitrosylation, resulting in neuroprotection by NO [17]. Thus, oxidative stress can bi-directionally lead to both cell death and cell protection, as a result of the net balance of redox states of cellular molecules.

MAP kinase pathways

About one decade ago, a family of 41–45 kDa serine/threonine kinases was identified that responded to various extracellular stimuli [18, 19]. These protein kinases were originally characterized by the ability to phosphorylate microtubule-associated protein-2 (MAP-2) or myelin basic protein as in vitro substrates. As a result, these kinases were first named MAP-2 or myelin basic protein kinases [20-22]. Later, these protein kinases were renamed mitogen-activated protein kinases (MAP kinases) or extracellular signal regulated kinases (ERKs) since a wide variety of mitogens and growth factors stimulated them [23, 24]. MAP kinases have been implicated in a variety of cellular functions, including cell division, regulation of embryonic development, and cell survival and differentiation. In contrast to many of well-characterized cell surface receptor-associated kinases such as protein kinase C that is activated by second small soluble messengers, MAP kinases are activated by phosphorylation on both threonine and tyrosine by dual-specificity MAP kinase kinases (MAPKK) or MAP kinase/ERK kinases (MEK), which in turn are activated by Raf.

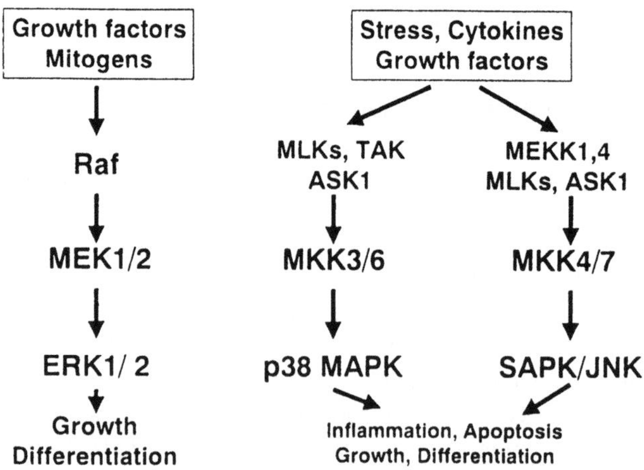

Fig. 1. MAP kinase pathways.

There have been three well-characterized mammalian MAPKs (Fig. 1): ERKs, c-JUN N-terminal protein kinases/stress activated kinases (JNKs/SAPKs), and p38 MAP kinases [25]. ERK1 (p44 MAP kinase) and ERK2 (p42 MAP kinase), and their direct activators MEK1 and MEK2, are stimulated by growth and mitogenic factors [e.g., epidermal growth factor (EGF), platelet-derived growth factor (PDGF), and nerve growth factor (NGF)]. On the other hand, JNKs/SAPKs and p38 MAP kinases are activated by lipopolysaccharides, cytokines, ionizing or ultraviolet radiation, heat shock, and hyperosmotic stress. These protein kinases have been implicated in cellular stress, inflammation, and apoptosis.

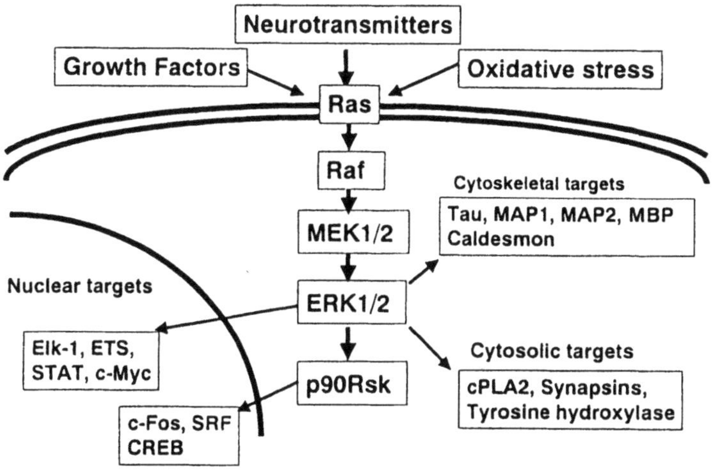

Fig. 2. The MEK/ERK pathway.

ERK1/2 phosphorylate a variety of molecules as substrates [26]. ERK1/2 phosphorylate not only transcription factors such as Elk-1 and ATF-2, but also other intracellular molecules (e.g., MAP-2, myelin basic protein, synapsins, Rsk, and CREB), which indicates the diverse biological functions of ERK1/2 (Fig. 2).

MAP kinases in oxidative stress

MAP kinases have been implicated in oxidative stress. Hypoxia and hypoxia/reoxygenation activate the MEK/ERK pathway in cultured cardiac myocytes [27]. In addition, hydrogen peroxide activates the MEK/ERK and p38 MAP kinase pathways. Inhibition of the MEK/ERK enhances apoptosis in cardiac myocytes [28]. Cisplatin, whose cytotoxicity is closely associated with increased generation of ROS, activates the MEK/ERK pathway [29-33]; however, observed effects by inhibition of this pathway are different from one study to another, which may reflect cell type specificity. Oxidative stimuli by using other modes also activate the MEK/ERK pathway in various cell types including neurons, as detailed below. While the MEK/ERK pathway is more often associated with survival, a pro-apoptotic function for the MEK/ERK pathway has also been suggested in several model systems. For example, an association between ERK2 activation and apoptosis was demonstrated in B lymphoma cells stimulated through the B-cell antigen receptor [34]. Cisplatin-induced apoptosis in HeLa cells requires ERK activation [33]. This dual function is also suggested in the JNK pathway. While JNK is more often associated with apoptosis [35], a protective role of it has also been demonstrated [36]. It would be important to study why the outcome differs from cell to cell, and from protocol to protocol.

MAP kinase activation in neuronal ischemia

ERK2 is widely expressed in adult brain, with the highest levels in neurons in the neocortex, hippocampus, striatum, and cerebellum, and with the lowest levels in oligodendrocyte [37]. ERKs are activated by growth factors as well as neurotransmitters. For example, brain derived neurotrophic factor (BDNF) activates ERKs in primary cultured cerebellar granule neurons [38]. Glutamate receptor activation stimulates ERKs in primary hippocampal cultures and cortical cultures [39, 40]. In addition, muscarinic receptor agonists or phorbol esters activate ERKs in hippocampal slices [41]. Moreover, electroconvulsive stimulation produces similar results in hippocampus in vivo [42-43]. Seizure activity phosphorylates ERK2 in primary hippocampal cultures after removal of kynurenate, a broad glutamate-receptor antagonist [44].

Tyrosine phosphorylation of ERK2 in brain ischemia was demonstrated by Campos-González and Kindy [45]. In the subsequent study by Kindy, general tyrosine kinase inhibitors such as genistein and lavendustin A prevented hippocampal delayed neuronal death caused by transient forebrain ischemia, suggesting a role of ERK2 in ischemic neuronal death [46]. Similar findings were obtained in other laboratories [47-49].

Recently, phospho-specific ERK1/2 antibodies have been available, which have facilitated identifying the localization of activated forms of ERK1/2. By using these antibodies, we demonstrated that reperfusion following focal cerebral ischemia resulted in a dramatic increase in ERK1/2 phosphorylation in the damaged brain area [50, 51]. Phospho-ERK1/2 immunoreactivity was predominantly observed in neurons. In addition, we also demonstrated that reperfusion activates ERK1/2 in the hippocampus after forebrain ischemia [52]. Phosphorylation of ERK1/2 is induced predominantly in the CA1 pyramidal, with very little phosphorylation of ERK1/2 in the CA3 pyramidal cells. The dentate granular cells and the mossy fibers, which originate from dentate granular cells, contain phospho-ERK1/2 immunoreactivity. This was also demonstrated by other laboratories [49, 53].

Ischemia mimicking stimuli such as NMDA receptor activation, exposure to NO, and hypoxia/reoxygenation phosphorylate ERK1/2 in primary cortical cultures [42, 54, 55]. Recovery after oxygen/glucose deprivation activates ERK1/2 in organotypic hippocampal cultures [56]. Activation of ERK1/2 was also demonstrated in HT22 cells, a hippocampal neuronal cell line, subjected to oxidative glutamate toxicity [57, 58]. ERK1/2 are activated in oligodendrocytes after cerebral ischemia [59], and are involved in oxidative damage in cultured oligodendrocytes [60].

MEK inhibitors

Recently, selective MEK inhibitors have been developed. One is PD98059 and the other is U0126 (Fig. 3), both of which have been used extensively to study the MEK/ERK pathway in a variety of experimental paradigms. Both compounds are selective MEK/ERK pathway inhibitors, and their mechanisms for inhibition is noncompetitive with respect to substrates. Although PD98059 and U0126 can both inhibit MEK1/2, the mode of inhibition by U0126 is distinct from that by PD98059. The inhibitory effects of PD98059 are due mainly to its binding directly to the inactive (nonphosphorylated) form of MEK and blocking its activation by Raf-mediated phosphorylation [61, 62]. On the other hand, U0126 does not affect MEK phosphorylation in vivo at concentrations sufficient to inhibit ERK phosphorylation [62]. In other words, U0126 inhibits MEK directly by blocking the catalytic activity of MEK even after activation; whereas PD98059 cannot efficiently inhibit the MEK activity once it is activated.

PD 98059 **U0126**

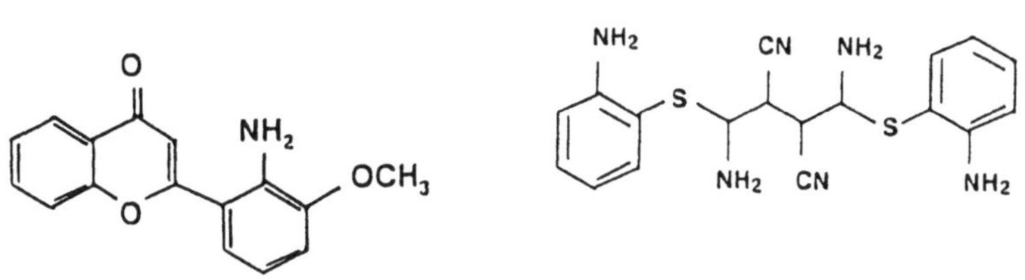

Fig. 3. MEK inhibitors.

Effects of MEK inhibitors on ischemic brain damage

Intracerebroventricular injection of PD98059 before ischemia is effective against transient focal cerebral ischemia (2 hours) in mice [50, 51]. U0126 is more effective against focal cerebral ischemia in mice. Intravenous (i.v.) injection of U0126 attenuates infarct size after permanent focal cerebral ischemia. Moreover, i.v. injection at 10 minutes before reperfusion is still protective against 3 hours transient focal cerebral ischemia. Irving and colleagues demonstrated attenuation of cerebral infarct by U0126 in rats [56]. More recently, another MEK1 inhibitor SL327 has been demonstrated to attenuate both infarct size and IL-1β production [63]. These data suggest that the MEK/ERK pathway also contributes to inflammation in ischemic brain.

Although the effect of PD98059 has not been established in global ischemia [49, 53], we found hippocampal protection by U0126 after 3.5 minutes of forebrain ischemia in the gerbil [52]. The protection by U0126 is closely correlated with inhibition of ERK1/2 phosphorylation. The neuroprotection by U0126 in vivo is consistent with in vitro data that show protection of pyramidal cells by U0126 in organotypic hippocampal cultures after oxygen/glucose deprivation [56].

MEK inhibitors are protective in neuronal cultures subjected to ischemia mimicking conditions. U0126 is protective against oxygen deprivation in rat and mouse primary cultured cortical neurons [52, 57]. In addition to U0126, PD98059 also enhances neuronal survivability after exposure to nitric oxide produced by sodium nitropruside (SNP) [52]. Both compounds are also protective against oxidative glutamate toxicity in the murine hippocampal cell line, HT22 [57, 58]. U0126 at the concentrations sufficient to inhibit both ERK2 phosphorylation and cell death does not block but rather enhances MEK1 phosphorylation in cultured cortical neurons [52]. This is evidence that neuroprotection by U0126 is not simply due to scavenging of free radicals because direct activation of Ras, an upstream effector of the MEK/ERK pathway, by NO is essential for NO-elicited ERK2 activation [54].

It has been shown that phospho-ERK1/2 immunostaining was localized in terminal boutons as well as processes and somata in cultured hippocampal neurons after seizure-like activity [44]. We also found strong phospho-ERK1/2 immunostaining in the mossy fibers that originate from dentate granule cells, and dendrite of CA1 pyramidal cells and cortical neurons after ischemia/reperfusion [52]. However, little is known about the functional meaning of ERK1/2 activation in the fiber and process of neurons. Synapsin I, a major phosphoprotein found in synaptic vesicles, is a substrate for ERK1/2 [64]. Phosphorylation of synapsin I leads to dissociation of the synaptic vesicles, resulting in neurotransmitter release that initiates neuronal injury. These data suggest that MEK inhibition may also contribute to brain protection by both postsynaptic and presynaptic mechanisms.

Ischemic preconditioning and MAP kinase

The role of the MEK/ERK pathway in ischemic preconditioning has been suggested both in cortical cultures and in an animal model [55, 65]. MEK1 and ERK2 inhibition by dominant negative forms of these genes abolishes the preconditioning effect in cortical neurons by 5 minutes oxygen/glucose deprivation 24 hours before 60 minutes oxygen/glucose deprivation [55]. Pretreatment with BDNF affords brain protection against hypoxic-ischemic injury in neonatal rats by the activation of ERK1/2 [65]. This protection is abolished by cotreatment with U0126. On the other hand, BDNF enhances neuronal necrosis resulting from oxygen/glucose deprivation [66]. Again, these studies indicate that the MEK/ERK pathway can lead cell death or cell survival, depending both on the timing of activation and on the status of other signaling pathways.

Clinical implication in reperfusion injury

As we demonstrated, reperfusion dramatically activates the MEK/ERK pathway, suggesting a role for MEK/ERK activation in reperfusion injury. Consistent with this view, U0126 given before reperfusion but during occlusion is protective. Thrombolysis therapy with i.v. injection of t-PA is limited within 3 hours of onset [1, 2]. Reperfusion injury may limit the therapeutic time window of t-PA therapy. Therefore, combined injection of MEK inhibitor and t-PA may afford additional effects, or may extend the therapeutic time window of t-PA beyond 3 hours.

Cerebral vasospasm

MAP kinases also play important roles in vascular structures. Significant activation of MAP kinases has been demonstrated in reperfusion injury of endothelial cells. Cerebral vasospasm may be another potential clinical entity that can be treated by MEK inhibitors. Cerebral vasospams is the major cause of mortality and morbidity after subarachnoidal hemorrhage. ERK1/2 MAP kinases activation has been demonstrated in association with cerebral vasospasm in a canine model [67]. In addition, PD98059 and U0126 both have been shown in rabbit basilar artery to diminish the contractile effect of endothelin-1, hemolysate, oxyhemoglobin, and blood containing CSF [68]. Thus, MEK/ERK inhibition may also provide a therapeutic intervention to treat cerebral vasospasm.

Limitations and cautions

Although the results with MEK inhibitors in animal stroke models are promising, further studies are needed. Kinetics of MEK inhibitors across the blood-brain barrier has not been fully established. In addition, systemic adverse effects such as immune-suppression and carcinogenicity remain to be examined. Before clinical studies, treatment studies in non-human primate stroke models will be important.

References

1. The National Institute of Neurological Disorders and Stroke rt-PA Stroke Study Group (1995) Tissue plasminogen activator for acute ischemic stroke. N Engl J Med 333:1581-1587
2. Hacke W, Kaste M, Fieschi C, et al (1995) Intravenous thrombolysis with recombinant tissue plasminogen activator for acute hemispheric stroke. The European Cooperative Acute Stroke Study (ECASS) JAMA 274:1017-1025
3. Cao W, Carney JM, Duchon A, et al (1988) Oxygen free radical involvement in ischemia and reperfusion injury to brain. Neurosci Lett 88:233-238
4. Malinski T, Bailey F, Zhang ZG, et al (1993) Nitric oxide measured by a porphyrinic microsensor in rat brain after transient middle cerebral artery. J Cereb Blood Flow Metab 13:355-358
5. Grammas P, Liu GJ, Wood K, et al (1993) Anoxia/reoxygenation induces hydroxyl free radical formation in brain microvessels. Free Radic Biol Med 14:553-557
6. Murakami K, Kondo T, Kawase M, et al (1998) Mitochondrial susceptibility to oxidative stress exacerbates cerebral infarction that follows permanent focal cerebral ischemia in mutant mice with manganese superoxide dismutase deficiency. J Neurosci 18:205-213
7. Fujimura M, Morita-Fujimura Y, Kawase M, et al (1999) Manganese superoxide dismutase mediates the early release of mitochondrial cytochrome C and subsequent DNA fragmentation after permanent focal cerebral ischemia in mice. J Neurosci 19:3414-3422
8. Yamaguchi T, Sano K, Takakura K, et al (1998) Ebselen in acute ischemic stroke: a placebo-controlled, double-blind clinical trial. Ebselen Study Group. Stroke 29:12-17
9. McCulloch J, Dewar D (2001) A radical approach to stroke therapy. Proc Natl Acad Sci USA 98:10989-10991
10. Huang Z, Huang PL, Panahian N, et al (1994) Effects of cerebral ischemia in mice deficient in neuronal nitric oxide synthase. Science 265:1883-1885
11. Iadecola C, Zhang F, Casey R, et al (1997) Delayed reduction of ischemic brain injury and neurological deficits in mice lacking the inducible nitric oxide synthase gene. J Neurosci 17:9157-9164
12. Kinouchi H, Epstein CJ, Mizui T, et al (1991) Attenuation of focal cerebral ischemic injury in transgenic mice overexpressing CuZu superoxide dismutase. Proc Natl Acad Sci USA 88:11158-11162

13. Chan PH, Kawase M, Murakami K, et al (1998) Overexpression of SOD1 in transgenic rats protects vulnerable neurons against ischemic damage after global cerebral ischemia and reperfusion. J Neurosci 18:8292-8299
14. Kondo T, Reaume AG, Huang T-T, et al (1997) Reduction of CuZn-superoxide dismutase activity exacerbates neuronal cell injury and edema formation after transient focal cerebral ischemia. J Neurosci 17:4180-4189
15. Ogawa A, Yoshimoto T, Kikuchi H, et al (1999) Ebselen in acute middle cerebral artery occlusion: a placebo-controlled, double-blind clinical trial. Cerebrovasc Dis 9:112-118
16. Kane DJ, Sarafian TA, Anton R, et al (1993) Bcl-2 inhibition of neural death: decreased generation of reactive oxygen species. Science 262:1274-1277
17. Lipton SA (1999) Neuronal protection and destruction by NO. Cell Death Differ 6:943-951
18. Blenis J (1991) Growth-regulated signal transduction by the MAP kinases and RSKs. Cancer Res 3:445-449
19. Cobb MH, Robbins DJ, Boulton TG. (1991) ERKs, extracellular signal-regulated MAP-2 kinases. Curr Opin Cell Biol 3:1025-1032
20. Hoshi M, Nishida E, Sakai H. (1988) Activation of a Ca2+-inhibitable protein kinase that phosphorylates microtubule-associated protein 2 in vitro by growth factors, phorbol esters, and serum in quiescent cultured human fibroblasts. J Biol Chem 263:5396-5401
21. Pelech SL, Tombes RM, Meijer L, et al (1988) Activation of myelin basic protein kinases during echinoderm oocyte maturation and egg fertilization. Dev Biol 130:28-36
22. Ray LB, Sturgill TW. (1987) Rapid stimulation by insulin of a serine/threonine kinase in 3T3-L1 and adipocytes that phosphorylate microtubule-associated protein 2 in vivo. Proc Natl Acad Sci USA 84:1502-1506
23. Boulton TG, Yancopoulos GD, Gregory JS, et al (1990) An insulin-stimulated protein kinase similar to yeast kinases involved in cell cycle control. Science 249:64-67
24. Boulton TG, Nye SH, Robbins DJ, et al (1991) ERKs: A family of protein-serine/threonine kinases that are activated and tyrosine phosphorylated in response to insulin and NGF. Cell 65:663-675
25. Nishida E, Gotoh Y. (1993) The MAP kinase cascade is essential for diverse signal transduction pathways. Trends Biochem Sci 18:128-131
26. Segar R, Krebs EG. (1995) The MAPK signaling cascade. FASEB J 9:726-735
27. Seko Y, Tobe K, Ueki K, et al (1996) Hypoxia and hypoxia/reoxygenation activate Raf-1, mitogen-activated protein kinase kinase, mitogen-activated protein kinases, and S6 kinase in cultured rat cardiac myocytes. Circ Res 78:82-90
28. Aikawa R, Komuro I, Yamazaki T, et al (1997) Oxidative stress activates extracellular signal-regulated kinases through Src and Ras in cultured cardiac myocytes of neonatal rats. J Clin Invest 100:1813-1821
29. Hayakawa J, Ohmichi M, Kurachi H, et al (1999) Inhibition of extracellular signal-regulated protein kinase or c-Jun N-terminal protein kinase cascade, differentially activated by cisplatin, sensitizes human ovarian cancer cell line. J Biol Chem 274:31648-31654
30. Persons DL, Yazlovitskaya EM, Cui W, et al (1999) Cisplatin-induced activation of mitogen-activated protein kinases in ovarian carcinoma cells: Inhibition of extracellular-signal-regulated kinase activity increases sensitivity to cisplatin. Clin Cancer Res 5:1007-1014

31. Gao XS, Asaumi J, Kawasaki S, et al (1995) Sensitivity of anticancer drugs in NIH3T3' cells transfected with oncogenes accompanied by pSV2neo vector. Anticancer Res 15:1911-1914
32. Fokstuen T, Rabo YB, Zhou JN, et al (1997) The Ras farnesylation inhibitor BZA-5B increases the resistance to cisplatin in a human melanoma cell line. Anticancer Res 17:2347-2352
33. Wang X, Martindale JL, Holbrook NJ (2000) Requirement for ERK activation in cisplatin-induced apoptosis. J Biol Chem 275:39435-39443
34. Sutherland CL, Heath AW, Pelech SL, et al (1996) Differential activation of the ERK, JNK, and p38 mitogen-activated protein kinases by CD40 and the B cell antigen receptor. J Immunol 157:3381-3390
35. Xia Z, Dickens M, Raingeaud J, et al (1995) Opposing effects of ERK and JNK-p38 MAP kinases on apoptosis. Science 270:1326-1331
36. Potapova O, Basu S, Mercola D, et al (2001) Protective role for c-Jun in the cellular response to DNA damage. J Biol Chem 276:28546-28558
37. Fiore RS, Bayer VE, Pelech SL, et a1 (1993) p42 mitogen-activated protein kinase in brain: Prominent localization in neuronal cell bodies and dendrites. Neuroscience 55:463-472
38. Bonni A, Brunet A, West AE, et al (1999) Cell survival promoted by the Ras-MAPK signaling pathway by transcription-dependent and –independent mechanisms. Science 286:1358-1362
39. Bading H, Greenberg ME (1991) Stimulation of protein tyrosine phosphorylation by NMDA receptor activation. Science 253:912-914
40. Fiore RS, Murphy TH, Sanghera JS, et al (1993) Activation of p42 mitogen-activated protein kinase by glutamate receptor stimulation in rat primary cortical cultures. J Neurochem 61:1626-1633
41. Stratton KR, Worley PF, Huganir RL, et al (1989) Muscarinic agonists and phorbol esters increase tyrosine phosphorylation of a 40-kilodalton protein in hippocampal slices. Proc Natl Acad Sci U S A 86:2498-2501
42. Baraban JM, Fiore RS, Sanghera J, et al (1993) Identification of p42 mitogen-activated protein kinase as a tyrosine kinase substrate activated by maximal electroconvulsive shock in hippocampus. J Neurochem 60:330-336
43. Stratton KR, Worley PF, Litz JS, et al (1991) Electroconvulsive treatment induces a rapid and transient increase in tyrosine phosphorylation of a 40-kilodalton associated with microtubule-associated protein 2 kinase activity. J Neurochem 56:147-152
44. Murray B, Alessandrini A, Cole AJ, et al (1998) Inhibition of the p44/42 MAP kinase pathway protects hippocampal neurons in a cell-culture model of seizure activity. Proc Natl Acad Sci USA 95:11975-11980
45. Campos-González R, Kindy MS (1992) Tyrosine phosphorylation of microtubule-associated protein kinase after transient ischemia in the gerbil brain. J Neurochem 59:1955-1958
46. Kindy MS (1993) Inhibition of tyrosine phosphorylation prevents delayed neuronal death following cerebral ischemia. J Cereb Blood Flow Metab 13:372-377
47. Hu B-R, Wieloch T (1994) Tyrosine phosphorylation and activation of mitogen-activated protein kinase in the rat brain following transient cerebral ischemia. J Neurochem 62:1357-1367

48. Ohtsuki T, Matsumoto M, Kitagawa K, et al (1996) Delayed neuronal death in ischemic hippocampus involves stimulation of protein tyrosine phosphorylation. Am J Physiol 271:C1085-C1097
49. Gu Z, Jiang Q, Zhang Z. (2001) Extracellular signal-regulated kinase 1/2 activation in hippocampus after cerebral ischemia may not interfere with postischemic cell death. Brain Res 901:79-84
50. Namura S, Alessandrini A, Bonventre JV, et al (1998) Inhibition of MEK1/ERK pathway reduces brain damage following focal cerebral ischemia and reperfusion in mice. Stroke 29:326
51. Alessandrini A, Namura S, Moskowitz MA, et al (1999) MEK1 protein kinase inhibition protects against damage resulting from focal cerebral ischemia. Proc Natl Acad Sci USA 96:12866-12869
52. Namura S, Iihara K, Takami S, et al (2001) Intravenous administration of MEK inhibitor U0126 affords brain protection against forebrain ischemia and focal cerebral ischemia. Proc Natl Acad Sci USA 98:11569-11574
53. Sugino T, Nozaki K, Takagi Y, et al (2000) Activation of mitogen-activated protein kinases after transient forebrain ischemia in gerbil hippocampus. J Neurosci 20:4506-4514
54. Yun HY, Gonzalez-Zulueta M, Dawson VL, et al (1998) Nitric oxide mediates N-methyl-D-aspartate receptor-induced activation of p21ras. Proc Natl Acad Sci U S A 95:5773-5778
55. Gonzalez-Zulueta M, Feldman AB, Klesse LJ, et al (2000) Requirement for nitric oxide activation of p21(ras)/extracellular regulated kinase in neuronal ischemic preconditioning. Proc Natl Acad Sci U S A 97:436-441
56. Irving EA, Ray AM, Staton PC, et al (2001) J Cereb Blood Flow Metab 21, Suppl. 1:S379
57. Satoh T, Nakatsuka D, Watanabe Y, et al (2000) Neuroprotection by MAPK/ERK kinase inhibition with U0126 against oxidative stress in a mouse neuronal cell line and rat primary cultured cortical neurons. Neurosci Lett 288:163-166
58. Stanciu M, Wang Y, Kentor R, et al (2000) Persistent activation of ERK contributes to glutamate-induced oxidative toxicity in a neuronal cell line and primary cortical neuron cultures. J Biol Chem 275:12200-12206
59. Irving EA, Barone FC, Reith AD, et al (2000) Differential activation of MAPK/ERK and p38/SAPK in neurones and glia following focal cerebral ischaemia in the rat. Brain Res Mol Brain Res 77:65-75
60. Bhat NR, Zhang P (1999) Hydrogen peroxide activation of multiple mitogen-activated protein kinases in an oligodendrocyte cell line: role of extracellular signal-regulated kinase in hydrogen peroxide-induced cell death. J Neurochem 72:112-119
61. Dudley DT, Pang L, Decker SJ, et al (1995) A synthetic inhibitor of the mitogen-activated protein kinase cascade. Proc Natl Acad Sci U S A 92:7686-7689
62. Favata MF, Horiuchi KY, Manos EJ, et al (1998) Identification of a novel inhibitor of mitogen-activated protein kinase kinase. J Biol Chem 273:18623-18632
63. Wang H, Xu L, Venkatachalam S, et al (2001) Differential regulation of IL-1β and TNF-α RNA expression by MEK1 inhibitor after focal cerebral ischemia in mice. Biochem Biophys Res Commun 286:869-874
64. Jovanovic JN, Czernik AJ, Fienberg AA, et al (2000) Synapsins as mediators of BDNF-enhanced neurotransmitter release. Nat Neurosci 3:323-329

65. Han BH, Holtzman DM. (2000) BDNF protects the neonatal brain from hypoxic-ischemic injury in vivo via the ERK path. J Neurosci 20:5775-5781
66. Koh J-Y, Gwag BJ, Lobner D, et al (1995) Potentiated necrosis of cultured cortical neurons by neurotrophins. Science 268:573-575
67. Tibbs R, Zubkov A, Aoki K, et al (2000) Effects of mitogen-activated protein kinase inhibitors on cerebral vasospasm in a double-hemorrhage model in dogs. J Neurosurg 93:1041-1047
68. Zubkov AY, Rollins KS, McGehee B, et al (2001) Relaxant effect of U0126 in hemolysate-, oxyhemoglobin-, and bloody cerebrospinal fluid-induced contraction in rabbit basilar artery. Stroke 32:154-161

Redox regulation in neuronal damage during brain ischemia

-The role of thioredoxin in ischemic neuronal death-

Yasushi Takagi[1], Itaro Hattori[1,2], Kazuhiko Nozaki[1], Nobuo Hashimoto[1], and Junji Yodoi[2]

[1]Department of Neurosurgery, Kyoto University Graduate School of Medicine, 54 Kawahara-cho, Shogoin, Sakyo-ku, Kyoto 606-8507, Japan
[2]Department of Biological Responses, Institute for Virus Research, Kyoto University, 53 Kawahara-cho, Shogoin, Sakyo-ku, Kyoto 606-8507, Japan

Summary: Reactive oxygen species has been proved not only to damage cells and tissues but to play as second messenger in signal transduction pathways. Increasing evidence has indicated that the cellular redox status modulates various aspects of cellular events, including proliferation and apoptosis. Thioredoxin (TRX) plays important biological roles both in intra- and extracellular compartments including regulation of various intracellular molecules via thiol redox control. We have described the role of TRX after brain ischemia. TRX was induced in neurons after middle cerebral artery occlusion. Moreover TRX overexpressing mice has the resistance against focal ischemic brain damage. In addition, we found about 20% reduction of infarct volume in recombinant human TRX-treated mice versus control animals. Neurological deficit was also ameriorated significantly in rhTRX-treated mice compared with control mice. In this section, we describe the role of TRX in ischemic neuronal death. TRX and the redox state modified by TRX play a crucial role in brain damage during stroke.

Key words: Thioredoxin, Redox regulation, Brain ischemia, Reactive oxygen species

Introduction

Thioredoxin (TRX) is a small multifunctional protein with a redox-active disulfide/dithiol within the conserved active site sequence: -Cys-Gly-Pro-Cys- [1,2]. Increasing evidence has indicated that cellular redox status modulates various aspects of cellular events, including proliferation and apoptosis. Human TRX has been identified as a highly expressed cytokine-like factor in activated T- and B- cells which upregulates the interlukin-2 receptor alpha-chain and interlukin-2 [3-5]. TRX regulates various intracellular molecules via thiol redox control involving transcription factors such as nuclear factor-kappaB (NF-kappaB), activator protein-1 (AP-1), myb and redox factor-1 (Ref-1) [6-10]. TRX has been reported to induce AP-1 through de novo transcription of the c-fos and c-jun [9]. TRX enhances the DNA-binding activity of Jun and Fos [7,9]. Hirota et al. [10] reported that AP-1 transcriptional activity regulated by a direct association between thioredoxin and Ref-1. Moreover TRX augmented the DNA-binding and transcriptional activities of the p50 subunit of NF-kappaB by reducing Cys-62 in its biding loop [8]. It has been indicated that TRX directly regulates apoptosis signaling kinase-1 (ASK-1) which is one of mitogen activated protein kinase kinase kinase (MAPKKK) enzymes and has anti-apoptotic function. [11] TRX is also a stress-inducible protein whose expression is enhanced by various types of stresses, e.g. viral infection, exposure to ultraviolet light, x-ray irradiation, and hydrogen peroxide [12-14]. Furthermore TRX is a scavenger of reactive oxygen species (ROS) [15], and recombinant TRX (rTRX) has protective activity against cytotoxicity, in which the generation of ROS seems to be involved in the cytotoxic mechanism [12,16,17]. These data suggest that TRX plays a number of important biological roles both in intra- and extracellular compartments. During ischemia or ischemia/reperfusion in the brain, excessive ROS alter or disrupt the balance of redox potential in cells and lead to protein oxidation, lipid peroxidation, and DNA damage. More recently oxidative stress is claimed to be one of crucial factor in the development of ischemic brain injury as well as excitatory amino acid toxicity, waves of spreading depolarization, and specific gene expression. Based on these considerations, we hypothesized that endogenous TRX functions as a regulator of ischemic injury. Firstly, we investigated TRX expression after middle cerebral artery occlusion (MCAO). We analyzed TRX and TRX mRNA by immunohistochemistry and hybridization experiment in rat brain after MCAO [18].

Induction of thioredoxin after brain ischemia

Male Wistar rats weighing 300-400 g were used. Under general anesthesia with mixture of 2% halothane, 30% oxygen, and 70% nitrous oxide, an 18.3 mm-long embolus made from a 4-0 nylon thread was inserted into the internal carotid artery through a small incision in the external carotid artery, so that MCA was obstructed [19]. The sections were immunohistochemically stained with polyclonal antibodies raised against a synthetic polypeptide of the C-terminal 10 amino acid of mouse thioredoxin. During ischemia, immunoreactivity for TRX decreased and dissapeared after MCAO in ischemic regions [18]. In the lateral striatum, TRX immunoreactivity rapidly decreased and nearly dissapeared 4 hours after MCAO [18]. In frontoparietal cortex, TRX immunoreactivity decreased and nearly dissapeared 16 hours after MCAO [18]. To the contrary, TRX immunoreactivity began to increase 4 hours after MCAO and increased till 24 hours in the perifocal ischemic region, which is called 'penumbra' [18] (Figure.1A, B). In addition, we performed in situ hybridization and northern blot analysis using antisense RNA probes manufactured from murine TRX cDNA [18]. In hybridization experiments, TRX mRNA also decreased and nearly dissapeared 4 hours after MCAO in the lateral striatum [18]. In frontoparietal cortex, TRX mRNA decreased till 24 hours after MCAO. In the perifocal ischemic region, TRX mRNA began to increase 4 hours after MCAO and increased till 24 hours [18] (Figure.1C, D).

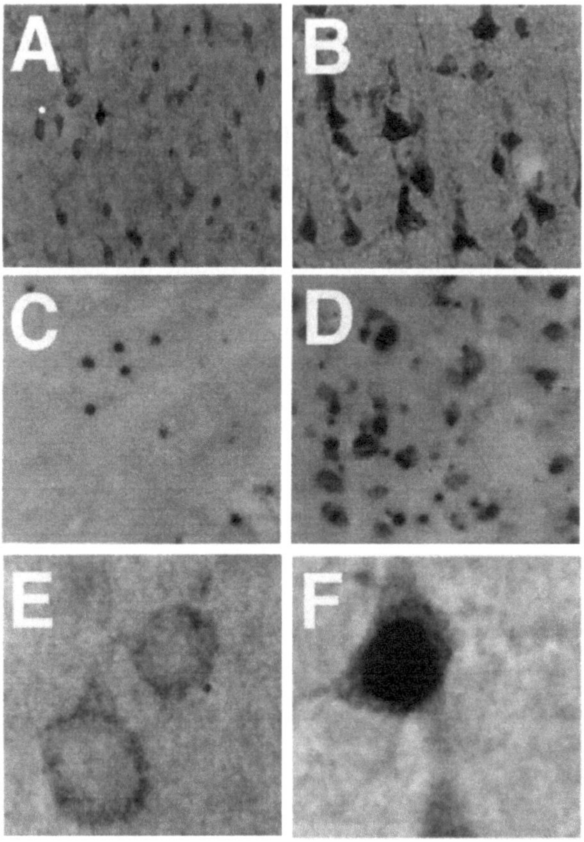

Fig. 1. Immunohistochemical staining for TRX indicates that TRX immunoreactivity was induced after ischemia in the perifocal ischemic cortex (A; sham control B; 24 hours after middle cerebral artery occlusion (MCAO)). Hybridization experiments indicated that TRX mRNA was induced after ischemia in the perifocal cortex. (C; sham control, D; 24 hours after MCAO. High power view of immunohistochemical study indicates that TRX translocates into the neuronal nuclei after tarnsient focal ischemia. (E; sham control F; 24 hours after 30 minutes of MCAO, A, B; frontoparietal cortex). Original magnification A-D; x 100, E-F; x 400. (modified from references [18,20], with permission)

Nothern blot analysis showed that TRX mRNA in the operated hemispheres increased until 24 hours after the surgical procedures [18]. Next, we assayed TRX expression in ischemia-reperfusion brain tissue. TRX was also induced in neurons and translocated into nuclei from cytoplasm [20] (Figure. 1E, F).

Overexpression of thioredoxin in transgenic mice has neuropretective effect

We produced TRX overexpressing mice and investigated TRX expression, brain anatomy and physiological state [21]. No anatomical abnormalities were found in TRX transgenic mice [21]. Western blot analysis indicated 4 times of TRX expression in the TRX transgenic mice brain when compared with wild-type mice [21]. We subjected these mice to MCAO and investigated their ischemic brain injury [21]. Physiologic parameters (blood pressure, PO_2, PCO_2, and blood pH) during surgery did not significantly differ in the two sets of mice [21]. Regional cerebral blood flow analyzed by laser-Doppler flowmetry revealed no significant differences during the ischemic insults (each n=6) between TRX transgenic and wild-type mice [21]. At 24 hours after the surgery, infarct volume was quantified with 2% 2,3,5-triphenyltetrazolium chloride (TTC) [21].

The infarct areas and volume was significantly smaller in TRX transgenic mice than in the wild-type mice [21]. Oxidative inactivation of enzymes and oxidative modification of proteins by metal-catalyzed oxidation reactions are accompanied by the generation of protein carbonyl derivatives that react with 2,4-dinitrophenylhydrazine (DNPH) to form protein hydrazone derivatives.

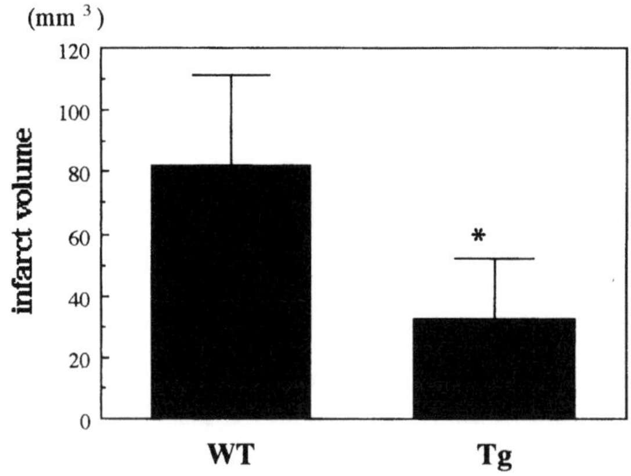

Fig. 2. Infarct volumes in TRX transgenic and in wild-type mice. Infarct size was analyzed 24 hours after MCA occlusion using 2,3,5-triphenyltetrazolium chloride (TTC) staining. Infarct volume was smaller in TRX transgenic mice than in wild-type mice (n=each 9). (Data are expressed as means ± SD, stastical analysis is performed using Student's t test; * $p< 0.01$) (modified from [21], with permission)

Using this property, we determined the protein carbonyl content of soluble fraction of crude brain cortical extract preparations from TRX transgenic and wild-type mice subjected to MCAO [21]. In sham-operated control mice, protein carbonyl contents were not singnificantly defferent [21]. The protein carbonyl content in sham-control animals were 57.0±45.1 in wild-type and 60.2±31.5 (% of control, mean ± SD, not significant) [21]. On the other hand, at 1 hour after the ischemic insult, the protein carbonyl contents did not increased in TRX transgenic mice compared with wild-type mice [21].The protein carbonyl content in sham-control animals were 230.0±116.0 in wild-type and 101.0±43.2 (% of control, mean ± SD, p<0.01) [21] (Figure.3). During ischemia, c-fos and c-jun family are known to be rapidly induced. Induction of c-fos, c-fos gene product is peaked at 1-4 hour after permanent MCAO according to previous observations [22,23]. We assayed c-fos level in the early stage of ischemia. First we performed western blot analysis. In sham controls, c-fos expression did not differ [21]. In contrast, 1 hour after ischemia, c-fos expression in TRX transgenic mice is stronger than in wild-type mice [21] (Figure.4). Moreover we performed immunohistochemical study of c-fos expression in wild-type and TRX transgenic mice [21].

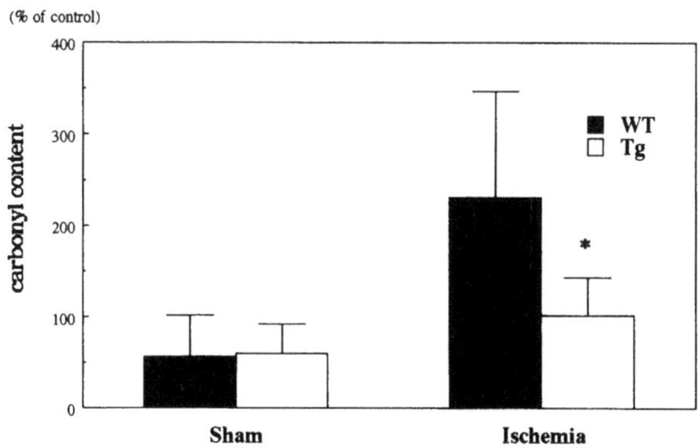

Fig. 3. Changes in protein carbonyl content after MCAO in TRX transgenic and wild-type mice. The DNP derivatized protein samples prepared from brains subjected to MCA occlusion were separated on a 15% SDS-polyacrylamide gel electrophoresis followed by Western blotting with primary antibody, specific to the DNP moiety of the proteins. In sham control animals, only a small amount of DNP moieties was detected, and no difference was detected between the two groups. At 1 hour after ischemia, more DNP moieties were detected in wild-type mice than in transgenic mice. The amount of carbonyl groups extracted from 18 mg of sample proteins was measured by an image analyzer (NIH image analysis system) compared with 2.5 ml of control DNP-lated proteins mixture (data are expressed as means ± SD, statistical analysis was performed using Student's t test; *p< 0.05) (WT: wild-type, TG: TRX transgenic mice, I: ischemia, S: sham).

The c-fos immunoreactivity in CA3 and penumbra was also stronger in TRX transgenic mice than in wild-type mice [21]. Another experiment of western blot analysis for c-jun level indicated that c-jun induction during ischemia did not differ in two sets of mice [21].

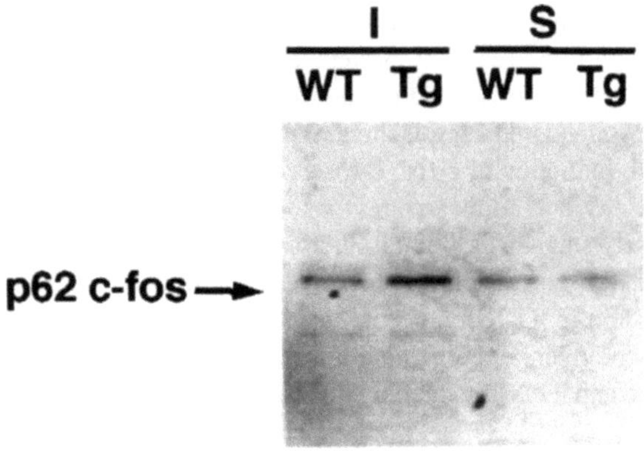

Fig. 4. Expression of c-fos in TRX transgenic and wild-type mice during MCAO. In sham-operated mice, c-fos expression was not different between the two groups. After ischemic insult, c-fos was induced more highly in TRX transgenic mice than in wild-type mice. In sham-operated animals, c-fos expression was not different between the two groups. After ischemic insult, c-fos expression was higher in transgenic mice than in wild-type mice (WT: wild-type, TG: TRX transgenic mice, I: ischemia, S: sham).

Intravenous administration of thioredoxin decreases brain damage following transient focal cerebral ischemia

Next, we examined the effects of intravenously-administrated TRX in a model of transient focal cerebral ischemia to clarify the possibility of clinical application. Mature male C57BL/6 mice received either continuous intravenous infusion of recombinant human TRX (rhTRX), bovine serum albumin, or vehicle alone for 2 hours after transient right MCAO (90 minutes). Twenty-four hours after MCAO, animals were evaluated neurologically and the volume of cerebral infarct was asscessed by image analysis. We found about 20% reduction in infarct volume in rhTRX-treated mice versus control animals ($p < 0.02$). Neurological deficit was also ameriorated significantly in rhTRX-treated mice compared with contorol mice (Hattori et al., in preparation).

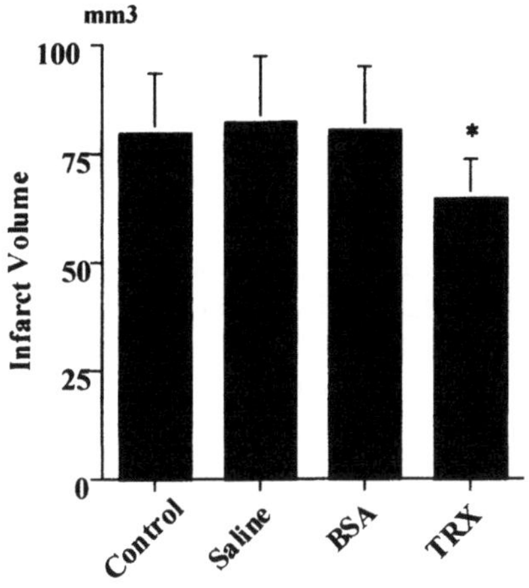

Fig. 5. Infarct volumes in mice subjected to 24 hours after MCAO assessed by TTC staining. Bar graph of mean ± SD infarct volume in brains of postischemic rats treated with rhTRX, BSA, saline, and non-treated (each n=8). Any value that is statistically significant different ($P < 0.05$) from the control value is indicated by an asterisk.

The role of thioredoxin and redox regulation in ischemic neuronal death

Redox regulation of intracellular molecules is an interesting and important issue. TRX is a small, ubiquitous protein with two redox-active half-cystine residues in active center. In the central nervous systems, rTRX has a neuroprotective effect on murine primary cultured neurons obtained from the striatum and cortex [24]. rTRX rescued primary cultured neurons from injury induced by serum-free medium. TRX functions like a neurotropic factor for central cholinergic neurons [25], and was upregulated in mechanical brain injury [26]. We have reported the proliferated astroglial induction of TRX in the CA1 region during transient forebrain ischemia [27]. In combination, these findings indicate that TRX and redox system modulated by TRX has a function in the cellular defense against oxidative stress in neurons as well as in other cell types and may play a role during brain injury.

Stress proteins such as heat shock proteins (HSPs), genes and several growth factors are induced in ischemic and periischemic lesions [28-32]. Induced stress proteins and growth factors enhance neuronal survival in vitro. c-fos and c-jun are immediate early genes that encoded c-fos and c-jun proteins, respectively. Homodimetric (Jun/Jun) or heterodimetric (Jun/Fos) complexes forms AP-1 which regulates various downstream molecules such as nerve growth factor (NGF), brain-derived neurotrophic factor (BDNF), and amyloid precurcer protein (APP). c-fos expression affects ischemic injury; in superoxide dismutase (SOD) transgenic mice during ischemia, prolonged and enhanced c-fos expression was reported [33]. Hyperglycemia, which increases brain damage, has been shown to suppress c-fos mRNA after transient cerebral ischemia [34,35]. In addition, KCl-induced spreading depression resulted in a widespread expression of c-fos mRNA in the ipsilateral cortex of rats and reduced neuronal cell death after ischemic challenge [36]. Moreover, intra-ischemic hypothermia, which protects the brain against ischemic injury, has been shown to increase the induction of c-fos mRNA after transient forebrain ischemia [37]. These data indicate that c-fos expression may influence attenuation of ischemic injury. TRX has been reported to directly activate the DNA-binding and transactivation abilities of AP-1. Recent invrstigation has indicated TRX regurated AP-1 transcriptional activity by a direct association with Ref-1 [10]. TRX has been reported to directly regulate ASK-1 in two-hybrid assay [11]. These reports have showed that TRX plays not only as one of antioxidants but has specific target molecules. TRX overexpressing mice expressed enhanced c-fos expression in the early stage of ischemia. Our findings coincide with the observation that in vitro, transient endogeneous TRX expression and extracellular TRX activate and enhance c-fos and c-jun expression [7,9]. However more studies on c-fos expression during ischemia are needed to further elucidate the role of AP-1 in the neuroprotective effect of TRX, but TRX may have neuroprotective function through the activation of AP-1.

Many factors are involved in the development of neuronal damage during ischemia. The neurotoxicity of excitatory amino acids, an overload of intracellular calcium (Ca^{++}), the suppression of protein synthesis, and free radical formation are thought to play detrimental roles in the pathogenesis of ischemic injury. The excitatory amino acids elevated cytosolic free Ca^{++}, and in pathological conditions, a Ca^{++} overload may occur, which can set off a cascade of events, such as phospholipase activation, potentially leading to free-radical production.

The formation of oxygen-derived free radicals may occur in the electron transport chain, in metabolic processes such as free fatty acids, and in purine and nitric oxide [38-41]. These oxidants destroy or inactivate cellular and subcellular proteins, and various enzymes. In this sense, oxygen-derived free radicals play an important role in neuronal death. This hypothesis is supported by the finding that SOD activity and immunoreactivity decline in the ischemic area during ischemia [42-44] and that several antioxidants (e.g. glutathione, ascorbic acid, a-tocopherol, and ubiquinone) significantly decrease brain damage during focal ischemia [45-47]. SOD and Bcl-2 transgenic animals were reported to be resistant to ischemic injury [48,49]. These findings reveal that ROS scavenging systems are important for the survival of neurons during ischemia.

Lipid and protein oxidation are both consequences of the damage caused by the production of free radicals during ischemia. Complete brain ischemia has been shown to cause severe acidosis which aggravates cell damage and impairs postischemic recovery. Oxidative modification of cellular proteins was reported to be occurred within 10 minutes and peaked at 1 or 2 hour after the ischemic insults [50,51]. Oxidative inactivation renders glutamine synthetase and other enzymes highly susceptible to proteolysis by proteases during ischemia [52]. The protein oxidation is an early intracellular indicator of tissue damage resulting from ischemia. Oxidative inactivation of enzymes could lead to disruption of cellular metabolism and seriously impair the ability of cells to repair this damage. In TRX transgenic mice, protein carbonyl content was suppressed at 1 hour after ischemia. The data presented here indicate that endogenous TRX prevents cellular protein from oxidation through its redox-active property.

Recombinant TRX exerts protective activity against a number of toxins and insults in in vitro studies, in which excessive ROS seems to be involved in the cytotoxic mechanism [53-55]. And it have been reported the cytoprotective effects of rhTRX against either ischemia/reperfusion-induced lung injury in animal models [56-59] and hypoxia-reoxigenation injury in in vitro [60].

In our study, protein carbonyl contents in the brain of hTRX-treated animals were significantly suppressed in comparison with the control animals after transient ischemia, which suggests that exogenous hTRX attenuates oxidative stress by exerting redox regulating activity including quenching ROS. In addition to the possibility that TRX scavenges ROS released from ischemic tissue, it is conceivable that TRX might cause increasing local CBF surrounding ischemic tissue and decreasing infarct size by preventing the adhesion of leukocytes to vascular endothelial membrane. Intravenous administration of rhTRX rescued the brain injury after stroke. In support of this, our recent studies showed that rhTRX suppresses the adhesion of neutrophils on human umbilical vein endothelial cells by adhesion assay [61] and that systemic administration of rhTRX suppress extravasation of leukocytes into the inflammatory site [61]. Regarding this possibility, further investigation is required.

In summary, we demonstrated that the roles of TRX in ischemic brain ijury. The redox regulating activity of TRX may contribute to neuroprotection by diminishing oxidative stress.

References

1. Holmgren A (1985) Thioredoxin. Annu Rev Biochem 54:237-271
2. Holmgren A (1989) Thioredoxin and glutaredoxin systems. J Biol Chem 264:13963-13966
3. Tagaya Y, Okada M, Sugie K, Kasahara T, et al (1988) IL-2 receptor (p55)/Tac inducing factor: purification and characterization of ATL-derived factor (ADF). J Immunol 140:2613-2620
4. Tagaya Y, Maeda Y, Mitsui A, et al (1989) ATL-derived factor (ADF), an IL-2 receptor/Tac inducer homologous to thioredoxin: possible involvement of ditiol-reduction in the IL-2 receptor induction. EMBO J 8:757-764
5. Yodoi J, Uchiyama T (1992) Diseases associated with HTLV-1: virus, IL-2 receptor dysregulation and redox regulation. Immunol Today 13:405-411
6. Abate C, Patel L, Rauscher III FJ, et al (1990) Redox regulation of Fos and Jun DNA-binding activity in vitro. Science 249:1157-1161
7. Meyer M, Schreck R, Baeuerle PA (1993) H_2O_2 and antioxidants have opposite effects on activation of NF-kappa B and AP-1 in intact cells: AP-1 as secondary antioxidant-responsive factor. EMBO J 12:2005-15

8. Okamoto T, Ogiwara H, Hayashi T, et al (1992) Human thioredoxin/adult T cell leukemia-derived factor activates the enhancer binding protein of human immunodeficiency virus type 1 by thiol redox control mechanism. Int Immunol 4:811-819
9. Schenk H, Klein M, Erdbrugger W, et al (1994) Distinct effects of thioredoxin and antioxidants on the activation of transcription factors NF-kappa B and AP-1. Proc Natl Acad Sci USA 91:1672-1676
10. Hirota K, Matsui M, Iwata S, et al (1997) AP-1 transcriptional activity regulated by a direct association between thioredoxin and Ref-1. Proc Natl Acad Sci USA 94:3633-3638
11. Saito M, Nishitoh H, Fujii M, et al (1998) Mammalial thioredoxin is a direct inhibitor of apoptosis signal-regulating kinase (ASK) 1. EMBO J 17:2596-2606
12. Nakamura H, Matsuda M, Furuke K et al (1994) Adult T cell leukemia derived factor/human thioredoxin protects endothelial F-2 cell injury caused by activated neutrophils or hydrogen peroxide. Immunol Lett 42:75-80
13. Ohira A, Honda O, Gauntt CD, et al (1994) Oxidative stress induces adult T cell leukemia derived factor/thioredoxin in the rat retina. Lab Invest 70:279-285
14. Sachi Y, Hirota K, Masutani H, et al (1995) Induction of ADF/TRX by oxidative stress in keratinocytes and lymphoid cells. Immunol Lett 44:189-193
15. Mitsui A, Hirakawa T, Yodoi J (1992) Reactive oxygen-reducing and protein-refolding activities of adult T cell leukemia-derived factor/human thioredoxin. Biochem Biophys Res Commun 186:1220-1226
16. Matsuda M, Masutani H, Nakamura H, et al (1992) Protective activity of ATL-derived factor (ADF) against tumor necrosis factor-dependent cytotoxicity on U937 cells. J Immunol 147:3837-3841
17. Sasada T, Iwata S, Sato N, et al (1996) Redox control of resistance to cis-diamminedichloroplatinum (II) (CDDP). J Clin Invest 97:2268-2276
18. Takagi Y, Tokime T, Gon Y, et al (1998) Redox control of neuronal damage during brain ischemia following middle cerebral artery occlusion in the rat: immunohistochemical and hybridization studies of thioredoxin. J Cereb Blood Flow Metab18:206-214
19. Longa EG, Weinstein PR, Carlson S, et al (1989) Reversible middle cerebral artery occlusion without craniectomy in rats. Stroke 20:84-91
20. Takagi Y, Horikawa F, Nozaki K, et al (1998) Expression and distribution of redox regulatory protein, thioredoxin during transient focal brain ischemia in the rat. Neurosci Lett 1998 251:25-28
21. Takagi Y, Mitsui A, Nishiyama A, et al (1999) Overexpression of thioredoxin in transgenic mice attenuates focal ischemic brain damage. Proc Natl Acad Sci USA 96:4131-4136
22. Kinouchi H, Sharp FR, Chan PH, et al (1994) Induction of c-fos, junB, and hsp70 mRNA in cortex, thalamus, basal ganglia and hippocampus following middle cerebral artery occlusion. J Cereb Blood Flow Metab 14:808-817
23. Shimazu M, Mizushima H, Sasaki K, et al (1994) Expression of c-fos in the rat cerebral cortex after focal ischemia and reperfusion. Brain Res Bull 33:689-697
24. Hori K, Katayama M, Sano N, et al (1994) Neuroprotection by glial cells through adult T cell leukemia-derived factor/human thioredoxin (ADF/TRX). Brain Res 652:304-310
25. Endoh M, Kunishita T, Tabira T (1993) Thioredoxin from activated macrophages as a trophic factor for central cholinergic neurons in vitro. Biochem Biophysi Res Comm 192:760-765
26. Lippoldt A, Padilla CA, Gerst H, et al (1995) Localization of thioredoxin in the rat

brain and functional implications. J Neurosci 15:6747-6756
27. Tomimoto H, Akiguchi I, Wakita H, et al (1993) Astroglial expression of ATL-derived factor, a human thioredoxin homologue, in the gerbil brain after transient global ischemia. Brain Res. 625:1-8
28. Kawagoe J, Abe K; Sato, S, et al (1992) Distributions of heat shock protein-70 mRNAs and heat shock cognate protein-70 mRNAs after transient global ischemia in gerbil brain. J Cereb Blood Flow Metab 12:794-801
29. Welsh FA, Moyer DJ, Harris VA (1992) Regional expression of heat shock protein-70 mRNA and c-fos mRNA following focal ischemia in rat brain. J Cereb Blood Flow Metab 12:204-212
30. Takeda A, Onodera H, Sugimoto A, et al (1993) Coordinated expression of messenger RNAs for nerve growth factor, brain-derived neurotrophic factor and neurotrophin-3 in the rat hippocampus following transient forebrain ischemia. Neuroscience 55:23-31
31. Honkaniemi J, Sharp FR (1996) Global ischemia induces immediate-early genes encoding zinc finger transcription factors. J Cereb Blood Flow Metab 16:557-565
32. Iihara K, Sasahara M, Hashimoto N, et al (1994) Ischemia induces the expression of the platelet-derived growth factor-B chain in neurons and brain macrophages in vivo. J Cereb Blood Flow Metab 14:818-824
33. Kamii H, Kinouchi H, Sharp FR, et al (1994) Expression of c-fos mRNA after a mild focal cerebral ischemia in SOD-1 transgenic mice. Brain Res 662:240-244
34. Combs DJ, Dempsey RJ, Donaldson D et al (1992) Hyperglycemia suppress c-fos mRNA expression following transient cerebral ischemia in gerbils. J Cereb Blood Flow Metab 12:169-172
35. Lin TN, Te J, Huang HC, et al (1997) Prolongation and enhancement of postischemic c-fos expression after fasting. Stroke 28:412-418
36. Kobayashi S, Harris VA, Welsh FA. (1995) Spreading depression induces tolerance of cortical neurons to ischemia in rat brain. J Cereb Blood Flow Metab 15:721-727
37. Kamme F, Campbell K, Wieloch T (1995) Biphasic expression of the fos and jun families of transcription factors following transient forebrain ischaemia in the rat. Effect of hypothermia. Eur J Neurosci 7:2007-2016
38. Kitagawa K, Matsumoto M, Oda T, et al (1990) Free radical generation during brief period of cerebral ischemia may trigger delayed neuronal death. Neuroscience 35:551-558
39. Lundgren J, Zhang H, Agardh CD, et al (1991) Acidosis-induced ischemic brain damage: are free radicals involved? J Cereb Blood Flow Metab 11:587-596
40. Dirnagl U, Lindauer U, Them A, et al (1995) Global cerebral ischemia in the rat: online monitoring of oxygen free radical production using chemiluminescence in vivo. J Cereb Blood Flow Metab 15:929-940
41. Chan PH (2001) Reactive oxygen radicals in signaling and damage in the ischemic brain. J Cereb Blood Flow Metab 21:2-14
42. Chan PH, Chu L, Fishman RA (1988) Reduction of activities of superoxide dismutase but not of glutathione peroxidase in rat brain regions following decapitation ischemia, Brain Res 439:388-390
43. Liu XH, Kato H, Araki T, et al (1994) An immunohistochemical study of copper/zinc superoxide dismutase and manganese superoxide dismutase following focal cerebral ischemia in the rat. Brain Res 644:257-266
44. Kato H, Kogure K, Araki T, et al (1995) Immunohistochemical localization of superoxide dismutase in the hippocampus following ischemia in a gerbil model of ischemic tolerance. J Cereb Blood Flow Metab 15:60-70
45. Abe K, Yoshida S, Watson B, et al (1983) Alpha-tocopherol and ubiquinones in rat brain subjected to decapitation ischemia, Brain Res. 273:166-169

46. Hara H, Kato H, Kogure K (1990) Protective effect of alpha-tocopherol on ischemic neuronal damage in the gerbil hippocampus. Brain Res 510:335-338
47. Sato PH, Hall ED (1992) Tirilazad mesylate protects vitamins C and E in brain ischemia-reperfusion injury. J Neurochem 58:2263-2268
48. Kinouchi H, Epstein CJ, Mizui T, et al (1991) Attenuation of focal cerebral ischemic injury in transgenic mice overexpressing CuZn superoxide dismutase. Proc Natl Acad Sci USA 88:11158-11162
49. Martinou JC, Dubois-Dauphin M, Staple JK, et al (1994) Overexpression of BCL-2 in transgenic mice protects neurons from naturally occurring cell death and experimental ischemia. Neuron 13:1017-30
50. Oliver CN, Starke-Reed PE, Stadtman ER, et al (1990) Oxidative damage to brain proteins, loss of glutamine synthetase activity, and production of free radicals during ischemia/reperfusion-induced injury to gerbil brain. Proc Natl Acad Sci USA 87:5144-5147
51. Hall NC, Carney JM, Cheng MS, et al (1995) Ischemia /reperfusion-induced changes in membrane proteins and lipids of gerbil cortical synaptosomes. Neuroscience 64:81-89
52. Smith CD, Carney JM, Starke-Reed PE, et al (1991) Excess brain protein oxidation and enzyme dysfunction in normal aging and in Alzheimer disease. Proc Natl Acad Sci USA 88:10540-3
53. Matsuda M, Masutani H, Nakamura H, et al (1991) Protective activity of adult T cell leukemia-derived factor (ADF) against tumor necrosis factor-dependent cytotoxicity on U937 cells. J Immunol 147:3837-3841
54. Nakamura H, Matsuda M, Furuke K et al (1994) Adult T cell leukemia-derived factor/human thioredoxin protects endothelial F-2 cell injury caused by activated neutrophils or hydrogen peroxide. Immunol Lett 42:75-80
55. Sasada T, Iwata S, Sato N, et al (1996) Redox control of resistance to cis-diamminedichloroplatinum (II) (CDDP): protective effect of human thioredoxin against CDDP-induced cytotoxicity. J Clin Invest 97:2268-2276
56. Fukuse T, Hirata T, Yokomise H, et al (1995) Attenuation of ischemia reperfusion injury by human thioredoxin. Thorax 50:387-391
57. Okubo K, kosaka S, Isowa N, et al (1997) Amelioration of ischemia-reperfusion injury by human thioredoxin in rabbit lung. J Thorc Cardiovasc Surg 113:1-9
58. Wada H, Hirata T, Decampos KN, et al (1995) Effect of the combination of human thioredoxin and L-cysteine on ischemia-reperfusion injury in isolated rat lung. Eur Surg Res 27:363-370
59. Yagi K, Liu CJ, Bando T, et al (1994) Inhibition of reperfusion injury by human thioredoxin (adult T-cell leukemia- derived factor) in canine lung transplantation. J Torac Cardiovasc Surg 108:913-921
60. Isowa N, Yoshimura T, Kosaka S, et al (2000) Human thioredoxin attenuates hypoxia-reoxygenation injury of murine endothelial cells in a thiol-free condition. J Cell Physiol 182:33-40
61. Nakamura H, Herzenberg LA, Bai Jie, et al (2001) Circulating thioredoxin suppress lipopolysaccharide-induced neutrophil chemotaxis. Proc Natl Acad Sci USA 98:15143-15148

Structure and functions of pituitary adenylate cyclase activating polypeptide (PACAP) as a neurotrophic factor

Atsuro Miyata[1] and Kenji Kangawa[2]

[1]Department of Pharmacology, Kagoshima University School of Medicine, 8-35-1 Sakuragaoka, Kagoshima 890-8520, Japan
[2]Department of Biochemistry, Research Institute of the NATIONAL CARDIO-VASCULAR CENTER, 5-7-1 Fujishirodai, Suita, Osaka 565-8565, Japan

Summary: Pituitary adenylate cyclase activating polypeptide (PACAP) is a neuropeptide that was first isolated from ovine hypothalamus extracts on the basis of its ability to increase cyclic AMP in cultured rat pituitary cells. PACAP belongs to the secretin/glucagon family, and shows highest homology (68%) with vasoactive intestinal polypeptide (VIP). The PACAP gene spans 6.5 kb and consists of 5 exons and 4 introns. Further in the mouse brain PACAP mRNA, a variety of the 5' untranslated region are present due to three independent promoters and alternative splicing of the transcripts, indicating that the expression of PACAP gene is regulated in dual mode, inducibly and constitutively. In the central nervous system, PACAP acts not only as a neurotransmitter or neuromodulator, but also as a neurotrophic factor that may play an important role during the development of the brain. In the adult brain, PACAP appears to function as a neuroprotective factor that attenuates the neuronal damages resulting from various insults like focal ischemia by middle cerebral artery occlusion (MCAO). Together with the fact that PACAP can easily cross the blood brain barrier, these suggest that PACAP may be a promising therapeutic agent in brain attack.

Key words: Neuropeptide, Gene, Neurotrophic factor, Neuroprotection, Review

Introduction

Pituitary adenylate cyclase activating polypeptide (PACAP) was isolated from ovine hypothalamic tissues based upon the ability to increase cyclic AMP in cultured rat pituitary cells [1]. As shown in Fig.1, two forms of PACAP, one with 38 residues (PACAP38) and truncated form with 27 residues (PACAP27) were isolated, and the carboxy-termini of both peptides were found to be amidated [1,2]. PACAP is a member of secretin/glucagon family, and shows highest homology (68%) with vasoactive intestinal polypeptide (VIP).

Among the mammalian species to be so far investigated, human, ovine, mouse, porcine and rat, the primary structure of PACAP38 is identical, indicating that in mammals the structure of PACAP38 is extremely well conserved [3-5]. PACAPs from lower vertebrates and protochordates were also identified. Frog and chicken PACAP38 appear to contain only one amino acid substitution [6,7]. Fish (Salmon & Catfish) PACAP38 differs from human PACAP38 by three or four amino acids [8,9]. In the tunicate, two genes of PACAP (PACAP1&2) were characterized [10]. The remarkable similarity between human and tunicate PACAP (96% homology to human PACAP27) suggests that the primary structure of PACAP remained virtually unchanged during an evolutionary period spanning more than 700 million years. Thus considerable homology of PACAP among different species, suggesting that the structure of PACAP has remained unchanged throughout phylogenetic development, may reflect its importance for the fundamental functions of life, particularly in the nervous system.

Since PACAP was first isolated from ovine hypothalamic extract, many efforts had been made to clarify the physiological function of PACAP as a novel hypophysiotropic hormone [1]. Then PACAP has been investigated in terms of neurotransmitter or neuromodulator in the central and peripheral nervous system [11,12]. PACAP elevates the cyclic AMP accumulation 1,000 to 10,000 times

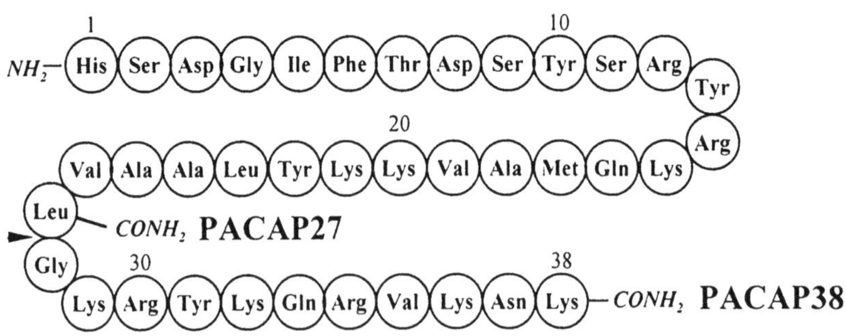

Fig. 1. The primary structure of mammalian PACAP27 & 38.

more potent than VIP as tested in pituitary cell, neuron, and astrocyte cultures [12]. Then the accumulated findings indicate that PACAP functions as a neurotrophic factor. As examined the potential role of PACAP as a survival-promoting factor in hippocampal cultures, the neutralizing antiserum against PACAP27 was incubate with the cultures to block the activity of endogenous peptide. Addition of the antiserum alone reduced the number of neurons. However the cell loss associated with the antiserum was prevented by cotreatment with PACAP27, indicating that endogenous PACAP plays a role in the survival of hippocampal neuron [13]. Therefore the clarification of the biosynthesis of PACAP as a survival-promoting factor could be very important and give some tips to develop novel therapeutic agents for brain attack, as well as the clarification of the neuroprotective action of PACAP.

This review will provide perspectives on the structure and function of this hypothalamic neuropeptide as a neurotrophic factor. Further we will discuss in some several important aspects of PACAP's neuroprotective effect.

Biosynthesis of PACAP

Primary structure and processing of PACAP precursor protein

PACAP exists in two amidated forms with 38 and 27 residues, designated as PACAP38 ad PACAP27, respectively. Complimentary DNAs for PACAP precursor were cloned from ovine hypothalamus and human testis [3]. The ovine cDNA encodes a protein of 176 amino acids, in which PACAP is proceeded by a putative signal peptide and a proregion (107 amino acids) and followed by a Gly-Arg-Arg sequence for proteolytic processing and amidation. PACAP38 is flanked, in its precursor, by dibasic processing sites and a carboxy-terminus amidation signal. Further the sequence of PACAP38 comprises an internal site for dibasic cleavage and amidation, suggesting that the PACAP precursor can generate a 27-residue α-amidated polypeptide (PACAP27). Subsequently, rat and mouse preproPACAP cDNA were cloned and these are similar to the human and ovine PACAP precursors (ranging from 81 to 91% sequence similarity) [4,5]. The rat, mouse, ovine and human PACAP precursor protein contains a peptide of 29 amino acid residues called PACAP-related peptide (PRP), which is also postulated to be cleaved out as a endogenous peptide. However physiological function of PRP has not been characterized so far. Further, the primary structure of the PACAP precursor reveals the existence of seven mono- or dibasic residues that can be cleaved by various prohormone overtaxes including PC1, PC2, PC4, and so on [14]. As shown Fig. 2, Together with the fact that PACAP38 is encoded in the last exon of single copy of PACAP gene, these indicate that the biosyntheses of

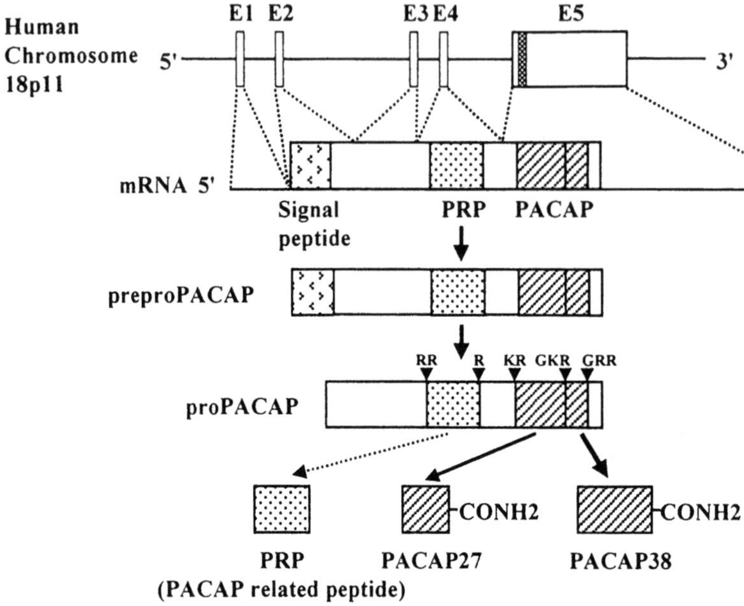

Fig. 2. The biosynthesis and processing of PACAP precursor protein.

PACAP27 and PACAP38 are not due to the presence of plural genes or alternative splicing of the transcript of the single copy of gene, but due to alternative processing at the dual amidation sites, as well as in the case of ACTH/αMSH biosynthesis [15].

PACAP gene structure

The gene encoding PACAP has been cloned in human and mouse [16,17]. PACAP genomic DNA were characterized to consist of five exons spanning 6.5 kb. The sequence of PRP is encoded by exon 4, and that of PACAP by exon 5. In mammals, the overall organization of the PACAP precursor exhibits strong similarities with that of the VIP precursor [18]. In particular, the VIP precursor encompasses a VIP-related peptide, called peptide histidine–methionine amide (PHM) in human or peptide histidine-isoleucine (PHI) amide in rat, sheep, mouse, which possesses moderate amino acid identity with VIP [19]. Interestingly the rat PRP is more similar to human growth hormone-releasing hormone (GHRH, 52% similarity) than to rat GHRH (41% similarity) and rat PHI (33% similarity). In contrast to PACAP, the structure of GHRH is not well conserved among species:

the peptides from seven mammalian species range in sequence homology with the human from 93% in the pig of 63% in the rat [11]. Thus it is assumed that intragenomic duplication of a VIP/PACAP ancestor sequence has occurred before duplication of the whole ancestor gene [21]. Incidentally in submammalian vertebrates, such as fish or birds, the PACAP precursor comprises both GHRH and PACAP [6-9]. In salmon and eel, salmon PACAP stimulated GH-release more potently than salmon GHRH [22]. A duplication of the GHRH like peptide/PACAP gene during evolution after divergence of fish and tetrapods could explain the separate genes and regulation for GHRH and PACAP in mammals [23]. In humans, the PACAP gene has been mapped to the p11 region of chromosome 18 by fluorescence in situ hybridization [16]. This region is associated with holoprosencephaly, the most common hereditary developmental defect of the forebrain in humans, suggesting that PACAP might be involved in the control of brain development [16,24].

The 5'-flanking region of the PACAP gene contains two cyclic AMP-response like elements, a 12-*O*-tetra-decanoylphorbol 13-acetate response element and a pair of sequences homologous to the consensus sequence for pituitary-specific growth hormone factor 1-binding sites, which are known to play a role in the tissue-specific expression of GH [20,25]. The detailed analysis of 5' upstream region of the mouse gene demonstrated the presence of a variety of 5' untranslated region in the brain mRNA, indicating that the transcription of the single-copy PACAP gene is regulated by three independent promoters, together with differential splicing of the transcripts (at least 5 types) [26]. As regards one of three promoter regions, in which two TATA like element are found, the luciferase reporter assay revealed that the distal TATA element functions more potently than proximal one as a promotor. However, other two promotor regions contain neither TATA nor CAAT box, instead several initiator (Inr)-like element, which is frequently observed in the promoter region of housekeeping genes. Thus the transcription of PACAP gene is regulated in dual mode, inducibly and constitutively [26].

The effects of PACAP on the CNS

The wide distribution of PACAP and its receptors suggests that the peptide may exert pleiotropic physiological functions. As a matter of fact, PACAP has now been shown to act as a hormone, a neurohormone, a neurotransmitter, and a trophic factor in a number of tissues. Two classes of PACAP binding sites have been characterized on the basis of their relative affinities for PACAP and VIP [27]. Type I binding sites exhibit high affinity for PACAP38 and PACAP27 and much lower affinity for VIP. Type II binding sites possess similar affinity for PACAPs and VIP. Then three PACAP receptors have been so far cloned and termed PAC1,

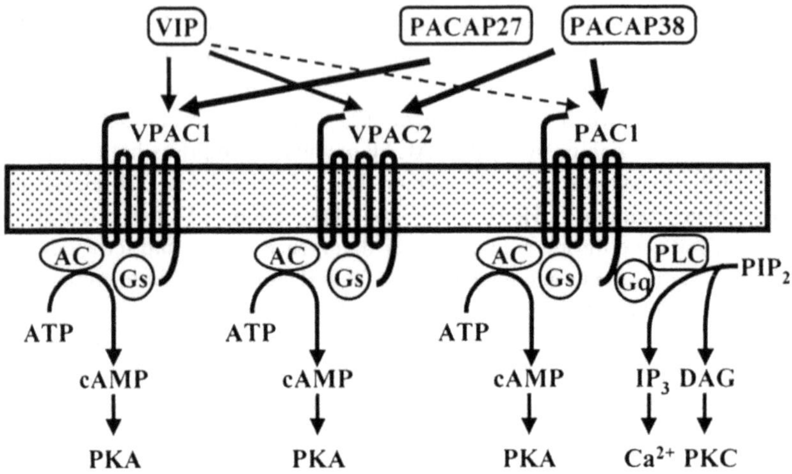

Fig. 3. Schematic representation of three subtypes of PACAP/VIP receptor.

VPAC1, VPAC2 receptors as shown in Fig. 3 [28]. These are a member of rhodopsin superfamily of G protein-coupled receptor with seven transmembrane domain and coupled with G proteins. In addition, eight subtypes of PAC1 receptor resulting from alternative splicing have been reported, but no subtype of either VPAC1 or VPAC2 has been found. All of them are coupled to a Gs protein and have effect on adenylyl cyclase. Further PAC1 is coupled with a Gq protein to activate phospholipase C (PLC). Most of the tissues possess various proportions of each receptor subtype.

Effects as a neurotransmitter, neuromodulator, or neurohormone

The most abundant population of PACAP-containing neurons and the highest density of PACAP binding sites are found in the hypothalamus [29,30]. In particular, a dense accumulation of PACAP-immunoreactive neurons and PACAP receptors are present in the magnocellular region of the PVN and SON where the neurosecretory Perikarya producing oxytocin and vasopressin are located [31-38]. Intracerebroventricular and intracisternal injection of PACAP causes a dose-dependent elevation of plasma vasopressin concentration [39,40]. In the neural lobe of the pituitary, PACAP stimulates the release of oxytocin and vasopressin through activation of the cAMP/protein kinase A signaling pathway [41]. PACAP has also been shown to modulate the activity of various other hypothalamic neuronal populations. For instance, central administration of PACAP produces significant increases in GnRH, somatostatin, and CRH gene expression [42,43].

Intracerebroventricular injection of PACAP stimulates the expression of PRL mRNA in the rat hypothalamus [44]. Similarly, injection of PACP in the medial basal hypothalamus suppresses luteinizing hormone (LH) secretion and LH pulse frequency [45]. Taken together, these data indicate that PACAP may act within the hypothalamus as a neurotransmitter or neuromodulator to regulate the secretion of neurohypophysial and hypophysiotropic neurohormones.

In rat, daily variations in the density of PAC1-R mRNA are observed in the suprachiasmatic and supraoptic nuclei with two peaks at noon and midnight, but not in the cingulate cortex [46]. Similar biphasic variations of VPAC2-R mRNA levels are observed in the suprachiasmatic nucleus [46,47]. These results indicate that PACAP receptors are differentially expressed in the rat brain across the 24-h cycle, suggesting that PACAP is involved in the circadian pacemaker clock.

Circadian variations in PACAP content occur in the rat pineal [48], and a high density of PACAP binding sites is present in the pineal gland [49,50], suggesting that PACAP is involved in the regulation of the rhythmicity of melatonin production. PACAP causes a dose-dependent increase in the activity of two key enzymes of the melatonin biosynthetic pathway, serotonin-N-acetyl-transferase [51] and hydroxyindole-0-methyltransferase [52]. Since melatonin suppresses the PACAP-induced stimulation of cyclic AMP production in the whole chicken hypothalamus and in the rat suprachiasmatic nucleus and pituitary cells, indicating that the hypothalamus is a site for a functional interaction between PACAP and the pineal hormone melatonin [53-56].

A number of neuropeptides have been shown to participate in the control of appetite and feeding behavior [57]. The high concentration of PACAP-expressing neurons in the PVN and ventromedial hypothalamic nuclei [29,30,35,37], two hypothalamic regions that play a role in the regulation of food intake [58,59], suggests that PACAP could be involved in the control of food consumption [60]. Indeed, i.c.v. injection of PACAP decreases food uptake [61-63] and antagonizes the orexigenic effect of NPY [61]. Concurrently, injection of PACAP in the vicinity of the perifornical lateral hypothalamus stimulates drinking [65]; reciprocally, water deprivation causes an increase in PACAP-LI in cell bodies and nerve fibers of the subfornical organ [66], suggesting that PACAP may play a role in the regulation of dipsic behavior.

The possible effect of PACAP in the transmission of noxious stimuli currently a matter of debate: PACAP has been found to reduce the instances of finching behavior in the formalin test, indicating that the peptide may possess antinociceptive properties [67], whereas other reports suggest that PACAP may play a facilitatory role in pain transmission [64].

Consistent with the occurrence of PACAP receptors astroglial cells, PACAP has been shown to mobilize intracellular calcium stores [68] in rat astrocytes. In brain slices from newborn rat, PACAP enhances the number of glial precursor cells that express the proenkephalin-A gene in the neocortical subventricular zone of the rat brain [69]. In cultured astrocytes, PACAP also stimulates the MAP kinase ERK2, suggesting that PACAP may regulate proliferation of astroglial cells [70]. In

Support of this notion, in vivo administration of a VIP antagonist induces a dramatic reduction of the density of astrocytes in the cortex of E17 mouse embryos, and this effect is reversed by cotreatment with PACAP or theVPAC2-R agonist RO 25-1553 [71], indicating that PACAP is actually involved in neocortical astrocytogenesis.

Neurotrophic actions

Soon after PACAP was identified, the peptide was found to stimulate the outgrowth of neurites from PC12 cells [72, 73] and to enhance the survival of sympathetic ganglion cells [18]. In cultured PC12 cells, 10nM PACAP caused a 1.5-fold and a 1.3-fold increase in cell diameter and cell protein, respectively. When cell survival was determined in serum-free medium in the absence and presence of PACAP27 from 0.01 to 100nM and NGF at 2nM after 5d in culture, the cell survival in the control media was <20%, 88% with NGF, 60% with 0.3-3nM PACAP27, and 100% with 10-300nM PACAP27. In the presence of 1% horse serum, 10nM PACAP27 supported neurite outgrowth from 70% of the cells at a nearly linear rate of 7.3 μm/d [18].

The effect of PACAP on naturally occurring neuronal cell death was examined in chick embryos by using experimental procedures similar to those described by Hamberger and Levi-Montalcini using fertilized white leghorn eggs [74]. The experiment was designed so that treatment began after the period of extensive neural proliferation in the embryo. This ensured that any increase in cell number was due to a prevention of natural cell death. not to a stimulation of mitosis. The administration of PACAP38 (25nM in the egg) daily from E (embryonic day) 3.5 to E8.5 significantly reduced the number of pyknotic cells in tile dorsomedial population of DRG18 on day E9 [13]. When chick embryos received 5 or 25nM PACAP38 daily from E6 to E9, the number of viable neurons in the lumbar motor column on E10 increased dose dependently. Twenty-five nanomolar VIP showed a neuroprotective effect similar to that induced by 5nM PACAP38 [13]. These findings suggest that PACAP38 functions as a neurotrophic factor during the development of sensory neurons and motoneurons in the chick spinal cord [13].

Sympathetic neurons (SN) of the chick embryo undergo apoptosis in culture when deprived of NGF. However, 30-100 nM PACAP added to NGF-free medium rescued a significant number of SN from apoptotic death. The SN rescued by PACAP maintained their physiological functions of transmitter uptake and release. When PACAP-supported SN were transferred to NGF-containing medium, their morphology and function were similar to those that remained in NGF all the time [75].

The presence of high concentrations of PACAP and PACAP receptors in germinative areas of the developing brain indicates that the peptide may exert important functions during ontogenesis of the CNS. Indeed, in cerebellar granule cells cultured in conditions promoting apoptosis, PACAP inhibits programmed cell death [76-80] and stimulates neurite outgrowth [79]. Second messenger studies have been conducted to investigate the mechanisms involved in the neurotrophic activity of PACAP [82]. Activation of PAC1-R induces a dose-dependent stimulation of cyclic AMP production and polyphosphoinositide hydrolysis [80,83-85].

Cultured cerebellar granule cells die rapidly in the absence of a high concentration of K^+ (25mM), resulting in massive neuronal apoptosis within I2h. The addition of PACAP38 or PACP27 prevented apoptosis resulting from K^+ deprivation. Those effects of PACAP were abolished on the transient transfection of cells with a dominant negative mutant of the cAMP dependent PKA [78]. Furthermore, PACAP38 increased survival of cerebellar neurons in a potassium deficient medium in a dose-dependent manner With an ED50 of 5nM. PACAP38 induced activation of the ERK-type of MAPK kinase through a cAMP-dependent pathway. PD98059, an inhibitor of MAPK kinase, completely abolished the antiapoptotic effect of PACAP38, suggesting that MAPK pathway activation is necessary for PACAP38 action [80]. Autoradiographic studies showed that type I PACAP binding sites are transiently expressed in the germinal matrix of the cerebellar cortex, in the external granule cell layer, and in the white matter. From postnatal days 8 to 25, a population of PACAP binding sites persisted in the internal granule cell layer in the mature cerebellum [86]. In cultured granule cells taken from 8-d-old rat cerebellum, PACAP not only increased the survival of granule cells, but also induced a transient increase in c-fos mRNA levels. Both effects of PACAP were mimicked by db-cAMP, but not by phorbol 12-myristate I3-acetate, and a PKA inhibitor suppressed PACAP-induced c-fos mRNA expression.

Thus it have been shown that the effect of PACAP on cell survival is mediated through activation of the adenylyl cyclase pathway, leading to phosphorylation of the extracellular signal-regulated (ERK)-type of mitogen-activated protein (MAP) kinase [80] and to an increase in *c-fos* gene expression [11,18]. In cultured granude cells, PACAP also stimulates calcium mobilization [87,88] and blocks transient potassium currents [89], two processes often involved in programmed cell death regulation [90-92]. The effect of PACAP on the development of the rat cerebellum has been investigated recently in vivo [81]. Injection of PACAP at the surface of the cerebellum of 8-day-old pups induces a transient enlargement of the volume of the cerebellar cortex with a maximum effect at P12, which can be accounted for by an increase in the number of granule cells in the EGL, the molecular layer, and the IGL. The effect of PACAP on the number of granule cells blocked by the antagonist PACAP(6-8). The fact that the PACAP antagonist produces by itself a slight inhibition of the number of granule cells in the IGL indicates that endogenous PACAP may exert a physiological role in the development of the rat cerebellum [18].

On cortical neuron precursors, PACAP decreases the proportion of mitotic cells and promotes neuroblast differentiation, indicating that the peptide is also involved in the development of the cerebral cortex [93-95]. After a week of culture in the presence of serum, cortical neuroblasts turn into nature neurons that express glutamate and its receptors. It should be recalled that micromolar concentrations of glutamate exert a slight protective action on cortical neurons in primary culture whereas millimolar doses of glutamate induce apoptotic cell death [96-98]. In this model, PACAP potentiates the effect of otherwise marginally effective concentrations of glutamate (1 μM) on c-fos expression [99], arachidonic acid release [100,101], and brain-derived neurotrophic factor production [102].

Neuroprotective effect

Most of the studies described above prompted the study of possible neuroprotection by PACAP. PACAP protects cultured cortical neurons from the cytotoxic effects of high (1 mM) concentrations of glutamate [103]. A neuroprotective effect of PACAP on glutamate-induced neurotoxicity also has been reported in cultured retinal neurons [104]. Most of the actions of PACAP on cortical neurons are mediated through the cyclic AMP pathway [99,103] although it has been reported that PACAP can directly modulate N-methyl-D-aspartate receptors independently of intracellular second messengers [105,106]. On these neurons, PACAP prevents the neurotoxic effect of lipopolysaccharide administration [107]. In mesencephalic dopaminergic neurons, PACAP counteracts the effects of 6-hydroxydopamine neurotoxicity [108].

It is generally accepted that the brain damage in AIDS patients is caused by indirect mechanisms of HIV-related toxicity rather than direct damage due to the viral infection of neurons. The major external envelope protein of HIV, gp120 was shown to produce neuronal toxicity in dissociated hippocampal [109]. Neuronal cell death associated with gp120 treatment of murine hippocampal cultures was first shown to be potently and completely prevented by VIP [109]. Because of the substantial sequence homology between VIP and PACAP, possible effect of PACAP on gp120-induced death in hippocampal neurons was examined under experimental conditions similar to those described for the VIP studies [109]. Both of PACAP38 and PACAP27 attenuated the neuronal cell death associated with gp120 treatment in bimodal dose-response curves with peaks at 0.1 pM and 0.1 nM. Previous results showed that 0.1 nM VIP prevented neuronal death in gp120-treated cultures [109]. The bimodal response for PACAP suggests a more complicated mechanism, probably involving more than one type of receptor, possibly PAC1-R and VPAC1- or VPAC2-R. In this regard VIP will bind to PAC1-R with an affinity that is 1,000 times less than that of PACAP. In contrast, PACAP binds to VPAC1- or VPAC2-R with an affinity similar to VIP [30]. It is possible that the PACAP-induced cytoprotective action observed at 0. 1 nM occurs through VPAC-R receptors, and the activity seen at 0.1 pM results from an interaction through PAC1-R. These results clearly show that developing hippocampal neurons exposed to lethal concentration of the HIV envelope protein survived in the presence of PACAP38 or PACAP27 at subpicomolar concentrations [13].

These neuroprotective findings of PACAP in vitro, in particular, dramatic neuroprotection by PACAP in gp120-induced neuronal cell death in cultured hippocampal neurons at subpicomolar concentrations, prompted the study of possible neuroprotection by PACAP in adult animals. Because neurons in the CA1 region of the hippocampus are vulnerable to global forebrain ischemia, this model has been widely used for evaluating neuroprotective agents [110]. Intracerebroventricular (I.C.V.) infusion of PACAP38 at increasing doses was given in adult rats over 7d, starting immediately after transient global ischemia induced by four-vessel occlusion [110]. In rats receiving I.C.V. PACAP38, a dose-dependent, statistically significant attenuation of neuronal death was seen on day 7, with a bell-shaped dose-response curve peaking at 1 pmol/h. PCAP38 prevented the otherwise total loss pyramidal cells and dendrite processes throughout CA1 [111]. Based on the results of distribution of I.C.V. infusion, it was calculated that an I.C.V. infusion of 1pmol/h would approximate the 0.1 pM concentration in the tissue, which was found to be optimal *in vitro* [13]. Furthermore, because PCAP38 was neuroprotective at such a low concentration as 0.1 pM in the brain and can cross the blood-brain-barrier (BBB) in a saturable manner [112], it was postulated that PACAP38 would be effective even when administered I.V. In fact I.V. infusion containing 16 and 160 pmol/μl of PACAP38 at 1 μl/h significantly protected CA1 neurons [111]. Moreover. Both 16 pmol/h and the 160 pmol/h I.V. infusions of PACAP38 over 1 week begun 24h after ischemia attenuated CA1 neuronal death [111]. Immunohistochemistry showed that only a small amount of PAC_1-R immunoreactivity was demonstrated in the CA1 pyramidal cell layer in the normal rat brain. After ischemia, astrocytes near the CA1 pyramidal cell layer expressed PAC_1-R immunoreactivity on day 1, then intensifying until day 7. Similarly, as detected by in situ hybridization, one day after ischemia, pyramidal cells and astrocytes had both increased their expression of PAC1-R mRNA. PACAP is still effective to protect cell death when treatment is started 24 h after the ischemia, which suggests that PACAP may have therapeutic potency in treating cerebral injuries. Since neuronal death is not evident 24h after global ischemia, the initiation of PACAP38 at this time may have prevented the further progress of cell death. After focal cerebral ischemia, the tumor suppressor P53 and the zinc finger protein Zac-1 (two genes responsible for cell cycle arrest and apoptosis control) are up-regulated [113,114]. The p53 and Zac proteins have been demonstrated to regulate the PAC1-R gene, which could, in the presence of its agonist, counteract the damages of ischemia. Consistent with this finding, PACAP and PAC1-A mRNA have been shown to) increase in the cortex and the hippocampus after traumatic brain injury [115].

In the dorsal root ganglions of embryos and newborn rats, the PACAP gene is expressed in sensory neurons [116], and the levels of PACAP and PAC1-R mRNAs are up-regulated by axotomy [117-119]. Treatment of cultured ganglion neurons with PACAP increases cell survival and promotes neurite outgrowth [116], supporting the view that PACAP exerts beneficial effects in nerve restoration after injury.

Further toward to therapeutic application, possible neuroprotective action of PACAP was examined in a model of transient focal ischemia produced by middle cerebral artery occlusion (MCAO) in rats [120]. Many substances have been shown to reduce brain damage in models of stroke, but mainly when given either before a shortly after the onset of ischemia. Since the delayed systemic administration of PACAP shows neuroprotection in a model of global ischemia as described above, PACAP38 was administrated as an intravenous bolus (20 nmol/kg body weight) followed by intravenous infusion, beginning 4, 8, 12 hours after a 2-hour transient MCAO using a filament model [121]. The administration of PACAP38 beginning 4 hours after MCAO significantly reduced the infarct size by 50.88% [120]. Treatment starting 8 or 12 hours after the onset of ischemia did not result in a significant reduction of the infarct size, although infarct volumes tended to be smaller than in the control group. Systemic administration of PACAP38 should be clinically useful for reducing brain damage resulting from stroke (brain attack) even when administration is delayed for several hours.

Conclusion

Most of the studies described above indicate that during development, PACAP function as a neurotrophic factor on developing neuronal cells, whereas, in the adult brain, the peptide appears to function as a neuroprotective agent that attenuates the neuronal damage resulting from various insults at nanomolar to subpicomolar concentrations. In addition, it should be emphasized that PACAP has been proven to cross the blood brain barrier (BBB): 0.118% of an intravenous dose of PACAP38 is taken up by brain when expressed by percent intravenous per gram, which 6 times the amount of morphine accumulated in the brain [112]. As shown in fig. 4, the cytoprotective effect of PACAP appears to be mediated by direct and indirect actions, via astrocytes partially as demonstrated for VIP [122].

In astrocytes, PACAP increases the production of neurotrophic factors that are responsible for neuronal proliferation and/or differentiation [123]. In this respect, PACAP has been shown to reduce ciliary neurotrophic factor mRNA level [124]. In contrast, PACAP activates brain-derived neurotrophic factor, a trophic peptide involved in neuronal plasticity [102] and stimulates the secretion of interleukin (IL)-6, which acts as atrophic cytokine in the CNS [125]. In addition, PACAP specific receptor exists in vascular walls and was demonstrated to involve in the proliferation of vascular cells as a trophic factor [126]. There is another possibility to exhibit indirect neuroprotection via vascular cells. It might be crucial to understand the cell-cell interaction between brain cells and vascular cells in order to pursue the novel concept of the therapeutic agents for cerebrovascular diseases. In summary, (i) PACAP is small molecule peptide, (ii) PACAP can easily

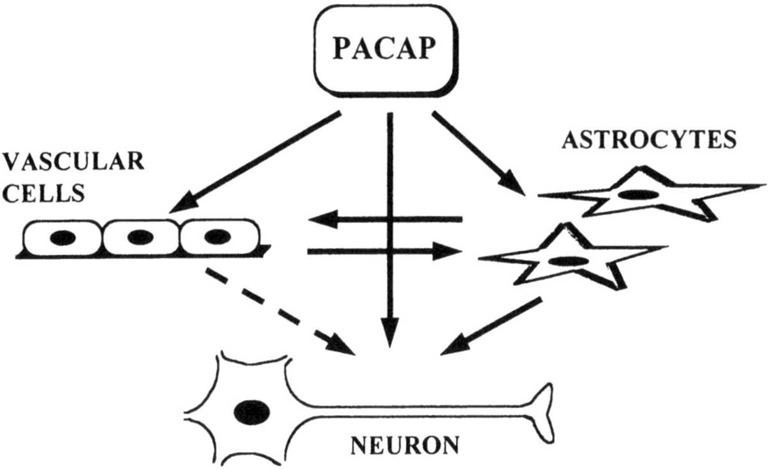

Fig. 4. Schematic representation of direct and indirect neuroprotection of PACAP.

cross BBB, (iii) PACAP exhibits neuroprotection in vitro and in vivo, (iv) PACAP is effective at very low concentration (subpicomolar order), (v) PACAP exhibits trophic effects on vascular cells. These findings strongly support PACAP as a candidate for therapeutic application for cerebrovascular diseases like stroke. However the nature of PACAP's neuroprotection still remains unclear. Further investigations are needed to clarify its molecular mechanism.

References

1. Miyata A, Arimura A, Dahl RR, et al (1989) Isolation of a novel 38 residue-hypothalamic polypeptide which stimulates adenylate cyclase in pituitary cells. Biochem Res Commun 164:567-574
2. Miyata A, Jiang L, Dahl RR, et al (1990) Isolation of a neuropeptide corresponding to the N-terminal 27 residues of the pituitary adenylate cyclase-activating polypeptide with 38 residues (PACAP38). Biochem Biophys Res Commun 170:643-648
3. Kimura C, Ohkubo S, Ogi K, et al (1990) A novel peptide which stimulates adenylate cyclase: Molecular cloning and characterization of the ovine and human cDNAs. Biochem Biophys Res Commun 166:81-89
4. Okazaki K, Itoh Y, Ogi K, et al (1995) Characterization of murine PACAP mRNA. Peptides 16:1295-1299

5. Ogi K, Kimura C, Onda H, et al (1990) Molecular cloning and characterization of cDNA for the precursor of rat pituitary adenylate cyclase-activating polypeptide (PACAP). Biochem Biophys Res Commun 173:1271-1279
6. McRory JE, Parker RL, Sherwood NM (1997) Expression and alternative processing of a chicken gene encoding both growth hormone-releasing hormone and pituitary adenylate cyclase-activating polypeptide. DNA and Cell Biol 16:95-102
7. Chartrel N, Tonon MC, Vaudry H, et al (1991) Primary structure of frog pituitary adenylate cyclase-activating polypeptide (PACAP) and effects of ovine PACAP on frog pituitary. Endocrinology 129-3367-3371
8. Parker DB, Coe IR, Dixon GH, et al (1993) Two salmon neuropeptides encoded by one brain cDNA are structurally related to members of the glucagons superfamily. Eur J Biochem 215:439-448
9. McRory JE, Parker DB, Ngamvongchon S, et al (1995) Sequence and expression of cDNA for pituitary adenylate cyclase-activating polypeptide (PACAP) and growth hormone-releasing hormone (GHRH) –like peptide in catfish. Mol Cell Endocrinol 108:169-177
10. McRory JE, Sherwood NM (1997) Two protochordate genes encode pituitary adenylate cyclase-activating polypeptide and related family members. Endocrinology 138:2380-2390
11. Arimura A (1998) Perspective on pituitary adenylate cyclase-activating polypeptide (PACAP) in the neuroendocrine, endocrine, and nervous systems. Jpn J Physiol 48:301-331
12. Arimura A (1993) Receptors for pituitary adenylate cyclase-activating polypeptide: comparison with vasoactive intestinal peptide receptors. Trends Endocrinol Metab 3: 288-294
13. Arimura A, Somgyvari VA, Weill C, et al (1994) PACAP function as a neurotrophic factor. Ann NY Acad of Sci 739: 228-243
14. Seidah NG, Day R, Hamelin J, et al (1992) Testicular expression of PC4 in the rat : molecular diversity of a novel germ cell-specific Kex2/subilisin-like proprotein convertase. Mol Endocrinol 6: 1559-1570
15. Loh Y, Peng S, Elkabes S, et al (1988) Regulation of pro-opiomelanocortin (POMC) biosynthesis in the amphibian and mouse pituitary intermediate lobe. In: The Melanotropic Peptides, Hadley ME (eds) CRC Press, Boca Raton, Fla., pp85-101
16. Hosoya M, Kimura C, Ogi K, et al (1992) Structure of the human pituitary adenylate cyclase-activating polypeptide (PACAP) gene. Biochem Biophys Acta 1129:199-206
17. Yamamoto K, Hashimoto H, Hagihara N, et al (1998) Cloning and characterization of the mouse pituitary adenylate cyclase-activating polypeptide (PACAP) gene. Gene 211:63-69
18. Vaudry D, Gonzalez BJ, Basille M, et al (2000) Pituitary adenylate cyclase-activating polypeptide and its receptors: from structure to functions. Pharmacol. Rev 52: 269-324
19. Itoh N, Obata K, Yanaihara N, et al (1983) Human preprovasoactive intestinal polypeptide contains a novel PHI-27-like peptide, PHM-27. Nature 304:547-549
20. Ohkubo S, Ogi K, Kimura C, et al (1994) Expression of the PACAP gene in a human neuroblastoma cell line: cDNA cloning and analyses of the upstream

regulatory region. Endocr J 2:135-145
21. Ohkubo S, Kimura C, Ogi K, et al (1992) Primary structure and characterization of the precursor to human pituitary adenylate cyclase-activating polypeptide. DNA Cell Biol 11:21-30
22. Parker DB, Power ME, Swanson P, et al (1997) Exon skipping in the gene encoding pituitary adenylate cyclase-activating polypeptide in salmon alters the expression of two hormone that stimulate growth hormone release. Endocrinology 138:414-423
23. Hoyle CH (1998) Neuropeptide families: Evolutionary perspectives. Regul Pept 73:1-33
24. Chang E, Welch S, Luna J, et al (1993) Generation of human chromosome 18-specific YAC clone collection and mapping of 55 unique YACs by FISH and fingerprinting. Genomics 17:393-402
25. Bodner M, Castrillo JL, Theill LE, et al (1988) The pituitary-specific transcription factor GHF-1 is a homeobox-containing protein. Cell 55:505-518
26. Miyata A, Sugawara H, Sano H, et al (2001) Characterization of the mouse PACAP gene promoter. Reg Peptides 102:61
27. Gottschall PE, Tatsuno I, Miyata A, et al (1990) Characterization and distribution of binding sites for the hypothalamic peptide, Pituitary adenylate cyclase-activating polypeptide. Endcrinology 127: 272-277
28. Harmar AJ, Arimura A, Gozes I, et al (1998) Nomenclature of receptors for vasoactive intestinal peptide (VIP) and pituitary adenylate cyclase-activating polypeptide (PACAP). Pharmacol Rev 50: 265-270.
29. Arimura A (1992) Pituitary adenylate cyclase-activating polypeptide (PACAP): Discovery and current status of research. Regul Pept 37:287-303
30. Arimura A, Shioda S (1995) Pituitary adenylate cyclase-activating polypeptide (PACAP) and its receptors: Neuroendocrine and endocrine interaction . Front Neuroendocrinol 16:53-88
31. Koves K, Arimura A, Somogyvari-Vigh A, et al (1990) Immunohistochemical demonstration of a novel hypothalamic peptide, Pituitary adenylate cyclase-activating polypeptide in the ovine hypothalamus. Endocrinology 127: 264-271
32. Koves K, Arimura A, Gorcs TG, et al (1990) Comparative distribution of immunoreactive pituitary adenylate cyclase-activating polypeptide ad vasoactive intestinal polypeptide in rat forebrain. Neuroendocrinology 54: 159-169
33. Masuo Y, Ohtaki T, Masuda Y, et al (1992) Binding sites for Pituitary adenylate cyclase-activating polypeptide (PACAP): Comparison with vasoactive intestinal polypeptide (VIP) binding site localization in rat brain sections Brain Res. 575: 113-123
34. Kimura S, Ohsige Y, Lin L, et al (1994) Localization of pituitary adenylate cyclase-activating polypeptide (PACAP) in the hypothalamus–pituitary system in rats: Light and electron microscopic immunocytochemical studies. J Neuroendocrinol. 6: 503-507.
35. Tamada T, Tanaka M, Ichitani Y, et al (1994) Pituitary adenylate cyclase-activating polypeptide (PACAP)-like immunoreactive neuronal elements in rat hypothalamus and median eminence with special reference to morphological background of its effect on anterior pituitary-light and electron microscopic immunocytochemistry Neurosci Lett 180: 105-108
36. Hannibal J, Mikkelsen JD, Clausen H, et al (1995a) Gene expression of pituitary adenylate cyclase-activating polypeptide (PACAP) in the rat hypothalamus. Regul

Pept 55:133-148
37. Shioda S, Yada T, Nakajo S, et al (1997) Pituitary adenylate cyclase-activating polypeptide (PACAP): A novel regulator of vasopressin-containing neurons. Brain Res 765: 81-90
38. Legradi G, Hannibal J, Lechan RM (1998) Pituitary adenylate cyclase-activating polypeptide-nerve terminals densely innervate corticotropin-releasing hormone-neurons in the hypothalamic paraventricular nucleus of the rat. Neurosci Lett 246: 145-148
39. MuraseT, Kondo K, Otake K, et al (1993) Pituitary adenylate cyclase-activating polypeptide stimulates arginine vasopressin release in conscious rats. Neuroendocrinology 57: 1092-1096
40. Seki Y, Suzuki Y, Baskaya MK, et al (1995) Central cardiovascular effects induced by intracisternal PACAP in dogs. Am J Physiol 269: H135-H139
41. Lutz-Bucher B, Monnier D, Koch B (1996) Evidence for the presence of receptors for pituitary adenylate cyclase-activating polypeptide in the neurohypophysis that are positively coupled to cyclic AMP formation and neurohypophyseal hormone secretion. Neuroendocrinology 64: 153-161
42. Li S. Grinevich V, Fournier A, et al (1996) Effect of pituitary adenylate cyclase-activating polypeptide (PACAP) on gonadotropin-releasing hormone and somatostatin gene expression in the rat brain. Mol Brain Res 41:157-162
43. Grinevich V, Fournier A, Pelletier G (1997) Effects of pituitary adenylate cyclase-activating polypeptide (PACAP) on corticotropin-releasing hormone (CRH) gene expression in the rat hypothalamic paraventricular nucleus. Brain Res 773: 190-196
44. Bredow S, Kacsoh B, Obal F Jr, et al (1994) Increase of prolactin mRNA in rat hypothalamus after intracerebroventricular injection of VIP or PACAP. Brain Res 660: 301-308
45. Anderson ST, Sawangiaroen K, Curlewis JD (1996) Pituitary adenylate cyclase-activating polypeptide acts within the medial basal hypothalamus to inhibit prolactin and luteinizing hormone secretion. Endocrinology 137: 3424-3429
46. Cagampang FR, Piggins HD, Sheward WJ, et al (1998) Circadian changes in PACAP type 1 (PAC1) receptor mRNA in the rat suprachiasmatic and supraoptic nuclei. Brain Res 813: 218-222
47. Shinohara K, Funabashi T, Kimura F (1999) Temporal profiles of vasoactive intestinal polypeptide precursor mRNA and its receptor mRNA in the rat suprachiasmatic nucleus. Brain Res Mol Brain Res 63: 262-267
48. Fukuhara C, Inouye SIT, Matsumoto Y, et al (1998) Pituitary adenylate cyclase-activating polypeptide rhythm in the rat pineal gland. Neurosci Lett 241: 115-119
49. Masuo Y, Ohtaki T, Masuda Y, et al (1992) Binding sites for pituitary adenylate cyclase-activating polypeptide (PACAP): Comparison with vasoactive intestinal polypeptide (VIP) binding site localization in rat brain sections. Brain Res 575: 113-123
50. Simonneaux V, Kienlen-Campard P, Loeffler JP, et al (1998) Pharmacological molecular and functional characterization of VIP/PACAP receptors in the rat pineal gland. Neuroscience 85: 887-896
51. Yuwiler A, Brammer GL, Bennett BL (1995) Interaction between adrenergic and peptide stimulation in the rat pineal: Pituitary adenylate cyclase-activating polypeptide. J Neurochem 64: 2273-2280
52. Ribelayga C, Pevet P, Simonneaux V (1997) Adrenergic and peptidergic regulations

of hydroxyindole-O-methyltransferase activity in rat pineal gland. Brain Res 777: 247-250
53. Von Gall C, Duffield GE, Hastings MH, et al (1998) CREB in the mouse SCN: A molecular interface coding the phase-adjusting stimuli light, glutamate, PACAP, and melatonin for clockwork access. J Neurosci 18: 10389-10397
54. Kopp MD, Schomerus C, Dehghani F, et al (1999) Pituitary adenylate cyclase-activating polypeptide and melatonin in the suprachiasmatic nucleus: Effects on the calcium signal transduction cascade. J Neurosci 19: 206-219
55. Nowak JZ, Kuba K, Zawiska JB (1999) PACAP-induced formation of cyclic AMP in the chicken brain: Regional variations and the effect of melatonin. Brain Res 830:195-199
56. Slanar O, Pelisek V, Vanecek J (2000) Melatonin inhibits pituitary adenylate cyclase-activating polypeptide increase of cyclic AMP accumulation and [Ca2+]I in cultured cells of neonatal rat pituitary. Neurochem Int 36: 213-219
57. Kalra SP, Dube MG, Pu S, et al (1999) Interacting appetite-regulating pathways in the hypothalamic regulation of body weight. Endocr Rev 20: 68-100
58. Luiten PG, ter Host GJ, Steffens AB (1987) The hypothalamus, intrinsic connections and outflow pathways to the endocrine system in relation the control of feeding and metabolism. Prog Neurobiol 28: 1-54
59. Leibowitz SF (1988) Hypothalamic paraventricular nucleus: Interaction between alpha 2-noradrenergic system and circulating hormone and nutrients in relation to energy balance. Neurosci Biobehav 12: 101-109
60. Christophe J (1998) Is there appetite after GLP-1 and PACAP? Ann N Y Acad Sci 865: 323-335
61. Morley JE, Horowitz M, Morley PMK, et al (1992) Pituitary adenylate cyclase-activating polypeptide reduces food intake in mice. Peptides13: 1133-1135
62. Chance WT, Thompson H, Thomas I, et al (1995) Anorectic and neurochemical effects of pituitary adenylate cyclase-activating polypeptide. Peptides 16: 1511-1516
63. Mizuno Y, Kondo K, Terashima Y, et al (1998) Anorectic effect of pituitary adenylate cyclase-activating polypeptide (PACAP) in rats: lack of evidence for involvement of hypothalamic neuropeptide gene expression. J Neuroendocrinol 10: 611-616
64. Narita M, Dun SL, Dun NJ, et al (1996) Hyperalgesia induced by pituitary adenylate cyclase-activating polypeptide in the mouse spinal cord. Eur J Pharmacol 311:121-126
65. Puig de Parada M, Parada M, Hernandez L (1995) Dispogenic effect of pituitary adenylate cyclase-activating polypeptide (PACAP38) injected into the lateral hypothalamus. Brain Res 696: 254-257
66. Nomura M, Ueta Y, Larsen PJ, et al (1997) Water deprivation increases the expression of pituitary adenylate cyclase-activating polypeptide gene in the rat subfornical organ. Endocrinology 138: 4096-4100
67. Yamamoto T, Tatsuno I (1995) Antinociceptive effect of intrathecally administered pituitary adenylate cyclase-activating polypeptide (PACAP) on the rat formalin test. Neurosci Lett 184: 32-35
68. Tatsuno I, Arimura A (1994) Pituitary adenylate cyclase-activating polypeptide (PACAP) mobilizes intracellular free calcium in cultures type-2, but not type-1, astrocytes. Brain Res 662: 1-10

69. Just L, Olenik C, Meyer DK (1998) Glial expression of the proenkephalin gene in slice cultures of the subventricular zone. J Mol Neurosci 11: 57-66
70. Moroo I, Tatsuno I, Uchida D, et al (1998) Pituitary adenylate cyclase-activating polypeptide (PACAP) stimulates mitogen-activated protein kinase (MAPK) in cultured rat astrocytes. Brain Res 765: 191-196
71. Zupan V, Hill JM, Brenneman DE, et al (1998) Involvement of pituitary adenylate cyclase-activating polypeptide II vasoactive intestinal peptide 2 receptor in mouse neocortical astrocytogenesis. J Neurochem 70: 2165-2173
72. Deutsch PJ, Schadlow V, Barzilai N (1992) 38-amino acid form of pituitary adenylate cyclase-activating polypeptide induces process outgrowth in human neuroblastoma cells. J Neurosci Res 35: 312-320
73. Deutsch PJ, Sun Y (1992) The 38 amino acid form of pituitary adenylate cyclase-activating polypeptide stimulates dual signaling cascades in PC12 cells and promotes neurite outgrowth. J Biol Chem 267: 5108-5113
74. Hamburger V, Levi-Montalcini R (1949) Proliferation, differentiation and degeneration in the spinal ganglia of the chick embryo under normal and experimental conditions. J Exp Zool 111: 457-502
75. Wakade AR (1997) Sympathetic neurons of chic embryo are rescued by PACAP from apoptotic death. Reg. Peptides 71:141
76. Cavallaro S, Copani A, D'Agata V, et al (1996) Pituitary adenylate cyclase-activating polypeptide prevents apoptosis in cultures cerebellar granule neurons. Mol Pharmacol 50:60-66
77. Chang JY, Korolev VV, Wang JZ (1996) Cyclic AMP and pituitary adenylate cyclase-activating polypeptide (PACAP) prevent programmed cell death of cultured rat cerebellar granule cells. Neurosci Let 206:181-184
78. Campard PK, Crochemore C, René F, et al (1997) PACAP type I receptor activation promotes cerebellar neuron survival through the cAMP/PKA signaling pathway. DNA Cell Biol 16:323-333
79. Gonzalez BJ, Basille M, Vaudry D, et al (1997) Pituitary adenylate cyclase-activating polypeptide promotes cell survival and neurite outgrowth in rat cerebellar neuroblasts. Neuroscience 78:419-430
80. Villalba M, Bockaert J, Journot L (1997) Pituitary adenylate cyclase-activating polypeptide (PACAP-38) protects cerebellar granule neurons from apoptosis by activating the mitogen-activating protein kinase (MAP kinase) pathway. J Neurosci. 17:83-90
81. Vaudry D, Gonzalez BJ, Basille M, et al (1999) Neurotrophic activity of pituitary adenylate cyclase activating polypeptide on rat cerebellar cortex during development. Proc Natl Acad Sci USA 96: 9415-9420
82. Gonzalez BJ, Vaudry D, Basille M, et al (1997) Rôle neurotrophique potential du pituitary adenylyl cyclase-activating polypeptide. Med/Sci 13:1331-1335
83. Gonzalez BJ, Leroux P, Basille M, et al (1994) Somatostatin and pituitary adenylate cyclase-activating polypeptide (PACAP):Two neuropeptides potentially involved in the development of the rat cerebellum. Ann Endocrinol 55:243-247
84. Basille M, Gonzalez BJ, Desrues L, et al (1995) Pituitary adenylate cyclase-activating polypeptide (PACAP) stimulates adenylyl cyclase and phospholipase C activity in rat cerebellar neuroblasts. J Neurochem 65:1318-1324
85. Favit A, Scapagnini U, Canonico PL (1995) Pituitary adenylate cyclase-activating polypeptide activates different signal transducing mechanism in cultured cerebellar

granule cells. Neuroendocrinology 61:377-382
86. Basille M, Gonzalez BJ, Leroux P, et al (1993) Localization and characterization of PACAP receptors in the rat cerebellum during development: evidence for a stimulatory effect of PACAP on immune cerebellar granule cells. Neuroscience 57: 329-338
87. Gonzalez BJ, Basille M, Mei YA, et al (1996) Ontogeny of PACAP and PACAP receptors in the rat brain: Role of PACAP in the cerebellum during development. Ann NY Acad Sci 805: 302-314
88. Mei YA (1999) High-voltage-activating calcium current and its modulation by dopamine D4 and pituitary adenylate cyclase-activating polypeptide receptors in cerebellar granule cells. Chung Kuo Yao Li Hsueh Pao 20: 3-9
89. Zerr P, Feltz A (1994) Forskolin blocks the transient K current of rat cerebellar granule neurons. Neurosci Lett 181: 153-157
90. Colom LV, Diaz ME, Beers DR, et al (1998) Role of potassium channels in amyloid-induced cell death. J Neurochem 70: 1925-1934
91. Kobayashi T, Mori Y (1998) Ca^{2+} channel antagonists and neuroprotection from cerebral ischemia. Eur J Pharmacol 363: 1-15
92. Krebs J (1998) The role of calcium in apoptosis. Biometals 11: 375-382
93. Lu N, DiCicco-Bloom E (1997) Pituitary adenylate cyclase-activating polypeptide is an autocrine inhibitor of mitosis in cultured cortical precursor cells. Proc Natl Acad Sci USA 94 :3357-3362
94. Lu N, Zhou R, DiCicco-Bloom E (1998) Opposing mitogenic regulation by PACAP in sympathetic and cerebral cortical precursors correlates with differential expression of PACAP receptor (PAC1-R) isoforms. J Neurosci Res 53: 651-662
95. DiCicco-Bloom E, Lu N, Pintar JE, et al (1998) The PACAP ligand/receptor system regulates cerebral cortical neurogenesis. Ann NY Acad Sci 865: 274-289
96. Choi DW, Maulucci-Gedde M, Kriegstein AR (1987) Glutamate neurotoxicity in cortical cell culture. J Neurosci 7: 357-368
97. Koh JY, Palmer E, Cotman CW (1991) Activation of the metabotropic glutamate receptor attenuates N-methyl-D-aspartate neurotoxicity in cortical cultures. Proc Natl Acad Sci USA 88: 9431-9435
98. Sagara Y, Schubert D (1998) The activation of metabotropic glutamate receptors protects nerve cells from oxidative stress. J Neurosci 18: 6662-6671
99. Martin JL, Gasser D, Magistretti PJ (1995) Vasoactive intestinal peptide and pituitary adenylate cyclase-activating polypeptide potentiate c-fos expression induced by glutamate in cultured cortical neurons. J Neurochem 65: 1-9
100. Stella N, Magistretti PJ (1996) Vasoactive intestinal peptide (VIP) and pituitary adenylate cyclase-activating polypeptide (PACAP) potential the glutamate-evoked release of arachidonic acid from mouse cortical neurons. Evidence for a cAMP-independent mechanism. J Biol Chem 271: 705-710
101. Magistretti PJ, Cardinaux JR, Martin JL (1998) VIP and PACAP in the CNS: Regulators of glial energy metabolism and modulators of glutamatergic signaling. Ann NY Acad Sci 865: 213-225
102. Pellegri G, Magistretti PJ, Martin JL (1998) VIP and PACAP potentiate the action of glutamate on BDNF expression in mouse cortical neurons. Eur J Neurosci 10: 272-280
103. Morio H, Tatsuno I, Hirai A, et al (1996) Pituitary adenylate-cyclase-activating polypeptide protects rat-cultured cortical neurons from glutamate-induced

cytotoxicity. Brain Res 741: 82-88
104. Shoge K, Mishima HK, Saitoh T, et al (1999) Attenuation by PACAP of glutamate-induced neurotoxicity in cultured retinal neurons. Brain Res 839: 66-73
105. Liu GL, Madsen BW (1997) PACAP38 modulates activity of NMDA receptors in cultured chick cortical neurons. J Neurophysiol 78: 2231-2234
106. Liu GJ, Madsen BW (1998) Modulatory action of PACAP27 on NMDA receptor channel activity in cultured chick cortical neurons. Brain Res 791: 290-294
107. Kong LY, Maderdrut JL, Jeohn GH, et al (1999) Reduction of lipopolysaccharide-induced neurotoxicity in mixed cortical neuron/glia cultures by femtomolar concentrations of pituitary adenylate cyclase-activating polypeptide. Neuroscience 91: 493-500
108. Takei N, Skoglösa Y, Lindholm D (1998) Neurotrophic and neuroprotective effects of pituitary adenylate cyclase-activating polypeptide (PACAP) on mesencephalic dopaminergic neurons. J Neurosci Res 54: 698-706
109. Brenneman DE, Westbrook GL, Fitzgeral SP, et al (1988) Neuronal cell killing by the envelop protein if HIV and its prevention by vasoactive intestinal peptide. Nature 335: 639-642
110. Pulsinelli WA, Brierly JB (1979) A new model of bilateral hemispheric ischemia in the unanesthetized rat. Stroke 10: 267-272
111. Uchida D, Arimura A, Somogyvari-Vigh A, et al (1996) Prevention of ischemia-induced death of hippocampal neurons by pituitary adenylate cyclase-activating polypeptide. Brain Res 736: 280-286
112. Banks WA, Kastin AJ, Komaki G, et al (1993) Passage of pituitary adenylate cyclase-activating polypeptide 1-27 and pituitary adenylate cyclase-activating polypeptide 1-38 across the blood-brain barrier. J Pharmacol Exp Ther 267: 690-696
113. Gillardon F, Hata R, Hossmann KA (1998) Delayed up-regulation of zacl and PACAP type I receptor after transient focal cerebral ischemia in mice. Brain Res Mol Brain Res 61: 207-210
114. Ciani E, Hoffman A, Schmidt P, et al (1999) Induction of the PAC1-R (PACAP-type I receptor) gene by p53 Zac. Brain Res Mol Brain Res 69: 290-294
115. Skoglösa Y, Lewen A, Takei N, et al (1999) Regulation of pituitary adenylate cyclase-activating polypeptide and its receptor type 1 after traumatic brain injury: Comparison with brain-derived neurotrophic factor and the induction of neuronal cell death. Neuroscience 90:235-247
116. Lioudyno M, Skoglösa Y, Takei N, et al (1998) Pituitary adenylate cyclase-activating polypeptide (PACAP) protects dorsal root ganglion neurons from death and induced calcitonin gene-related peptide (CGRP) immunoreactivity in vivo. J Neurosci Res 51: 243-256
117. Zhang Y, Danielsen N, Sundler F, et al (1998) Pituitary adenylate cyclase-activating peptide is unregulated in sensory neurons by inflammation. NeuroReport 9: 2833-2836
118. Zhang YZ, Hannibal J, Zhao Q, et al (1996) Pituitary adenylate cyclase-activating peptide expression in the rat dorsal root ganglia: Up-regulation after peripheral nerve injury. Neuroscience 74: 1099-1110
119. Zhou X, Rodriguez WI, Casillas RA, et al (1999b) Axotomy-induced changes in pituitary adenylate cyclase activating polypeptide (PACAP) and PACAP receptor gene expression in the adult rat facial motor nucleus. J Neurosci Res 57: 953-961

120. Reglodi D, Somogyvari VA, Vigh S, et al (2000) Delayed systemic administration of PACAP38 is neuroprotective in transient middle cerebral artery occlusion in the rat. Stroke 31: 1411-1417
121. Longa EZ, Weinstein PR, Carlson S, et al (1989) Reversible middle cerebral artery occlusion without craniectomy in rats. Stroke 20: 84-91
122. Brenneman DE, Neale EA, Foster GA, et al (1987) Nonneuronal cells mediate neurotrophic action of vasoactive intestinal polypeptide. J Cell Biol 104: 1603-1610
123. Ashur-Fabian O, Giladi E, Brennemam DE, et al (1997) Identification of VIP/PACAP receptors on rat astrocytes using antisense oligodeoxynucleotides. J Mol Neurosci 9:11-22
124. Nagao H, Matsuoka I, Kurihara K (1995) Effects of adenylyl cyclase-linked neuropeptides on the expression of ciliary neurotrophic factor-mRNA in cultured astrocytes. FEBS Lett 362: 75-79
125. Gottschall PE, Tatsuno I, Arimura A (1994) Regulation of interleukin-6 (IL-6) secretion in primary cultured rat astrocytes: Synergism of interleukin-1 (IL-1) and pituitary adenylate cyclase-activating polypeptide (PACAP). Brain Res 637:197-203
126. Miyata A, Sato K, Hino j, et al ((1998) Rat aortic smooth-muscle cell proliferation is bidirectionally regulated in a cell cycle-dependent manner via PACAP/VIP type 2 receptor. Ann N Y Acad Sci 865: 73-81

Neurite outgrowth-promoting prostaglandins that act as neuroprotective agents against brain ischemia and may enhance recovery of higher neuronal functions

Takumi Satoh[1], Ryuzo Shingai[1], Kyoji Furuta[2], Masaaki Suzuki[2], and Yasuyoshi Watanabe[3]

[1]Department of Welfare Engineering, Faculty of Engineering, Iwate University, 4-3-5 Ueda, Morioka, Iwate 020-8551, Japan
[2]Department of Biomolecular Science, Faculty of Engineering, Gifu University, Gifu 501-1193, Japan
[3]Department of Physiology, Osaka City University, Graduate School of Medicine, Osaka 545-8585, Japan

Summary: A large number of compounds have been reported to prevent ischemia-induced neuronal death, whereas there are few described to enhance recovery of brain functions. Since neurotrophins do not only prevent neuronal death but also protect neuronal circuits, they may be potential candidates. However, their poor penetration of the blood-brain-barrier hampers their development as therapeutic agents. In this context, low-molecular-weight compounds that possess neurite outgrowth- and neuronal survival-promoting activities may be alternative candidates. Neurite outgrowth-promoting prostaglandins, which were recently-synthesized based on the chemical structure of anti-tumor cyclopentenone prostaglandin derivatives, have been characterized by their neurotrophic effects on neurons in the central nervous system. In this paper, we present a review of these compounds as therapeutic agents against brain ischemia.

Key words: Neurotrophin, Cyclopentenone prostaglandin, Neuronal survival, Neurite outgrowth, NEPP

Introduction

Neurotrophins play an essential role in the maintenance of populations of neuronal cells from development through adulthood. The administration of neurotrophins may be an effective treatment for disorders of neurons in the peripheral nervous system (PNS) (McMahon and Priestly, 1995). Treatment for degeneration of neurons in the central nervous system (CNS) with neurotrophins is also possible both *in vivo* and *in vitro* models (Barde 1998). In fact, brain-derived neurotrophic factor (BDNF) and neurotrophin-4/5 promoted neurite outgrowth and survival of CNS neurons (Schabitz et al., 1997; Rabacchi et al., 1999) and prevented the death of neuronal somas and promoted axon regeneration in response to axotomy of CNS neurons (Kobayashi et al., 1997). In CNS neurons, not only distal axons but also afferent somas undergo severe degeneration, called "retrograde degeneration", in response to nerve transection (Williams et al., 1986; Hefti and Wainer, 1986). This fact suggests that the administration of some agent, such as BDNF, that promotes neurite outgrowth/regeneration of CNS neurons might prevent their death. However, as proteins, neurotrophins do not make ideal drug candidates due to the low permeability of the blood-brain barrier for these factors. Therefore, much effort has been made in the search for non-peptidyl low molecular weight compounds that have neurotrophic effects on desired neurons (Snyder et al, 1998; Pollack et al., 1999; Saragovi and Gehring, 2000; Furuta K., 2000; Satoh et al., 2001).

Compounds that activate Trk receptor (neurotrophin receptor)-signaling pathways may, e.g., NB506, have neurite outgrowth- and neuronal survival-promoting activities (Pollack et al., 1999). Strictly speaking, this compound should qualify as a neurotrophin-like compound since it utilizes the same intracellular signaling pathway as neurotrophins. However, the purpose of the present review was not to clarify the intracellular signaling pathways of neurotrophins but to examine the development of molecular probes or drugs against brain ischemia and to report on the identification of trophic mechanisms other than those of neurotrophins. Thus, we do not adopt the limited definition given above. A compound that simply has neurite outgrowth- and neuronal survival-promoting activities is defined as a neurotrophin-like compound in this review. Although NB506 reportedly had neurite outgrowth- and neuronal survival-promoting activities in PNS neurons (Pollack et al., 1999), it was strongly toxic toward cultured CNS neurons within the concentrations required for activation of Trk receptor-signaling pathways (Wilkie et al., 2001). It might have other non-specific toxic activities. Otherwise, excessive activation of Trk signaling pathways itself by any compound might lead to cell death of CNS neurons, especially under oxidative conditions. It has been clarified that oxidative stress plays a central role in several types of neuronal death (Gleenlund et al., 1995; Satoh et al., 1996; Schulz et al., 1996). Neurotrophins were reported to enhance the oxidative stress-induced death of CNS neurons in a Trk-dependent manner (Gwag et al., 1995; Ishikawa et al., 2000) although they have anti-apoptotic effects in some systems (Bonni et al., 1999; Kubo et al., 1995). This may be a serious disadvantage for *in vivo* use of NB506 as a neuroprotective agents for CNS neurons since oxidative stress may play some role in the neurodegenerative process (Coyle and Puttfarcken, 1993; Satoh et al.,1999a). We consider that such a compound might not be the best for therapeutic agents because of their intrinsic activation of oxidative stress-induced neuronal death by excessive activation of Trk-signaling pathways. Are there any compounds which induce neurite outgrowth- and neuronal survival-promoting activities but do not activate Trk-signaling pathways?

One possible candidate for such a neurotrophin-like compound for CNS neurons is the neuroimmunophilin ligand, GPI1046 (Snyder et al., 1998). GPI1046 was elaborated based on the chemical structure of an immunosupressant drug, FK506 (Snyder et al, 1998). GPI1046 was reported to possess neurite outgrowth- and neuronal survival-promoting activities toward both CNS and PNS neurons (Snyder et al., 1998). However, these neurotrophic effects have been challenged on the ground of unreproducibility by other groups. For example, Harper et al. (1999) failed to obtain evidence in support of the notion of a general neuroprotective effect and effect on morphologic nerve regeneration *in vivo*, and they concluded that GPI1046 had only a marginal effect on neurite outgrowth and neuronal survival.

Recently, we accumulated several lines of evidences that NEurite outgrowth-Promoting Prostaglandins (NEPP's) are candidate compounds having neurotrophin-like and Trk-independent actions on CNS neurons. NEPP's [Δ^7-prostaglandin (PG) A_1 methyl ester derivatives] were originally designed on the basis of the chemical structure of Δ^{12}-PGJ_2, which was used for the development of anti-cancer drugs (Suzuki et al., 1997 and 1998). The cyclopentenone-structured PGA's and PGJ's exhibit anti-tumor activity both *in vivo* and *in vitro* (Honn et al., 1981; Fukushima, 1992; Suzuki et al., 1997 and 1998). They accumulate in the nuclear fraction, bind to some unknown nuclear proteins (Narumiya and Fukushima, 1986; Narumiya et al., 1986 and 1987; Parker, 1995), and thereby modulate the expression of various genes (Holbrook et al., 1992; Gorspe et al., 1996a and 1996b; Tanikawa et al., 1998; Ishikawa et al., 1998). Although PGJ_2 metabolites have been identified as natural ligands for peroxisome proliferator-activated receptor γ (PPARγ) and promote adipocyte differentiation (Forman et al., 1995; Kliewer et al., 1995), the expression of PPARγ is highly restricted to adipose tissue (Chawala et al., 1994), suggesting that the involvement of PPARγ activation in the neuronal function of PGJ_2 metabolites is very small. Because PGD_2, a precursor of PGJ_2 metabolites (Fukushima, 1992), is one of the most abundant arachidonic acid metabolites in the brain (Yoshida et al. 1983), CNS neurons are possibly exposed to PGJ_2 metabolites. Recently, several physiological functions of PGJ_2 metabolites in the nervous system independent of PPARγ activation were reported (Petrova et al., 1999; Satoh et al., 1999b). For example, PGJ_2 metabolites inhibited the expression of iNOS by activated microglia, which may lead to down-regulation of these activated cells, through inhibition of an NFκB-mediated signaling pathway, but not through PPARγ activation, suggesting that these cyclopentenone PG's function as anti-inflammatory factors in the brain (Petrova et al., 1999). However, the direct actions of PGJ_2 metabolites on neurons remain largely unknown possibly because their cytotoxicity masks their intrinsic biological functions or because they are extremely unstable in a neutral solution (Fukushima, 1992). We found that PGJ_2 metabolites promoted neurite outgrowth induced by nerve growth factor (NGF) in PC12 cells independently of PPARγ activation (Satoh et al., 1999b). This result suggests that PGJ_2 metabolites function as neurite outgrowth-promoting factors in neurons. Thus the development of drugs that mimic the neurite outgrowth-promoting activity of PGJ_2 metabolites for treatment of neurodegenerative diseases may be possible. However, instability and the complicated chemical synthesis of them have hampered the study of their structure-function relationship and the development of such drugs (Fukushima, 1992; Suzuki et al., 1997 and 1998). The use of Δ^7-PGA_1 methyl ester derivatives (NEPP's) can overcome these problems of PGJ_2 metabolites (Suzuki et al., 1997 and 1998), since they are easily and rapidly synthesized by 3 component chemical synthesis (Noyori and Suzuki, 1993).

Previous experiments in our laboratories demonstrated that NEPP's are a novel type of neuroprotective compounds characterized by their dual biological effects of promoting neurite outgrowth and preventing the death of CNS neurons (Satoh et al., 1999b, 2000a, 2000c, 2001). Our results suggest that NEPP's accumulate in nuclei and bind covalently to unknown nuclear proteins, thereby increasing the expression of chaperone molecules, to induce neurotrophic effects on CNS neurons (Fig. 2).

Promotion of neurite outgrowth by NEPP's

PGJ_2 metabolites (PGJ_2, Δ^{12}-PGJ_2 and *15-deoxy-*$\Delta^{12,14}$-PGJ_2) promoted neurite outgrowth from PC12 cells (Satoh et al., 1999b). It occurred to us that NEPP's may promote neurite outgrowth since NEPP's share similar biological activities with PGJ_2 metabolites (Fukushima, 1992; Suzuki et al., 1997 and 1998). We examined neurite outgrowth-promoting effects of NEPP's on PC12 cells and dorsal root ganglia (DRG) explants (Satoh et al., 2000a). Although NGF itself slightly enhanced neurite outgrowth from PC12 cells at 24 hr (Fig. 3A), the presence of NEPP10 in addition to NGF potently promoted the outgrowth (Fig. 3B). Although NEPP1 to NEPP6 (NEPP1-6) promoted dose-dependent neurite outgrowth to a level comparable to that obtained with NEPP10, NEPP1-6 showed more potent toxic effects than NEPP10 (Satoh et al., 2000a and 2000c). Thus, NEPP10 was selected as the best candidate for the development of a drug with high biological activity and low cytotoxicity. The neurite outgrowth-promoting activity of NEPP10 was also examined in DRG explants from chick embryos at embryonic day 8. In this system, the presence of NGF is reported to promote neurite regeneration/outgrowth (Levi-Montalcini and Angeletti, 1968). The presence of NEPP10 potently promoted NGF-induced neurite outgrowth from DRG explants (Satoh et al., 2000a). Similar neurite outgrowth-promoting effect on CNS neurons in culture was also observed in the presence of BDNF (data not shown). These results suggest that the promotion of neurite outgrowth induced by

NEPP's is a general consequence in the case of both CNS and PNS neurons. However, we later found that NEPP10 does not qualify as a neurotrophin-like compound since it did not protect neuronal cells (Satoh et al., 2001).

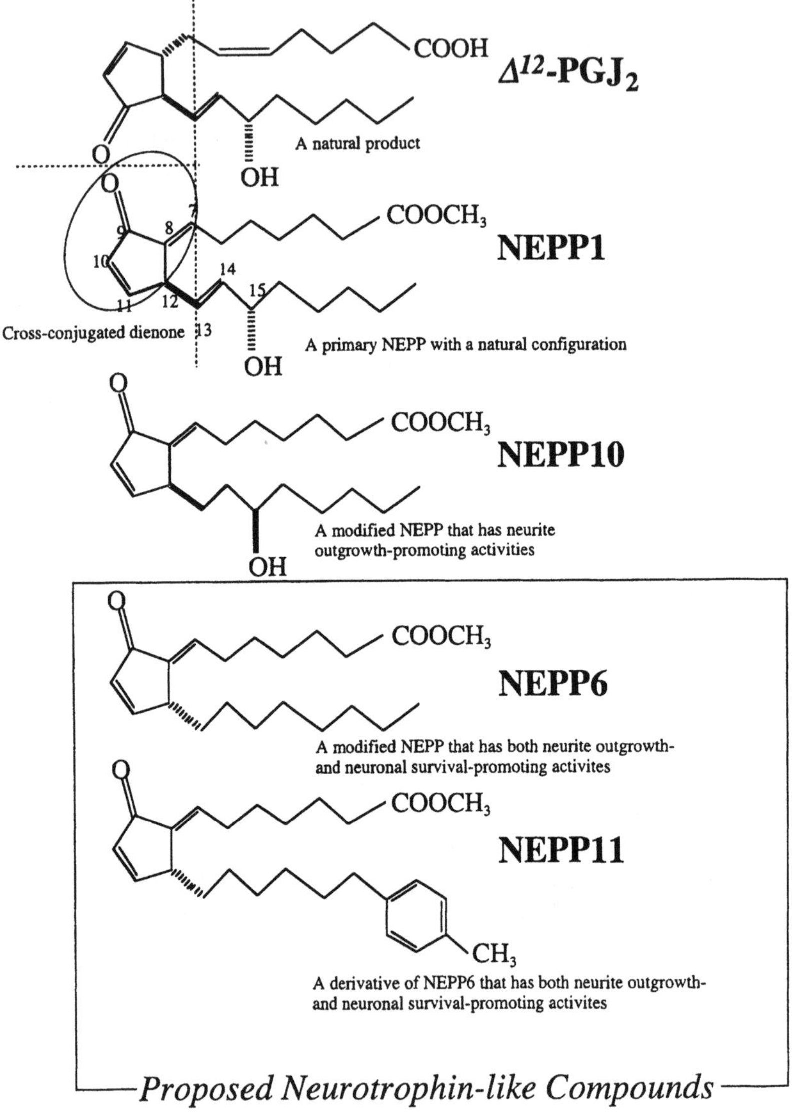

Fig. 1. Chemical structures of Δ^{12}-PGJ_2 and NEPP's. A characteristic chemical structure of NEPP's, "cross-conjugated dienone" at C(7)-C(11) is demonstrated in the chemical structure of NEPP1. All NEPP's have "cross-conjugated dienone" in their chemical structures.

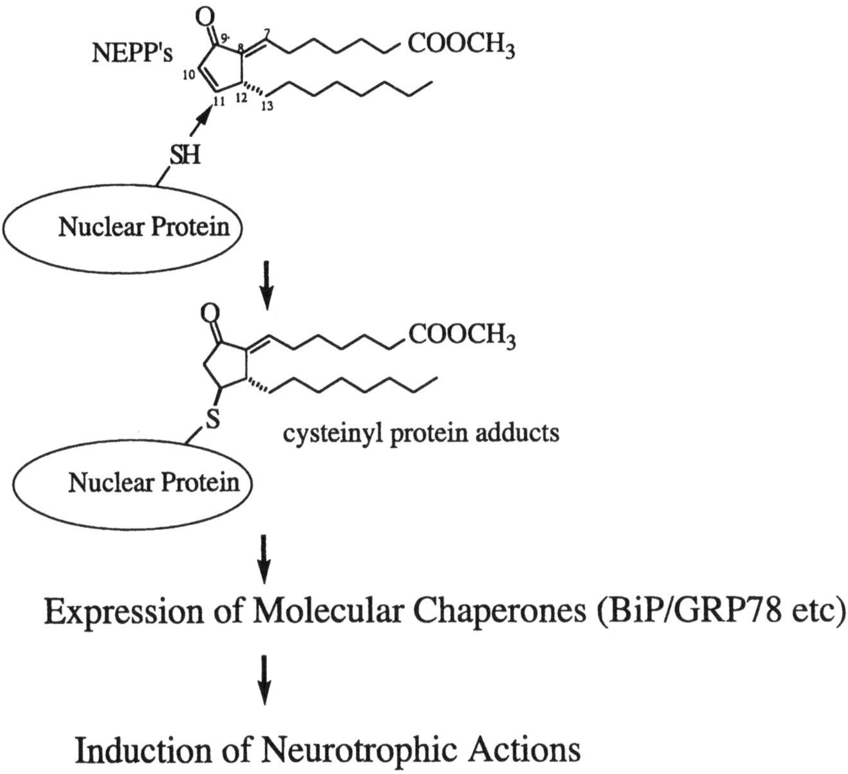

Fig. 2. A possible molecular mechanism of neurotrophic actions of NEPP's. Since C(11) of NEPP's is an electrophilic carbon, it is easily attacked by nucleophilic SH group-containing molecules such as free glutathione and cysteine residues in proteins (Suzuki et al., 1997). They might initiate upregulation of some chaperone molecules to induce their neurotrophic actions.

Although NEPP's enhanced the NGF-induced neurite outgrowth from PC12 cells, they enhanced the basic fibroblast growth factor (bFGF)-induced neurite outgrowth to a much lesser extent (Fig. 4). This action may be a big advantage of NEPP's since NEPP's might have neurite outgrowth-promoting effects in the presence of neurotrophins, but not in the presence of other growth factors. In contrast to the clear dependence of NEPP's on the presence of neurotrophins, other neurotrophin-like compounds such as GPI1046 and NB506 themselves enhanced neurite outgrowth, suggesting that they might non-specifically enhance it in the absence of neurotrophin. Since expression of neurotrophins in the CNS is strictly regulated (Barde, 1998), the actions of NEPP's may be restricted to the sites where neurotrophin is upregulated. These sites of adult brain may correspond to those where neurons are damaged or where rearrangement of neuronal circuits is urgently needed in the brain. NEPP's might specifically act on these sites *in vivo*. What is the molecular basis by which NEPP's discriminate the neurite outgrowth by NGF from that by bFGF? It is likely that NEPP's discriminate NGF from bFGF independently of Extracellular-signal-Responsive Kinases 1/2-mediated pathways since NEPP's did not affect the activities of these kinases (Satoh et al., 2000a). We found that induction of immunoglobulin heavy chain binding protein/glucose-regulated protein 78 (BiP/GRP78) was critical for the neurite outgrowth-promoting activities of NEPP's (Satoh et al., 2000a), suggesting that the upregulation of BiP/GRP78 is more prominent in the presence of NGF than in the presence of bFGF. However, it remains to be investigated how BiP/GRP78 regulates neurite outgrowth.

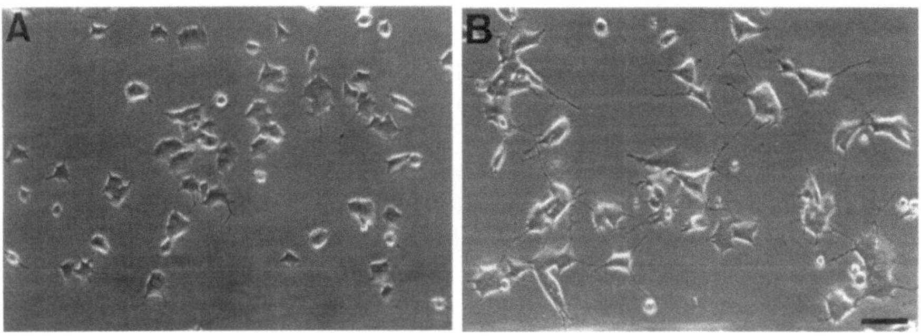

Fig. 3. NEPP10-mediated NGF-induced promotion of neurite outgrowth from PC12 cells. PC12h cells, a subclone of PC12 cells (Greene and Tischler, 1976), were used throughout the experiments and cultured as described previously (Hatanaka et al., 1981). PC12 cells (10^4 cells/cm^2) were cultured in serum-free 1:1 mixture of Dulbecco's Modified Eagle medium and F12 medium (DF medium) in the presence of the NGF (50 ng/ml) for 24 hr (**A** and **B**). NEPP10 (0.5 μM) was added (**B**) or not (**A**) 30 min before NGF. The bar represents 10 μm.

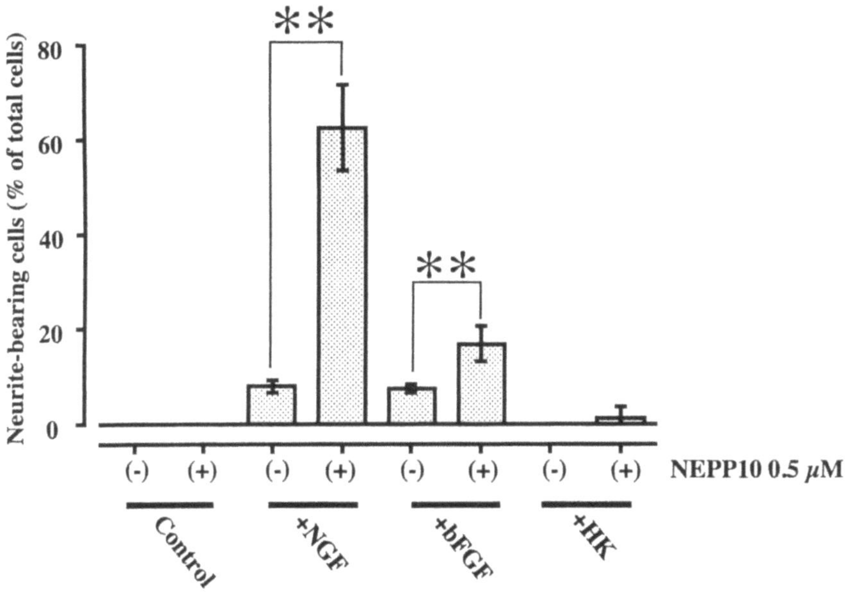

Fig. 4. Promotion of neurite outgrowth by NEPP10 in the presence of NGF, bFGF and high potassium solution. PC12 cells (10^4 cells/cm^2) were cultured in serum-free DF medium in the presence of NGF (50 ng/ml), bFGF (50 ng/ml) or high potassium (50 mM) solution for 24 hr. 0.5 μM of NEPP10 was added or not 30 min before NGF, bFGF or the high potassium solution. The cells were subsequently incubated for 24 hr and neurite (>10 μm)-bearing cells in a defined area of each well were then counted under microscopic observation. The values are means ± SD (n=4). Significance of difference values at any concentrations of NEPP11 v.s. those in the absence of NEPP11 was determined by ANOVA (** $p < 0.01$).

Promotion of neuronal survival by NEPP's

In order to generate neurotrophin-like compounds, we examined NEPP's1-10 for neuronal survival-promoting activity (Satoh et al., 2001). We found that NEPP6 and 11 had a potent protective effect on neurronal cells. NEPP11 (1.0 μM) significantly protected HT22 cells against oxidative glutamate toxicity (Fig. 5C) to the comparable level of cycloheximide (3.0 μM) (Fig. 5**D**). Furthermore, NEPP11 prevented the death against focal ischemia in mice (Satoh et al., 2001). These results suggested that it works *in vivo* that it is a candidate for a neurotrophin-like compound for CNS neurons.

Next, we measured the time at which NEPPs' action was necessary to inhibit neuronal death (Fig. 6). In this experiment, NEPP11 or ebselen was added to HT22 culture at various times after the glutamate addition. Ebselen, a seleno-organic compound, is an anti-oxidant, that is supposed to interfere with the activation phase of cell death (Deshmukh and Johnson, 1997; Tan et al., 1998). Ebselen was reported to effectively suppress focal ischemia-induced neuronal death in mice (Namura et al., 2001).

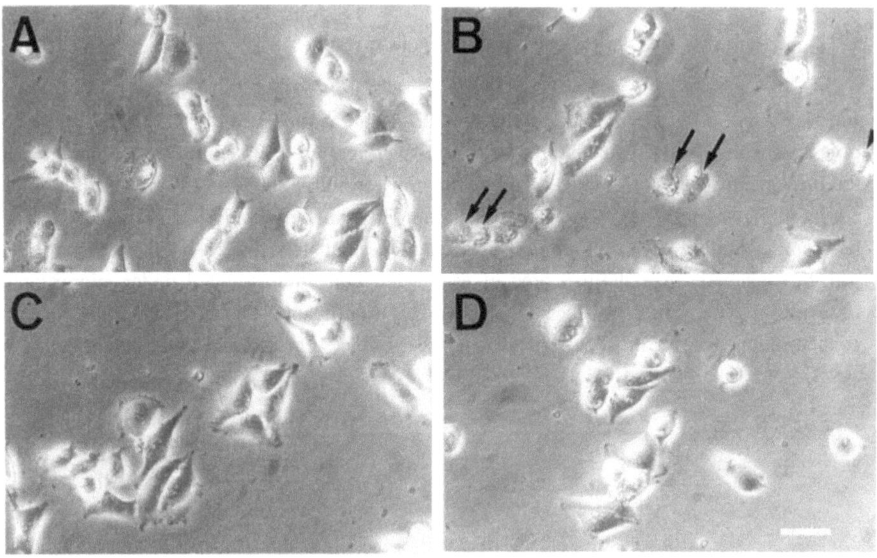

Fig. 5. Protection of HT22 cells by NEPP11 against oxidative glutamate toxicity. HT22 cells were seeded into 24-well plates at a density of 4 x 10^4 cells/cm^2. After a 5-hr incubation, 1.0 μM NEPP11 (C) or 3.0 μM cycloheximide (D) was added to the cultures. Thirty minutes later, vehicle (A) or 5 mM glutamate (B, C and D) was added; and the cells were incubated further for 10 hr. Arrows in B showed degenerated cells. The bar represents 25 μm.

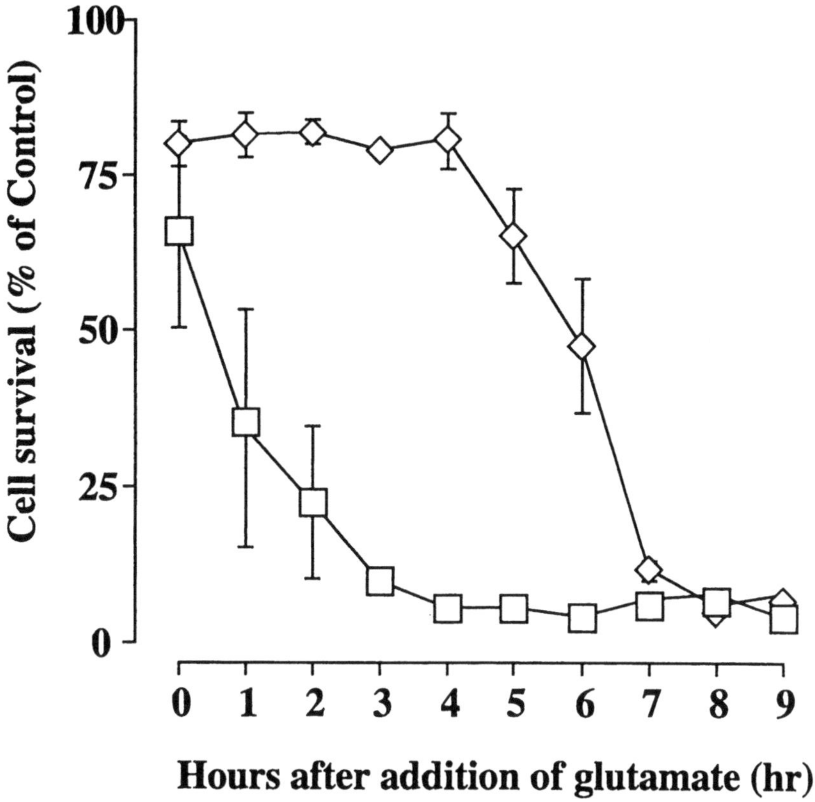

Fig. 6. Commitment to inhibition of neuronal death by NEPP11 and ebselen. HT22 cells were cultured as described previously (Satoh et al., 2000b). Briefly, HT22 cells were seeded into 24-well plates at a density of 4 x 10^4 cells/cm^2. After a 5-hr incubation, 5 mM of glutamate were added to the cultures. At indicated times after glutamate addition, NEPP11 (squares) or ebselen (diamonds) was added; and the cells were then incubated further for 24 hr. To evaluate cell survival of HT22 cells, we performed the MTT assay according to a modified procedure (Kubo et al., 1996). The values representing % of the MTT activity of control cells are reported as means $\pm$ SD (n=4).

During the course of oxidative glutamate toxicity in HT22 cells, the cell death mechanism is initiated by a decrease in the levels of reduced glutathione associated with an increase in those of intracellular reactive oxygen species (Davis and Maher, 1994; Tan et al., 1998). This event occurs at 4-7 hr during the activation phase (Tan et al., 1998). Consistent with these previous reports, the commitment time of ebselen was 4-7 hr (Fig. 6). In contrast to the case of ebselen, the presence of NEPP11 before initiation of the cell death mechanism was necessary for its inhibition of cell death. Since NEPP's enter the cells and make a covalent bond with nuclear proteins within 10 min by the experiment with biotinylated NEPP's (data not shown), it did not take so much time to reach site of action. This result strongly suggests that NEPP11 itself does not interfere in the cell death pathway as ebselen dose. A cellular event, presumably transcription of some gene(s), seems to be required for the inhibition of cell death by NEPP's. This speculation is fully justified by the previous works with anti-tumor PG's (Fukushima, 1992; Narumiya et al., 1987). They discussed that anti-tumor PG's enter the cells and make a covalent bond with unknown nuclear protein(s) to induce transcription of genes and arrest of cell cycle. At present, we consider that this speculation is applicable to the neurotrophic actions of NEPP's as shown in Fig. 2. A big question what gene's transcription is responsible for the inhibition of cell death remains to be addressed. Furthermore, the abilities of NEPP11 to regenerate neurites from CNS neurons both *in vivo* and *in vitro* and to recover higher neuronal functions are next issues to be examined.

Requirement of intracellular SH group for the cellular accumulation

Enone and dienone structures were reported to bind covalently to intracellular SH compounds (Suzuki et al., 1997). To test the hypothesis, we examined the effect of N-ethylmaleimide (NEM), which irreversibly masks SH groups under physiological conditions (Fig. 7). In this experiment, fixed cells were used because of the high cytotoxicity of NEM. The cells were fixed with 4% paraformaldehyde for 5 min and then subjected to treatment with 30 μM (Fig. 7E-F) or 100 μM (Fig. 7G-H) NEM. Thirty minutes later, the cells were treated with vehicle (Fig. 7A-B) or 10 μM NEPP6-biotin (Fig. 7C-H) for 1 hr and thereafter stained with Alexa-conjugated streptavidin and Hoechst 33,258. Cellular signals of NEPP6-biotin were significantly suppressed by a low concentration (30 μM) of NEM than were cytoplasmic signals (Fig. 7E-F). The signals of NEPP6-biotin were more reduced by treatment with 100 μM NEM (Fig. 7G-H), suggesting that the binding of NEPP6-biotin to the cells requires intracellular SH groups. Since NEPP's exist not only in nuclei but also in cytosol (Satoh et al., 2001), we could not identify their sites of action. Nuclear existence of NEPP's may suggest that activation of transcription of specific genes in nuclei mediates the protective effects of NEPP's. The possibility of covalent binding of dienone-structured cyclopentenone PG's to nuclear proteins was also proposed from the results of a biochemical experiment: a dienone PG (Δ^{12}-PGJ_2), but not enone PG (PGA_2) bound to the nuclear fractions, and the binding was resistant to extraction with acidic ethyl acetate but sensitive to treatment with proteases, suggesting that a dienone PG had formed a covalent bond with nuclear proteins (Narumiya et al., 1987). The requirement of cysteine residues in the targeted protein of cyclopentenone PG's was reported by Rossi et al. (2000) and Straus et al. (2000): *15-deoxy-*$\Delta^{12,14}$-PGJ_2 directly bound to IκB kinase β (IKKβ), and the transcription

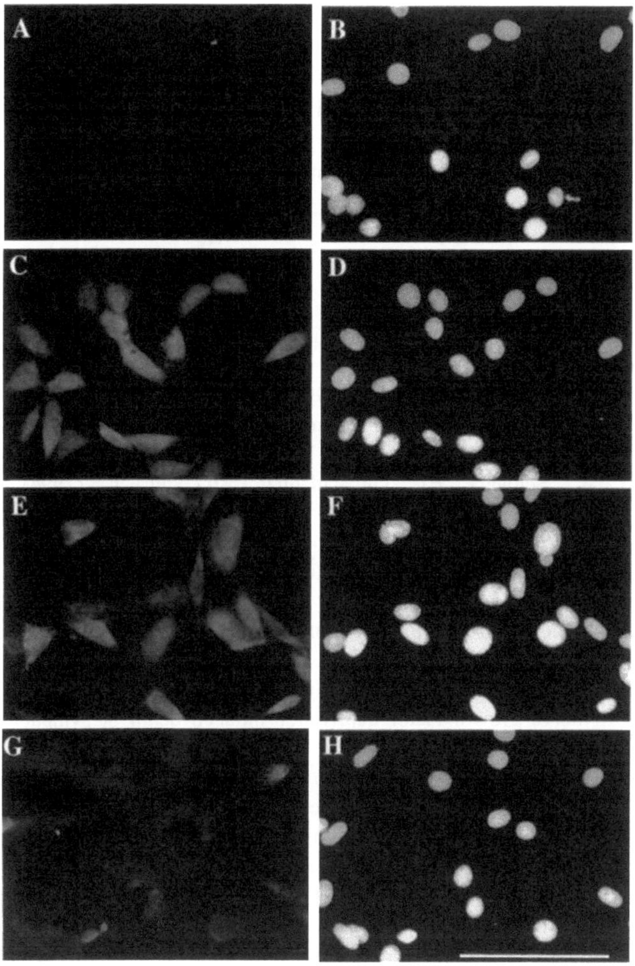

Fig. 7. NEM blocked cellular accumulation of NEPP6-biotin. HT22 cells were seeded at a density of 4 x 10^4 cells/cm^2. After a 5-hr incubation, the cells were fixed and treated with vehicle (A-D), NEM 30 μM (E-F) or NEM 100 μM (G-H). After a 30-min incubation, vehicle (A-B) or 10 μM NEPP6-biotin (C-H) was added to the cultures, and the cultures were then stained with Alexa-conjugated streptavidin and Hoechst 33,258. The stained cells were observed under a fluorescence microscope with excitation at wavelengths of 480 nm (Alexa) and 380 nm (Hoechst 33,258). A-B, C-D, E-F, and G-H are the same fields. A, C, E, and G are Alexa (NEPP6-biotin) signals. B, D, F, and H are Hoechst 33,258 signals. The bar represents 100 μm.

complex of NFκB. The cysteine residues in IKKβ and p65 of this transcription complex were essential for the inhibition of NFκB-mediated TNFα signaling by the PG, suggesting that a covalent bond was formed between the SH group of proteins and *15-deoxy-*$\Delta^{12,14}$-PGJ_2. These and our results suggest that neuroprotective NEPP6 and NEPP11 are transported to nuclei and bind to nuclear proteins in order to exhibit their neuroprotective effects.

References

1. Barde YA (1998) Biological roles of neurotrophins, in Neurotrophic Factors (Hefti F., ed.), pp1-31, Springer, Berlin
2. Bonni A, Brunet A, West AE, et al (1999) Cell survival promoted by the Ras-MAPK signaling pathway by transcription-dependent- and -independent mechanisms. Science 286:1358–1362
3. Chawala A, Schwarz EJ, Dimaculangan DD, et al (1994) Peroxisome proliferator-activated receptor (PPAR) γ: adipocyte-predominant expression and induction early in adipocyte differentiation. Endocrinology 135:798-800
4. Coyle JT, Puttfarcken P (1993) Oxidative stress, glutamate and neurodegenerative disorders. Science 262:689–695
5. Davis JB, Maher P (1994) Protein kinase C activation inhibits glutamate-induced cytotoxicity in a neuronal cell line. Brain Res 652:169–173
6. Deshmukh M, Johnson EMJr (1997) Programmed cell death in neurons: Focus on the pathway of nerve growth factor deprivation-induced death of sympathetic neurons. Mol Pharamcol 51:897–906
7. Forman BM, Tontonoz P, Chen J, et al (1995) *15-deoxy-*$\Delta^{12,14}$-prostaglandin J_2 is a ligand for the adipocyte determination factor PPARγ. Cell 83: 803-812
8. Fukushima M (1992) Biological activities and mechanism of action of PGJ_2 and related compounds: an update. Prostagl Leukotri Essen Fatty acids 47:1-12
9. Furuta K, Tomokiyo K, Satoh T, et al (2000) Designed prostaglandins with neurotrophic activities. Chem BioChem 1:283-286
10. Gorospe M, Liu Y, Xu Q, et al (1996a) Inhibition of G_1 cyclin-dependent kinase activity during growth arrest of human breast carcinoma cells by prostaglandin A_2. Mol Cell Biol 16:762-770
11. Gorospe M, Wang X, Guyton KZ, et al (1996b) Protective role of $p21^{Waf1/Cip1}$ against prostaglandin A_2-mediated apoptosis of human colorectal carcinoma cells. Mol Cell Biol 16:6654-6660
12. Greene LA, Tischler AS (1976) Establishment of a noradrenergic clonal line of rat adrenal pheochromocytoma cells which respond to nerve growth factor. Proc Natl Acad Sci USA 73: 2424-2428
13. Greenlund LJ, Deckwerth TI, Johnson EMJr (1995) Superoxide dismutase delays neuronal apoptosis: a role for reactive oxygen species in programmed neuronal death. Neuron 14:303-315
14. Gwag BJ, Koh JY, Chen MM, et al (1995) BDNF or IGF-I potentiates free radical-mediated injury in cortical neurons. Neuroreport 29:93–96

15. Harper S, Bilsland J, Young L, et al (1999) Analysis of the neurotrophic effects of GPI-1046 on neuron survival and regeneration in culture and in vivo. Neurosci 88:257–267
16. Hefti F, Weiner WJ (1986) Nerve growth factor and Alzheimer's disease. Ann Neurol 20:275–281
17. Hatanaka H (1981) Nerve growth factor-mediated differentiation of nerve cell line cultured in a hormone-supplemented serum-free medium. Dev Brain Res 222:225-233
18. Honn KV, Bockman RS, Marnett LJ (1981) Prostaglandins and cancer: a review of tumor initiation through tumor metastasis. Prostaglandins 21:833-864
19. Holbrook NJ, Carlson SG, Choi AMK., et al (1992) Induction of HSP70 gene expression by antiproliferative prostaglandin PGA_2: a growth-dependent response mediated by activation of heat shock transcription factor. Mol Cell Biol 12:1528-1538
20. Ishikawa T, Akimaru K, Nakanishi M, et al (1998) Anticancer prostaglandin-induced cell cycle arrest and its modulation by GS-X pump inhibitor. Biochem J 336:569–576
21. Ishikawa Y, Ikeuchi T, Hatanaka H (2000) Brain-derived neurotrophic factor accelerates nitric oxide donor-induced apoptosis of cultured cortical neurons. J Neurochem 75:494–502
22. Kobayashi NR, Fan DP, Giehl KM, et al (1997) BDNF and NT-4/5 prevent atrophy of rat rubrospinal neurons after cervical axotomy, stimulate GAP-43 and Talpha1-tublin mRNA expression, and promote axonal regeneration. J Neurosci 15:9583–9595
23. Kliewer SA, Lenhard JM, Willson TM, et al (1995) A prostaglandin J_2 metabolite binds peroxisome proliferator-activated receptor γ and promotes adipocyte differentiation. Cell 83:813-819
24. Kubo T, Nonomura T, Enokido Y, et al (1995) Brain-derived neurotrophic factor (BDNF) can prevent apoptosis of rat cerebellar granule neurons in culture. Dev Brain Res 85:249–258
25. Levi-Montalcini R, Angeletti PU (1968) Nerve growth factor. Physiol Rev 48:534-569
26. McMahon SB, Priestly JV (1995) Peripheral neuropathies and neurotrophic factors: animal model and clinical perspectives. Curr Opin Neurbiol 5:614-616
27. Namura S, Nagata I, Takami S, et al (2001) Ebselen reduces cytochrome c release from mitochondria and subsequent DNA fragmentation after transient focal cerebral ischemia in mice. Stroke 32:1906-1911
28. Narumiya S, Fukushima M (1986) Site and mechanism of growth inhibition by prostaglandins. I. Active transport and intracellular accumulation of cyclopentenone prostaglandins, a reaction leading to growth inhibition. J Pharmacol Exp Ther 238:500-505
29. Narumiya S, Ohno K, Fujiwara M, et al (1986) Site and mechanism of growth inhibition by prostaglandins. II. Temperature-dependent transfer of a cyclopentenone prostaglandin to nuclei. J Pharmacol Exp Ther 238:506-511
30. Narumiya S, Ohno K, Fukushima M, et al (1987) Site and mechanism of growth inhibition by prostaglandins. III. Distribution and binding of prostaglandin A_2 and Δ^{12}-prostaglandin J_2 in nuclei. J Pharmacol Exp Ther 242:306-311
31. Noyori R, Suzuki M (1993) Organic synthesis of prostaglandin: advancing biology. Science 259:44-45
32. Parker J. (1995) Prostaglandin A_2 protein interactions and inhibition of cellular proliferation. Prostaglandins 50:359-375

33. Petrova TV, Akama KT, VanEldik LJ (1999) Cyclopentenone prostaglandins suppress activation of microglia: down-regulation of inducible nitric-oxide synthase by *15-deoxy-*$\Delta^{12,14}$-prostaglandin J_2. Proc Natl Acad Sci USA 96:4668-4673
34. Pollack S, Young L, Bilsland J, et al (1999) The staurosporine-like compound L-753,000 (NB-506) potentiates the neurotrophic effects of neurotrophin-3 by acting selectively at the TrkA receptor. J Pharmacol Exp Ther 56:185–195
35. Rabacchi SA, Kruk B, Hamilton J, et al (1999) BDNF and NT-4/5 promote survival and neurite outgrowth of protocerebellar mossy fiber neurons. J Neurosci 40:254–269
36. Rossi A, Kapahi P, Natoli G, et al (2000) Anti-inflammatory cyclopentenone prostaglandins are direct inhibitors of I-kappa-B kinase. Nature 403:103-108
37. Saragovi HU, Gehring K (2000) Development of pharmacological agents for targeting neurotrophins and their receptors. Trends Phamacol Sci 21:93-98
38. Satoh T, Sakai N, Enokido Y, et al (1996) Survival factor-insensitive generation of reactive oxygen species induced by serum deprivation in neuronal cells. Brain Res 733:9–14
39. Satoh T, Enokido Y, Kubo K, et al (1999a) Oxygen toxicity induces apoptosis in neuronal cells. Cell Mol Neurobiol 18: 649-666
40. Satoh T, Furuta K, Suzuki M, et al (1999b) Prostaglandin J_2 and its metabolites promoted neurite outgrowth induced by nerve growth factor in PC12 cells. Biochem Biophys Res Comm 258:50–53
41. Satoh T, Furuta K, Tomokiyo K, et al (2000a) Facilitatory roles of novel compounds designed from cyclopentenone prostaglandins on the neurite outgrowth-promoting activities of NGF. J Neurochem 75:1092-1102
42. Satoh T, Nakatsuka D, Watanabe Y, et al (2000b) Neuroprotection by MAPK/ERK kinase inhibition with U0126 against oxidative stress in a mouse neuronal cell line and rat primary cultured cortical neurons. Neurosci Lett 288:163-166
43. Satoh T, Furuta K, Tomokiyo K, et al (2000c) Designed cyclopentenone prostaglandin derivatives as neurite outgrowth-promoting compounds for CAD cells, a rat catecholaminergic neuronal cell line of the central nervous system. Neurosci Lett 291:167-70
44. Satoh T, Furuta K, Tomokiyo K, et al (2001) Neurotrophic actions of novel compounds designed from cyclopentenone prostaglandins. J Neurochem 77: 50-62
45. Schabitz WR, Schwab S, Spragnger M, et al (1997) Intraventricular brain-derived neurotrophic factor reduces infarct size after focal cerebral ischemia in rats. J Cereb Blood Flow Metab 17:500–506
46. Schulz JB, Weller M, Klockgether T (1996) Potassium deprivation-induced apoptosis of cerebellar granule neurons: a sequential requirement for new mRNA and protein synthesis, ICE-like protease activity, and reactive oxygen species. J Neurosci 16:4696-4706
47. Snyder SH, Sabatini DM, Lai MM, et al (1998) Neural action of immunophilin ligands. Trends Pharmacol Sci 19:21–26
48. Straus DS, Pascual G, Li M, et al (2000) *15-deoxy-*$\Delta^{12,14}$-prostaglandin J_2 inhibits multiple steps in the NF-κB signaling pathway. Proc Natl Aacd Sci USA 97:4844–4849
49. Suzuki M, Mori M, Niwa T, et al (1997) Chemical implication for antitumor antiviral prostaglandins: reaction of Δ^7-prostaglaindin A_1 and prostaglandin A_1 methyl esters with thiol. J Am Chem Soc 119:2376-2385

50. Suzuki M, Kiho T, Tomokiyo K, et al (1998) Rational design of antitumor prostaglandins with high biological stability. J Med Chem 41:3084–3090
51. Tan S, Sagara Y, Liu Y, et al (1998) The regulation of reactive oxygen species production during programmed cell death. J Cell Biol 141:1423–1432
52. Tanikawa M, Yamada K, Tominaga K, et al (1998) Potent prostaglandin A_1 analogs that suppress tumor cell growth through induction of p21 and reduction of cyclin E. J Biol Chem 273:18522-18527
53. Wilkie N, Wingrove PB, Bilsland JB, et al (2001) The non-peptidyl fungal metabolite L-783,281 activate TRK neurotrophin receptors. J Neurochem 78:1135-1145
54. Williams LR, Varon S, Peterson GM, et al (1986) Continuous infusion of nerve growth factor prevents basal forebrain neuronal death after fimbria fornix transection. Proc Natl Acad Sci USA 83:9231–9235
55. Yoshida S, Inoh S, Asano T, et al (1983) Brain free fatty acids, edema, and mortality in gerbils subjected to transient, bilateral ischemia, and effect of barbiturate anesthesia. J Neurochem 40:1278-1286

3. Strategies using survival or death signals in neurons

Molecular mechanisms of neuronal survival;
Roles of kinases in ischemic cell death

Yukiko Gotoh

Institute of Molecular and Cellular Biosciences, University of Tokyo, 1-1-1 Yayoi, Bunkyo-ku, Tokyo 113-0032, Japan

Summary: During the course of development, neural cells are generated in excess, and damaged cells and developmentally unwanted cells are eliminated through a process called apoptosis. Once the overall neuronal architecture is established, most of the neurons must survive for a lifetime, decades in the case of humans, as de novo neurogenesis rarely takes place in adult. Susceptibility of neurons to apoptosis is determined by a balance between pro-apoptotic and anti-apoptotic (survival) signals. Mature neurons are normally protected by potent survival signals, but neuronal loss does occur when acute (e.g. ischemia) and chronic (e.g. Alzheimer's diseases) neurotoxic insults provide enough apoptotic signals that override survival signals. This review focuses on the signaling molecules that regulate neuronal survival and death after ischemia and in general, with an emphasis on the roles of kinases.

Key words: Survival, Apoptosis, Akt, p38, MAP kinase

Introduction

Mature neurons require trophic support for their survival. Almost a half century ago, Rita Levi-Montalcini and Viktor Hamburger described that the survival of projecting neurons is related to the innervation towards their targets [1]. These observations led to establish the neurotrophic theory, which proposed that neurons compete for a limited amount of target-derived trophic factors, and that those neurons with incorrect synaptic connection are eliminated by apoptosis due to insufficient trophic support [2]. The concept of the neurotrophic support has been expanded, and the trophic factors now include not only the classical neurotrophic factors such as NGF, BDNF, NT-3 and NT-4/5, but also growth factors/cytokines and neurotransmitters released from afferent terminals. The spectrum of factors required for survival varies among cell types, depending on which receptors are expressed. For example, NGF and its receptor TrkA are necessary for the survival of a subset of sympathetic neurons, as revealed by gene targeting *in vivo* as well as *in vitro* culture experiments [3, 4]. BDNF and its receptor TrkB have been implicated in the survival of cerebellar granule cells both *in vivo* and *in vitro* [5, 6].

The levels of neurotrophic factors affect susceptibility of neurons to apoptosis in pathological contexts in addition to physiological contexts. In several models of ischemia, exogenous administration of neurotrophic factors has been shown to protect neurons. These neurotrophic factors include BDNF, basic FGF, acidic FGF, IGF-I, PDGF, EGF, NGF, CSF-1, VEGF, CNTF, Epo, PACAP, TGFbeta and Midkine [7-19]. Some of these factors can reduce ischemic brain damage even when they are introduced several hours after ischemia [12-17]. It is possible that the increase in the mRNA levels of BDNF, its receptor TrkB, NT-3, HB-EGF and basic FGF after transient (preconditioning) ischemia or cortical spreading depression contributes to the tolerance against ischemic cell death [8, 20-22]. This also tells us that mimicking the effects of those neurotrophic factors would be a promising clinical strategy to protect neurons from ischemic cell death. Thus it is important to investigate how neurotrophic factors promote survival and how neurons die in the absence of trophic support. Recent studies have indeed revealed the signaling pathways mediating neuronal survival, most notably the PI3K-Akt pathway, as detailed below.

The PI3K-Akt pathway

PI3K phosphorylates the 3'-OH position of the inositol ring in inositol phospholipids, generating 3'-phosphoinositides. Inside a cell, it produces three lipid products, phosphatidylinositol (PtdIns)3P, PtdIns(3,4)P_2 and PtdIns(3,4,5)P_3. Resting cells contain substantial levels of PtdIns3P and PtdIns(4,5) P_2, but low levels of PtdIns(3,4) P_2 and PtdIns(3,4,5) P_3 PI3K recruitment to the plasma membrane takes place upon activation of receptor tyrosine kinases such as TrkA and TrkB or non-receptor tyrosine kinases such as src and fyn, and thus leads to the generation of PtdIns(3,4) P_2 and PtdIns(3,4,5) P_3, the lipids crutial for the activation of PI3K effectors [23].

The identification of the pleckstrin homology domain (PH domain) as a specialized PtdIns(3,4) P_2 and PtdIns(3,4,5) P_3 -binding module has been a breakthrough towards the understanding of how PI3K works [24, 25]. PH domain can be found in a wide variety of molecules, and a subset of those PH domains have actually been proven to bind these lipids. Among them are the PH domains of Akt and PDK1. Akt, also called protein kinase B (PKB), was first identified as a protein kinase with high homology with protein kinase A (PKA) and protein kinase C (PKC), and as the cellular homolog of the viral oncoprotein v-Akt [26, 27]. Mammalian cells have three Akt genes (Akt1-3), whose structures are closely related. Akt is localized in the cytoplasm in unstimulated cells, and upon activation of PI3K, translocates to the plasma membrane, where it becomes active by phosphorylation of two critical sites, Thr308 and Ser473. Thr308 phosphorylation is catalyzed by PDK1, which is also recruited to the plasma membrane upon PI3K activation. Once Akt becomes activated, it translocates to the cytoplasm and in part to the nucleus, and phosphorylates its targets.

The roles of the PI3K-Akt pathway in survival

The involvement of PI3K in survival was first demonstrated by Yao and Cooper, who have shown that inhibition of PI3K abrogates the ability of NGF to promote survival of PC12 cells [28]. PI3K was subsequently found to be essential for a wide range of survival signaling, elicited by growth factor/cytokine stimulation and cell attachment. In addition, PI3K activity is sufficient for promoting cell survival in the absence of trophic support and to block apoptosis induced by toxic insults [24, 25, 28-30]. A genetical deletion of PTEN, a lipid phosphatase that dephosphorylates PI3K-generated products, causes a failure in developmental apoptosis and embryonic lethality, further suggesting that PI3K products promote cell survival *in vivo* [31, 32].

There are a number of downstream targets of PI3K, including small GTP-binding proteins, p70S6K, atypical PKCs, SGK and Akt [24, 25]. Although some of them are implicated in mediating survival signaling, Akt appears to play a central role in PI3K promotion of cell survival in most of the systems. Expression of an active form of Akt promotes cell survival potently, and inhibition of Akt suppresses cell survival supported by growth factor, depolarization, cell attachment or active PI3K [26, 27, 33, 34]. The PI3K-Akt pathway activated by neurotrophic factors or preconditioning has also been implicated in protection of neurons from ischemic injury (see below).

Other kinases also mediate survival

The survival of cerebellar granule neurons provides a well-characterized model for studying extracellular signal-regulated survival, since their survival is supported by secreted polypeptides such as insulin-like growth factor (IGF-I) and BDNF. In addition, their survival can be supported by membrane-depolarizing concentrations of KCl (high KCl), which lead to increased concentrations of intracellular Ca^{2+} through voltage-gated channels, and may therefore mimic neuronal (synaptic) activation. Furthermore, pharmacological reagents which elevate intracellular cAMP promote their survival efficiently in the absence of trophic factors and high KCl. Recent studies on intracellular signal transduction pathways have shown that PI3K and Akt play an essential role in IGF-I-mediated neuronal survival [33]. It is not clear, on the other hand, if Ca^{2+}-mediated survival is dependent on the PI3K-Akt pathway. In our hand, inhibition of PI3K had only a marginal effect on high KCl-induced survival in cerebellar granule cells (unpublished results). Agonists which increase Ca^{2+} levels such as NMDA have been reported to activate Akt in a PI3K-independent manner through the Ca^{2+}/calmodulin-dependent protein kinase kinase (CaMKK), and thus promote survival [35]. This study reported that CaMKK phsophorylates Akt on Thr308 in the absence of PtdIns(3,4,5)P3. However, another group has found that CaMKK cannot phosphorylate Akt efficiently [36], and others have found that an increase in Ca^{2+} levels does not correlate with activation of Akt [27].

Proteins dependent on Ca^{2+}/calmodulin are likely involved in depolarization-induced survival, as calmodulin inhibitors such as trifluoperazine, calmidazolium and W7 block the high KCl and glutamate-induced survival of cerebellar granule cells and sympathetic neurons [37-39]. Changes in intracellular cAMP levels after depolarization, due to Ca^{2+}/calmodulin-dependent adenylate cyclase, may play a role in survival [40]. Ca^{2+}/calmodulin-dependent kinases (CaMKs) may also promote survival in response to depolarization, since CaMK inhibitors partially block high KCl- and glutamate-induced survival [38]. In neurons, there is accumulating evidence that increased levels of intracellular Ca^{2+} induce neurotrophic factors, especially BDNF and NGF [41, 42]. Ca^{2+} entry activates the Ras-MAP kinase pathway (see below) and the CaMK pathway, which both contribute to the expression of BDNF mRNA. The depolarization-induced Ca^{2+} entry also activates p38, a member of the MAP kinase superfamily, which catalyzes phosphorylation and activation of MEF2, that may be involved in the induction of BDNF [43]. These neurotrophic factors might contribute to the depolization-induced survival.

MAP kinase is a serine/threonine kinase, that is commonly activated by a variety of growth factors, tumor promoters and differentiation factors [44]. It is well established that MAP kinase mediates mitogenic signals and differentiation signals emanating from tyrosine kinase receptors. MAP kinase has also been reported to contribute to cell survival. For example, activation of both MAP kinase and PI3K is necessary to promote survival in BDNF-treated cerebellar granule cells [45]. RSK is a serine/threonine kinase activated by MAP kinase-catalyzed phosphorylation, and has been shown to promote survival via transcription-dependent and –independent manners [45].

Interestingly, cAMP promotes survival even in the presence of PI3K inhibitors and low concentrations of extracellular Ca^{2+} [29, 30, 46]. Therefore, cAMP may function either independently or downstream of PI3K and Ca^{2+} in promoting survival. There are at least three direct targets for cAMP; PKA, cAMP-dependent guanine-nucleotide exchange factor (cAMP-GEF, also called Epac) and the cAMP-gated ion channel [47-49]. It is likely that PKA mediates the cAMP-mediated survival, because ectopic expression of PKA promotes survival of sympathetic neurons and cerebellar granule cells, and because PKA inhibitors block depolarization-induced survival partially [50-52]. cAMP-GEF is a small GTP-binding protein exchanging factor, which is highly specific to Rap1. Binding of cAMP activates cAMP-GEF and leads to activation of the Rap1-B-raf-MEK-MAP kinase pathway. Therefore it is possible that the MAP kinase pathway mediates the cAMP-induced survival. PKA is also reported to be capable of activating the Rap1-B-raf-MEK-MAP kinase pathway [53]. However, in cerebellar granule cells, MEK inhibitors did not block the survival-promoting effects of forskolin or IBMX, which elevate intracellular levels of cAMP, suggesting that cAMP promotes survival in a MAP kinase- and PI3K-independent manner (unpublished results).

IGF-I promotion of survival in cerebellar granule cells can be completely blocked by a PI3K inhibitor, suggesting an essential role of PI3K [33]. On the other hand, H89 or KT5720, PKA inhibitors, or U126 or PD98059, MEK inhibitors had little effect on the IGF-I-mediated survival (unpublished results). Therefore, the PI3K (and Akt)-mediated survival signaling is independent of the PKA and MAP kinase pathways. Taken together, there results clearly indicate the existence of parallel survival pathways.

Crosstalk between apoptosis and survival signals

Bcl-2 family

The regulation of mitochondrial membrane integrity and the release of cytochrome c from mitochondria are important processes during apoptosis, and are controlled by the Bcl-2 family. The Bcl-2 family includes both pro- and anti- apoptotic members, that possess upto four conserved Bcl-2 homology domains designated BH1, BH2, BH3 and BH4 [54]. Many of the anti-apoptotic members, including Bcl-2 and Bcl-X_L, contain all four domains, while the pro-apoptotic members, including Bax and Bak, lack the BH4 domain, and the pro-apoptotic members, so-called "BH3 domain only proteins", including Bid, Bim, and Bad, contain only the BH3 domain. One of the intriguing aspects of the Bcl-2 family is their subcellular localization and translocation. For example, anti-apoptotic members such as Bcl-2 and Bcl-X_L, and pro-apoptotic members such as Bak localize predominantly at mitochondria, and regulate the mitochondrial membrane integrity and cytochrome c release. On the other hand, other members such as Bax, Bid and Bad reside in cytoplasm in healthy cells. In response to apoptotic stimuli, these cytosolic pro-apoptotic members redistribute to mitochondria and promote cytochrome c release. For example, active caspase-8 cleaves p22 Bid into p15 Bid, which translocates to mitochondria [55, 56]. For Bad, the localization is regulated by phosphorylation: survival signals induce phosphorylation of Bad at Ser112, Ser136 and Ser155, which results in 14-3-3 binding and sequestration from its mitochondrial target, Bcl-X_L [57, 58]. Therefore, the loss of survival signals translocates Bad to mitochondria through dephosphorylation.

There are several kinases reported to catalyze Bad phosphorylation. Akt activity was found to be both necessary and sufficient for IGF-I-induced Ser136 phosphorylation in cerebellar granule cells [59, 60]. Constitutively active Akt effectively blocks Bad-induced apoptosis, but is unable to promote survival of cells co-transfected with Bad in which Ser136 has been mutated to Ala [59, 60]. On the other hand, PKA and RSK can suppress Bad function in vivo through phosphorylation of Ser112 [61-65]. CaMKs and PAK have also been shown to phosphorylate Bad [66, 67]. Therefore it is likely that Bad represents a convergence point for a number of survival signals.

After translocation to mitochondria, Bax induces cytochrome c release either by forming a pore through oligomerization or by opening a channel called voltage-dependent anion channel (VDAC) via direct interaction [68, 69]. Bax translocation to mitochondria may serve as a key integration point for various apoptosis signalings, because Bax translocation takes place in response to a wide variety of apoptotic stimuli including staurosporine, dexamethasone, etoposide, nitric oxide, Fas, cell detachment and γ-irradiation, and because the essential roles of Bax in inducing apoptosis have been revealed by gene disruption of Bax alone and of both Bax and Bak. NGF treatment of sympathetic neurons inhibits Bax translocation [70] to mitochondria, suggesting that some survival signals also regulate Bax translocation. Indeed, we found that the PI3K-Akt pathway blocks Bax translocation (unpublished results). Sympathetic neurons as well as facial motor neurons from Bax-deficient mice are resistant to cell death induced by NGF withdrawal and axotomy, respectively [71]. Therefore, trophic factors protect neurons from the activation of Bax, a critical step for neuronal cell death induced by injury.

Caspase cascade

The central component of apoptosis is a proteolytic system involving a family of proteases called caspases [72]. The caspases reside in cells as inactive proforms (procaspases), and in most cases can be activated by caspase-mediated cleavage. The release of cytochrome c from mitochondria induces cytochrome c-mediated oligomerization of Apaf-1, which in turn recruits and activates procaspase-9, the "initiator caspase". The active caspase-9 then cleaves and activates "executor caspases" such as caspase-3 and caspase-7, and leads to the cleavage of key cellular substrates that orchestrate the death process.

Neurotrophic factors can suppress apoptotic pathway at several steps, both upstream and downstream of cytochrome c release from mitochondria [73, 74]. It has been shown that NGF and IGF-I are capable of inhibiting apoptosis induced by cytochrome c injection into neuronal cells [75], demonstrating that survival pathways must have a target(s) downstream of cytochrome c. Since the activation of the caspase cascade is an irreversible and amplifying process through sequential proteolysis, it would be effective to inhibit the caspase cascade at the initial steps. In fact, we found that activation of Akt can block activation of Apaf-1/caspase-9 in cerebellar granule cells. In *in vitro* reconstitution experiments, Akt blocks cytochrome c activation of caspase-9 in the presence of dATP and Apaf-1 (unpublished results). Furthermore, Akt is capable of phosphorylating caspase-9 directly. Cardon et al. has shown that Akt phosphorylates caspase-9 on Ser196 [76], but the mutation of this site had no effect on its inhibition by Akt [77]. More studies will be required to clarify the mechanisms by which Akt inhibits the Apaf-1/caspase-9 complex. Activation of the Raf-MAP kinase pathway has also been shown to block cytochrome c-induced apoptosis in fibroblasts, although its underlying mechanism is unclear.

Death and survival signaling during ischemia

It appears that there are several distinct modes of cell death that participate in ischemic cell death. Focal ischemic stroke results in brain damage characterized by an infarct with a necrotic core, in which all cells die immediately, and a surrounding ischemic penumbra, in which neurons die over days to weeks [78, 79]. As the penumbra can progress to infarction, a main goal of neuroprotection is to salvage the ischemic penumbra. Neurons in the ischemic penumbra exhibit morphological and molecular changes consistent with apoptosis, including expression of pro-apoptotic genes, release of cytochrome c and caspase activation [78, 79]. In addition to necrotic and apoptotic modes of cell death, another mode of cell death called autophagocytotic cell death (or type II cell death according to Clarke [80]) may also take place during ischemia [81-83]. Autophagocytotic cell death, characterized by the appearance of autophagosomes and perinulearly condensed chromatin, is now thought to participate in active (suicidal) elimination of cells physiologically and pathologically, and may involve caspase-independent mechanisms [80].

For neuroprotection, it is important to understand how ischemia results in apoptosis in the penumbra. There are several main triggers of apoptosis during ischemia. Among them are calcium homeostasis, excitotoxicity, metabolic stress (hypoxia, low glucose), free radicals, mitochondrial dysfunction and inflammation, which most likely crosstalk to each other (see reviews [78, 79, 84]). For example, limited supply of oxygen and glucose leads to the energy depletion in neurons, resulting in membrane depolarization, influx of Ca^{2+}, Na^{+} and Cl^{-}, release of glutamate, and impairment of glutamate uptake. Activation of glutamate receptors, through the attendant failure of ion homeostasis and increase in intracellular Ca^{2+} concentration, is a major factor in initiating ischemic cell death. Antagonists of NMDA receptor can protect neurons in models of permanent or temporary ischemia, demonstrating the important role of glutamate-mediated excitotoxicity during ischemic stroke. Excitotoxicity contributes to acute necrosis and delayed types of cell death (mostly apoptosis), and induces expression of genes initiating post-ischemic inflammation, which also contribute to ischemic injury.

Mitochondria is thought to be important in transmitting apoptotic signals during ischemia, in providing both free radicals and cytochrome c release leading to caspase activation. Caspase-3 activation has widely been observed in ischemic brain, and caspase inhibitors or gene disruption of caspases significantly attenuate ischemic neuronal injury, establishing the involvement of caspase in ischemia. Free radicals also play key roles during the ischemic damage. Activation of phospholipase A2 and cyclooxygenase has been detected commonly in ischemic brain, which results in generation of free-radicals. Free-radicals trigger inflammation, apoptosis as well as caspase-independent cell death with a swollen morphology. Nitric oxide (NO) synthesized by Ca^{2+}-activated NO synthase (NOS) reacts with a superoxide anion to generate peroxynitrite, a potent inducer of cellular damages. Restoration of blood flow upon reperfusion, not just reduction of blood flow, produces free radicals by bringing oxygen into the damaged brain.

Some aspects of ischemic cell death can only been investigated in animal models, but it would also be informative to use cultured neuron models to figure out basic molecular mechanisms by which a certain death trigger induces apoptosis. Previous studies have revealed a possible involvement of stress-activated kinases in excitotoxicity and other ischemia-related cell death, and the role of these kinases in ischemia has now been under investigation by animal models.

Stress-activated MAP kinases in ischemia

P38 and JNK classes of the MAP kinase superfamily are preferentially activated by cellular stresses and proinflammatory stimuli [85, 86]. Four isoforms of p38 MAP kinases (p38α, β, γ and δ) and three isoforms of JNK MAP kinases (JNK1, 2 and 3) have been identified, which are all phosphorylated and activated by the MAP kinase kinase superfamily (MKK3 and MKK6 for p38, and MKK4 and MKK7 for JNK). We found that p38 and JNK are activated in response to glutamate treatment in cerebellar granule cells [87]. The concentrations of glutamate effective for inducing apoptosis cerrelated well with those for p38 activation. Furthermore, SB203580, a specific p38 inhibitor, blocked glutamate-induced apoptosis, suggesting that p38 activation may be a prerequisite step for excitotoxicity [87].

Excitotoxic injury leads to increased NO formation as well as p38 activation. NO has been implicated as a critical mediator of neuronal injury in association with ischemia [88-90]. Inhibitors of neuronal NOS (nNOS) have been shown to significantly reduce lesions after focal ischemia [91]. Moreover, nNOS-deficient mice exhibit marked protection against cerebral ischemia [92, 93]. Interestingly, sodium nitroprusside (SNP), an NO donor, induces activation of p38, and p38 inhibitor blocks SNP-induced caspase activation and cell death in cortical neurons [94]. p38 inhibitor also blocks translocation of Bax from cytoplasm to mitochondria after treatment with SNP [94]. Since Bax-deficient cortical neurons are resistant to SNP, Bax translocation might be a primary target for p38 in NO-mediated neuronal death [95]. The importance of p38 has further been demonstrated in low potassium-induced apoptosis in cerebellar granule cells, and oxygen/glucose deprivation-induced apoptosis in hippocampal slice cultures [96-98].

Recent studies demonstrated that phosphorylation of p38 occurs after ischemia and ischemia-reperfusion in mice, rats and gerbils [98-103]. Importantly, p38 inhibitors significantly attenuate neuronal death after ischemia. For example, oral administration of SB239063 resulted in neuroprotection against middle cerebral artery occlusion [98, 101]. Intravenous administration of SB239063 was effective even 15 min after ischemic stroke (the reagent exhibited enough brain penetration [98]). Transient global ischemia causes delayed neuronal death (DND) in the CA1 region of hippocampus in gerbil, which accompanies p38 phosphorylation [100]. In this case also, a p38 inhibitor reduced ischemic cell death in the CA1 region [100]. The roles of p38 in ischemic cell death are not fully understood, but they may involve the Bax translocation-mediated apoptosis as described above, as well as inflammation through the expression of p38 target genes such as TNFα and MAO [104].

JNK is also implicated in neuronal apoptosis. JNK is essential for apoptosis induced by neurotrophic factor deprivation in sympathetic neurons. The role for JNK in stress-induced neuronal cell death has been confirmed in studies of mice with targeted disruption of JNK3; in these mice, hippocampal neurons are significantly resistant to kainate, an excitotoxin [105]. In this case, it is likely that JNK mediates excitotoxic cell death via phosphorylation of c-Jun, since the gene knock-in of c-Jun with phosphorylation site mutation resulted in similar resistance against excitotoxin [106]. c-Jun in turn induces pro-apoptotic genes such as Bim and FasL [107]. The effect of JNK on apoptosis is not limited to the phosphorylation of c-Jun, since JNK activation can induce the mitochondrial pathway without regulation of transcription [108]. JNK may also participate in caspase-independent cell death [109]. JNK phosphorylation can be detected after ischemia, but it is not clear whether JNK is involved in ischemic cell death.

ERK members of the MAP kinase superfamily are also phosphorylated in response to ischemic injury [27, 99, 100, 103, 110, 111]. Namura and colleagues have found that intravenous administration of U126, an inhibitor for ERK activator MEK, reduces neuronal damage against bilateral carotid artery occlusion and middle cerebral artery occlusion in gerbils [110, 112]. In addition, U126 protects cultured cortical neurons against hypoxia and NO. Although the effect of U126 appears to depend on the model and the protocol of administration [100, 111, 113, 114], it is worthy pursuing the MEK/MAP kinase pathway as a promising target to protect brain from ischemic injury. MAP kinase may enhance the inflammation via phosphorylation of phospholipaseA2 and ischemic release of glutamate, the latter could be blocked by administration of PD98059, another MEK inhibitor.

The roles of the PI3K-Akt pathway in inhibition of ischemic cell death

Neurotrophic factors can prevent neuronal death induced by glutamate or NO. For example, bFGF and EGF can prevent hippocampal neuronal cell death during NO exposure [115]. As described above, a number of neurotrophic factors can prevent neuronal apoptosis after cerebral ischemia [7-19] and in its *in vitro* culture model [115]. Importantly, in some of these experiments, it has been shown that PI3K inhibitors can block these neuroprotective effects. VEGF- and Epo-mediated neuroprotection against hypoxia and low glucose was canceled by the addition of PI3K inhibitors [116, 117]. Induction of ischemic tolerance resulting from a sublethal ischemic insult may require PI3K-Akt activation, since intracerebral ventricular infusion of wortmannin, a PI3K inhibitor, before the preconditioning blocked the neuroprotective effect of preconditioning [118]. More work has be done to ensure that the activation of Akt is sufficient for neuroprotection, but it would be a good strategy to activate the PI3K-Akt pathway to pursue neuroprotection, considering the potent survival-promoting activity of this pathway [119-123].

References

1. Hamburger V, Levi-Montalcini R (1949) Proliferation, differentiation and degeneration in the spinal ganglia of the chick embryo under normal and experimental conditions. J Exp Zool 111: 457-501
2. Korsching S (1993) The neurotrophic factor concept: a reexamination. J Neurosci 13: 2739-2748
3. Crowley C, Spencer SD, Nishimura MC, Chen KS, Pitts-Meek S, Armanini MP, Ling LH, MacMahon SB, Shelton DL, Levinson AD, et al. (1994) Mice lacking nerve growth factor display perinatal loss of sensory and sympathetic neurons yet develop basal forebrain cholinergic neurons. Cell 76: 1001-1011
4. Smeyne RJ, Klein R, Schnapp A, Long LK, Bryant S, Lewin A, Lira SA, Barbacid M (1994) Severe sensory and sympathetic neuropathies in mice carrying a disrupted Trk/NGF receptor gene. Nature 368: 246-249
5. Minichiello L, Klein R (1996) TrkB and TrkC neurotrophin receptors cooperate in promoting survival of hippocampal and cerebellar granule neurons. Genes Dev 10: 2849-2858
6. Schwartz PM, Borghesani PR, Levy RL, Pomeroy SL, Segal RA (1997) Abnormal cerebellar development and foliation in BDNF-/- mice reveals a role for neurotrophins in CNS patterning. Neuron 19: 269-281
7. Beck T, Lindholm D, Castren E, Wree A (1994) Brain-derived neurotrophic factor protects against ischemic cell damage in rat hippocampus. J Cereb Blood Flow Metab 14: 689-692

8. Tsukahara T, Yonekawa Y, Tanaka K, Ohara O, Wantanabe S, Kimura T, Nishijima T, Taniguchi T (1994) The role of brain-derived neurotrophic factor in transient forebrain ischemia in the rat brain. Neurosurgery 34: 323-331; discussion 331
9. MacMillan V, Walton-Roche K, Davis J (1993) Acidic fibroblast growth factor infusion reduces ischemic CA1 hippocampal damage in the gerbil. Can J Neurol Sci 20: 37-40
10. Sasaki K, Oomura Y, Suzuki K, Hanai K, Yagi H (1992) Acidic fibroblast growth factor prevents death of hippocampal CA1 pyramidal cells following ischemia. Neurochem Int 21: 397-402
11. Shigeno T, Mima T, Takakura K, Graham DI, Kato G, Hashimoto Y, Furukawa S (1991) Amelioration of delayed neuronal death in the hippocampus by nerve growth factor. J Neurosci 11: 2914-2919
12. Jiang N, Finklestein SP, Do T, Caday CG, Charette M, Chopp M (1996) Delayed intravenous administration of basic fibroblast growth factor (bFGF) reduces infarct volume in a model of focal cerebral ischemia/reperfusion in the rat. J Neurol Sci 139: 173-179
13. Zhang Y, Pardridge WM (2001) Neuroprotection in transient focal brain ischemia after delayed intravenous administration of brain-derived neurotrophic factor conjugated to a blood-brain barrier drug targeting system. Stroke 32: 1378-1384
14. Tsuzuki N, Miyazawa T, Matsumoto K, Nakamura T, Shima K, Chigasaki H (2000) Hepatocyte growth factor reduces infarct volume after transient focal cerebral ischemia in rats. Acta Neurochir Suppl 76: 311-316
15. Wang JM, Hayashi T, Zhang WR, Sakai K, Shiro Y, Abe K (2000) Reduction of ischemic brain injury by topical application of insulin- like growth factor-I after transient middle cerebral artery occlusion in rats. Brain Res 859: 381-385
16. Ay I, Sugimori H, Finklestein SP (2001) Intravenous basic fibroblast growth factor (bFGF) decreases DNA fragmentation and prevents downregulation of Bcl-2 expression in the ischemic brain following middle cerebral artery occlusion in rats. Brain Res Mol Brain Res 87: 71-80
17. Uchida D, Arimura A, Somogyvari-Vigh A, Shioda S, Banks WA (1996) Prevention of ischemia-induced death of hippocampal neurons by pituitary adenylate cyclase activating polypeptide. Brain Res 736: 280-286
18. Sadamoto Y, Igase K, Sakanaka M, Sato K, Otsuka H, Sakaki S, Masuda S, Sasaki R (1998) Erythropoietin prevents place navigation disability and cortical infarction in rats with permanent occlusion of the middle cerebral artery. Biochem Biophys Res Commun 253: 26-32
19. Yanamoto H, Nagata I, Sakata M, Zhang Z, Tohnai N, Sakai H, Kikuchi H (2000) Infarct tolerance induced by intra-cerebral infusion of recombinant brain-derived neurotrophic factor. Brain Res 859: 240-248
20. Lindvall O, Ernfors P, Bengzon J, Kokaia Z, Smith ML, Siesjo BK, Persson H (1992) Differential regulation of mRNAs for nerve growth factor, brain-derived neurotrophic factor, and neurotrophin 3 in the adult rat brain following cerebral ischemia and hypoglycemic coma. Proc Natl Acad Sci USA 89: 648-652
21. Merlio JP, Ernfors P, Kokaia Z, Middlemas DS, Bengzon J, Kokaia M, Smith ML, Siesjo BK, Hunter T, Lindvall O, et al. (1993) Increased production of the TrkB protein tyrosine kinase receptor after brain insults. Neuron 10: 151-164
22. Takeda A, Onodera H, Sugimoto A, Kogure K, Obinata M, Shibahara S (1993) Coordinated expression of messenger RNAs for nerve growth factor, brain- derived

neurotrophic factor and neurotrophin-3 in the rat hippocampus following transient forebrain ischemia. Neuroscience 55: 23-31
23. Stephens LR, Jackson TR, Hawkins PT (1993) Agonist-stimulated synthesis of phosphatidylinositol(3,4,5)- trisphosphate: a new intracellular signalling system? Biochim Biophys Acta 1179: 27-75
24. Leevers SJ, Vanhaesebroeck B, Waterfield MD (1999) Signalling through phosphoinositide 3-kinases: the lipids take centre stage. Curr Opin Cell Biol 11: 219-225
25. Rameh LE, Cantley LC (1999) The role of phosphoinositide 3-kinase lipid products in cell function. J Biol Chem 274: 8347-8350
26. Coffer PJ, Jin J, Woodgett JR (1998) Protein kinase B (c-Akt): a multifunctional mediator of phosphatidylinositol 3-kinase activation. Biochem J 335: 1-13
27. Vanhaesebroeck B, Alessi DR (2000) The PI3K-PDK1 connection: more than just a road to PKB. Biochem J 346 Pt 3: 561-576
28. Yao R, Cooper GM (1995) Requirement for phosphatidylinositol-3 kinase in the prevention of apoptosis by nerve growth factor. Science 267: 2003-2006
29. Miller TM, Tansey MG, Johnson EM, Jr., Creedon DJ (1997) Inhibition of phosphatidylinositol 3-kinase activity blocks depolarization- and insulin-like growth factor I-mediated survival of cerebellar granule cells. J Biol Chem 272: 9847-9853
30. Crowder RJ, Freeman RS (1998) Phosphatidylinositol 3-kinase and Akt protein kinase are necessary and sufficient for the survival of nerve growth factor-dependent sympathetic neurons. J Neurosci 18: 2933-2943
31. Stambolic V, Suzuki A, de la Pompa JL, Brothers GM, Mirtsos C, Sasaki T, Ruland J, Penninger JM, Siderovski DP, Mak TW (1998) Negative regulation of PKB/Akt-dependent cell survival by the tumor suppressor PTEN. Cell 95: 29-39
32. Suzuki A, de la Pompa JL, Stambolic V, Elia AJ, Sasaki T, del Barco Barrantes I, Ho A, Wakeham A, Itie A, Khoo W, Fukumoto M, Mak TW (1998) High cancer susceptibility and embryonic lethality associated with mutation of the PTEN tumor suppressor gene in mice. Curr Biol 8: 1169-1178
33. Dudek H, Datta SR, Franke TF, Birnbaum MJ, Yao R, Cooper GM, Segal RA, Kaplan DR, Greenberg ME (1997) Regulation of neuronal survival by the serine-threonine protein kinase Akt. Science 275: 661-665
34. Vaillant AR, Mazzoni I, Tudan C, Boudreau M, Kaplan DR, Miller FD (1999) Depolarization and neurotrophins converge on the phosphatidylinositol 3- kinase-Akt pathway to synergistically regulate neuronal survival. J Cell Biol 146: 955-966
35. Yano S, Tokumitsu H, Soderling TR (1998) Calcium promotes cell survival through CaM-K kinase activation of the protein-kinase-B pathway. Nature 396: 584-587
36. Pullen N, Dennis PB, Andjelkovic M, Dufner A, Kozma SC, Hemmings BA, Thomas G (1998) Phosphorylation and activation of p70s6k by PDK1. Science 279: 707-710
37. Gallo V, Kingsbury A, Balazs R, Jorgensen OS (1987) The role of depolarization in the survival and differentiation of cerebellar granule cells in culture. J Neurosci 7: 2203-2213
38. Hack N, Hidaka H, Wakefield MJ, Balazs R (1993) Promotion of granule cell survival by high K+ or excitatory amino acid treatment and Ca2+/calmodulin-dependent protein kinase activity. Neuroscience 57: 9-20
39. Franklin JL, Sanz-Rodriguez C, Juhasz A, Deckwerth TL, Johnson EM, Jr. (1995) Chronic depolarization prevents programmed death of sympathetic neurons in vitro

but does not support growth: requirement for Ca2+ influx but not Trk activation. J Neurosci 15: 643-664
40. Franklin JL, Johnson EM, Jr. (1992) Suppression of programmed neuronal death by sustained elevation of cytoplasmic calcium. Trends Neurosci 15: 501-508
41. Lipton SA (1986) Blockade of electrical activity promotes the death of mammalian retinal ganglion cells in culture. Proc Natl Acad Sci USA 83: 9774-9778
42. Ghosh A, Carnahan J, Greenberg ME (1994) Requirement for BDNF in activity-dependent survival of cortical neurons. Science 263: 1618-1623
43. Mao Z, Bonni A, Xia F, Nadal-Vicens M, Greenberg ME (1999) Neuronal activity-dependent cell survival mediated by transcription factor MEF2. Science 286: 785-790
44. Nishida E, Gotoh Y (1993) The MAP kinase cascade is essential for diverse signal transduction pathways. Trends Biochem Sci 18: 128-131
45. Bonni A, Brunet A, West AE, Datta SR, Takasu MA, Greenberg ME (1999) Cell survival promoted by the Ras-MAPK signaling pathway by transcription-dependent and -independent mechanisms. Science 286: 1358-1362
46. D'Mello SR, Galli C, Ciotti T, Calissano P (1993) Induction of apoptosis in cerebellar granule neurons by low potassium: inhibition of death by insulin-like growth factor I and cAMP. Proc Natl Acad Sci USA 90: 10989-10993
47. Kawasaki H, Springett GM, Mochizuki N, Toki S, Nakaya M, Matsuda M, Housman DE, Graybiel AM (1998) A family of cAMP-binding proteins that directly activate Rap1. Science 282: 2275-2279
48. de Rooij J, Zwartkruis FJ, Verheijen MH, Cool RH, Nijman SM, Wittinghofer A, Bos JL (1998) Epac is a Rapl guanine-nucleotide-exchange factor directly activated by cyclic AMP. Nature 396: 474-477
49. Downward J (1998) Signal transduction. New exchange, new target. Nature 396: 416-417
50. Tanaka J, Koshimura K, Murakami Y, Sohmiya M, Yanaihara N, Kato Y (1997) Neuronal protection from apoptosis by pituitary adenylate cyclase- activating polypeptide. Regul Pept 72: 1-8
51. Buckmaster EA, Tolkovsky AM (1994) Expression of the cyclic AMP-dependent protein kinase (PKA) catalytic subunit from a herpes simplex virus vector extends the survival of rat sympathetic neurons in the absence of NGF. Eur J Neurosci 6: 1316-1327
52. Campard PK, Crochemore C, Rene F, Monnier D, Koch B, Loeffler JP (1997) PACAP type I receptor activation promotes cerebellar neuron survival through the cAMP/PKA signaling pathway. DNA Cell Biol 16: 323-333
53. Vossler MR, Yao H, York RD, Pan MG, Rim CS, Stork PJ (1997) cAMP activates MAP kinase and Elk-1 through a B-Raf- and Rap1-dependent pathway. Cell 89: 73-82
54. Gross A, McDonnell JM, Korsmeyer SJ (1999) BCL-2 family members and the mitochondria in apoptosis. Genes Dev 13: 1899-1911
55. Li H, Zhu H, Xu CJ, Yuan J (1998) Cleavage of BID by caspase 8 mediates the mitochondrial damage in the Fas pathway of apoptosis. Cell 94: 491-501
56. Luo X, Budihardjo I, Zou H, Slaughter C, Wang X (1998) Bid, a Bcl2 interacting protein, mediates cytochrome c release from mitochondria in response to activation of cell surface death receptors. Cell 94: 481-490

57. Datta SR, Katsov A, Hu L, Petros A, Fesik SW, Yaffe MB, Greenberg ME (2000) 14-3-3 proteins and survival kinases cooperate to inactivate BAD by BH3 domain phosphorylation. Mol Cell 6: 41-51
58. Zha J, Harada H, Yang E, Jockel J, Korsmeyer SJ (1996) Serine phosphorylation of death agonist BAD in response to survival factor results in binding to 14-3-3 not BCL-X(L). Cell 87: 619-628
59. Datta SR, Dudek H, Tao X, Masters S, Fu H, Gotoh Y, Greenberg ME (1997) Akt phosphorylation of BAD couples survival signals to the cell- intrinsic death machinery. Cell 91: 231-241
60. del Peso L, Gonzalez-Garcia M, Page C, Herrera R, Nunez G (1997) Interleukin-3-induced phosphorylation of BAD through the protein kinase Akt. Science 278: 687-689
61. Virdee K, Parone PA, Tolkovsky AM (2000) Phosphorylation of the pro-apoptotic protein BAD on serine 155, a novel site, contributes to cell survival. Curr Biol 10: 1151-1154
62. Lizcano JM, Morrice N, Cohen P (2000) Regulation of BAD by cAMP-dependent protein kinase is mediated via phosphorylation of a novel site, Ser155. Biochem J 349: 547-557
63. Tan Y, Demeter MR, Ruan H, Comb MJ (2000) BAD Ser-155 phosphorylation regulates BAD/Bcl-XL interaction and cell survival. J Biol Chem 275: 25865-25869
64. Zhou XM, Liu Y, Payne G, Lutz RJ, Chittenden T (2000) Growth factors inactivate the cell death promoter BAD by phosphorylation of its BH3 domain on Ser155. J Biol Chem 275: 25046-25051
65. Harada H, Becknell B, Wilm M, Mann M, Huang LJ, Taylor SS, Scott JD, Korsmeyer SJ (1999) Phosphorylation and inactivation of BAD by mitochondria-anchored protein kinase A. Mol Cell 3: 413-422
66. Wolf D, Witte V, Laffert B, Blume K, Stromer E, Trapp S, d'Aloja P, Schurmann A, Baur AS (2001) HIV-1 Nef associated PAK and PI3-Kinases stimulate Akt-independent Bad- phosphorylation to induce anti-apoptotic signals. Nat Med 7: 1217-1224
67. Schurmann A, Mooney AF, Sanders LC, Sells MA, Wang HG, Reed JC, Bokoch GM (2000) p21-activated kinase 1 phosphorylates the death agonist bad and protects cells from apoptosis. Mol Cell Biol 20: 453-461
68. Saito M, Korsmeyer SJ, Schlesinger PH (2000) BAX-dependent transport of cytochrome c reconstituted in pure liposomes. Nat Cell Biol 2: 553-555
69. Shimizu S, Narita M, Tsujimoto Y (1999) Bcl-2 family proteins regulate the release of apoptogenic cytochrome c by the mitochondrial channel VDAC. Nature 399: 483-487
70. Putcha GV, Deshmukh M, Johnson EM, Jr. (1999) BAX translocation is a critical event in neuronal apoptosis: regulation by neuroprotectants, BCL-2, and caspases. J Neurosci 19: 7476-7485
71. Deckwerth TL, Elliott JL, Knudson CM, Johnson EM, Jr., Snider WD, Korsmeyer SJ (1996) BAX is required for neuronal death after trophic factor deprivation and during development. Neuron 17: 401-411
72. Wang X (2001) The expanding role of mitochondria in apoptosis. Genes Dev 15: 2922-2933
73. Zhou H, Li XM, Meinkoth J, Pittman RN (2000) Akt regulates cell survival and apoptosis at a postmitochondrial level. J Cell Biol 151: 483-494

74. Kennedy SG, Kandel ES, Cross TK, Hay N (1999) Akt/Protein kinase B inhibits cell death by preventing the release of cytochrome c from mitochondria. Mol Cell Biol 19: 5800-5810
75. Deshmukh M, Johnson EM, Jr. (1998) Evidence of a novel event during neuronal death: development of competence-to-die in response to cytoplasmic cytochrome c. Neuron 21: 695-705
76. Cardone MH, Roy N, Stennicke HR, Salvesen GS, Franke TF, Stanbridge E, Frisch S, Reed JC (1998) Regulation of cell death protease caspase-9 by phosphorylation. Science 282: 1318-1321
77. Fujita E, Jinbo A, Matuzaki H, Konishi H, Kikkawa U, Momoi T (1999) Akt phosphorylation site found in human caspase-9 is absent in mouse caspase-9. Biochem Biophys Res Commun 264: 550-555
78. Dirnagl U, Iadecola C, Moskowitz MA (1999) Pathobiology of ischaemic stroke: an integrated view. Trends Neurosci 22: 391-397
79. Lipton P (1999) Ischemic cell death in brain neurons. Physiol Rev 79: 1431-1568
80. Clarke PG (1990) Developmental cell death: morphological diversity and multiple mechanisms. Anat Embryol 181: 195-213
81. Glaumann H, Ericsson JL, Marzella L (1981) Mechanisms of intralysosomal degradation with special reference to autophagocytosis and heterophagocytosis of cell organelles. Int Rev Cytol 73: 149-182
82. Marzella L, Glaumann H (1981) Effects of in vivo liver ischemia on microsomes and lysosomes. Virchows Arch B Cell Pathol Incl Mol Pathol 36: 1-25
83. Nitatori T, Sato N, Waguri S, Karasawa Y, Araki H, Shibanai K, Kominami E, Uchiyama Y (1995) Delayed neuronal death in the CA1 pyramidal cell layer of the gerbil hippocampus following transient ischemia is apoptosis. J Neurosci 15: 1001-1011
84. Mattson MP (2000) Apoptosis in neurodegenerative disorders. Nat Rev Mol Cell Biol 1: 120-129
85. Davis RJ (2000) Signal transduction by the JNK group of MAP kinases. Cell 103: 239-252
86. Nebreda AR, Porras A (2000) p38 MAP kinases: beyond the stress response. Trends Biochem Sci 25: 257-260
87. Kawasaki H, Fujii H, Gotoh Y, Morooka T, Shimohama S, Nishida E, Hirano T (1999) Requirement for mitogen-activated protein kinase in cerebellar long term depression. J Biol Chem 274: 13498-13502
88. Beal MF (1996) Mitochondria, free radicals, and neurodegeneration. Curr Opin Neurobiol 6: 661-666
89. Dawson VL, Dawson TM (1996) Nitric oxide neurotoxicity. J Chem Neuroanat 10: 179-190
90. Heales SJ, Bolanos JP, Stewart VC, Brookes PS, Land JM, Clark JB (1999) Nitric oxide, mitochondria and neurological disease. Biochim Biophys Acta 1410: 215-228
91. Yoshida T, Limmroth V, Irikura K, Moskowitz MA (1994) The NOS inhibitor, 7-nitroindazole, decreases focal infarct volume but not the response to topical acetylcholine in pial vessels. J Cereb Blood Flow Metab 14: 924-929
92. Ayata C, Ayata G, Hara H, Matthews RT, Beal MF, Ferrante RJ, Endres M, Kim A, Christie RH, Waeber C, Huang PL, Hyman BT, Moskowitz MA (1997) Mechanisms of reduced striatal NMDA excitotoxicity in type I nitric oxide synthase knock-out mice. J Neurosci 17: 6908-6917

93. Huang Z, Huang PL, Panahian N, Dalkara T, Fishman MC, Moskowitz MA (1994) Effects of cerebral ischemia in mice deficient in neuronal nitric oxide synthase. Science 265: 1883-1885
94. Ghatan S, Larner S, Kinoshita Y, Hetman M, Patel L, Xia Z, Youle RJ, Morrison RS (2000) p38 MAP kinase mediates bax translocation in nitric oxide-induced apoptosis in neurons. J Cell Biol 150: 335-347
95. Cao G, Minami M, Pei W, Yan C, Chen D, O'Horo C, Graham SH, Chen J (2001) Intracellular Bax translocation after transient cerebral ischemia: implications for a role of the mitochondrial apoptotic signaling pathway in ischemic neuronal death. J Cereb Blood Flow Metab 21: 321-333
96. Yamagishi S, Yamada M, Ishikawa Y, Matsumoto T, Ikeuchi T, Hatanaka H (2001) p38 mitogen-activated protein kinase regulates low potassium-induced c- Jun phosphorylation and apoptosis in cultured cerebellar granule neurons. J Biol Chem 276: 5129-5133
97. Nath R, McGinnis K, Dutta S, Shivers B, Wang KK (2001) Inhibition of p38 kinase mimics survival signal-linked protection against apoptosis in rat cerebellar granule neurons. Cell Mol Biol Lett 6: 173-184
98. Barone FC, Irving EA, Ray AM, Lee JC, Kassis S, Kumar S, Badger AM, White RF, McVey MJ, Legos JJ, Erhardt JA, Nelson AH, Ohlstein EH, Hunter AJ, Ward K, Smith BR, Adams JL, Parsons AA (2001) SB 239063, a second-generation p38 mitogen-activated protein kinase inhibitor, reduces brain injury and neurological deficits in cerebral focal ischemia. J Pharmacol Exp Ther 296: 312-321
99. Irving EA, Barone FC, Reith AD, Hadingham SJ, Parsons AA (2000) Differential activation of MAPK/ERK and p38/SAPK in neurones and glia following focal cerebral ischaemia in the rat. Brain Res Mol Brain Res 77: 65-75
100. Sugino T, Nozaki K, Takagi Y, Hattori I, Hashimoto N, Moriguchi T, Nishida E (2000) Activation of mitogen-activated protein kinases after transient forebrain ischemia in gerbil hippocampus. J Neurosci 20: 4506-4514
101. Legos JJ, Erhardt JA, White RF, Lenhard SC, Chandra S, Parsons AA, Tuma RF, Barone FC (2001) SB 239063, a novel p38 inhibitor, attenuates early neuronal injury following ischemia. Brain Res 892: 70-77
102. Takagi Y, Nozaki K, Sugino T, Hattori I, Hashimoto N (2000) Phosphorylation of c-Jun NH(2)-terminal kinase and p38 mitogen- activated protein kinase after transient forebrain ischemia in mice. Neurosci Lett 294: 117-120
103. Ozawa H, Shioda S, Dohi K, Matsumoto H, Mizushima H, Zhou CJ, Funahashi H, Nakai Y, Nakajo S, Matsumoto K (1999) Delayed neuronal cell death in the rat hippocampus is mediated by the mitogen-activated protein kinase signal transduction pathway. Neurosci Lett 262: 57-60
104. De Zutter GS, Davis RJ (2001) Pro-apoptotic gene expression mediated by the p38 mitogen-activated protein kinase signal transduction pathway. Proc Natl Acad Sci USA 98: 6168-6173
105. Yang DD, Kuan CY, Whitmarsh AJ, Rincon M, Zheng TS, Davis RJ, Rakic P, Flavell RA (1997) Absence of excitotoxicity-induced apoptosis in the hippocampus of mice lacking the Jnk3 gene. Nature 389: 865-870
106. Behrens A, Sibilia M, Wagner EF (1999) Amino-terminal phosphorylation of c-Jun regulates stress-induced apoptosis and cellular proliferation. Nat Genet 21: 326-329

107. Whitfield J, Neame SJ, Paquet L, Bernard O, Ham J (2001) Dominant-negative c-Jun promotes neuronal survival by reducing BIM expression and inhibiting mitochondrial cytochrome c release. Neuron 29: 629-643
108. Tournier C, Hess P, Yang DD, Xu J, Turner TK, Nimnual A, Bar-Sagi D, Jones SN, Flavell RA, Davis RJ (2000) Requirement of JNK for stress-induced activation of the cytochrome c- mediated death pathway. Science 288: 870-874
109. Ura S, Masuyama N, Graves JD, Gotoh Y (2001) MST1-JNK promotes apoptosis via caspase-dependent and independent pathways. Genes Cells 6: 519-530
110. Namura S, Iihara K, Takami S, Nagata I, Kikuchi H, Matsushita K, Moskowitz MA, Bonventre JV, Alessandrini A (2001) Intravenous administration of MEK inhibitor U0126 affords brain protection against forebrain ischemia and focal cerebral ischemia. Proc Natl Acad Sci USA 98: 11569-11574
111. Gu Z, Jiang Q, Zhang G (2001) Extracellular signal-regulated kinase 1/2 activation in hippocampus after cerebral ischemia may not interfere with postischemic cell death. Brain Res 901: 79-84
112. Stanciu M, Wang Y, Kentor R, Burke N, Watkins S, Kress G, Reynolds I, Klann E, Angiolieri MR, Johnson JW, DeFranco DB (2000) Persistent activation of ERK contributes to glutamate-induced oxidative toxicity in a neuronal cell line and primary cortical neuron cultures. J Biol Chem 275: 12200-12206
113. Gonzalez-Zulueta M, Feldman AB, Klesse LJ, Kalb RG, Dillman JF, Parada LF, Dawson TM, Dawson VL (2000) Requirement for nitric oxide activation of p21(ras)/extracellular regulated kinase in neuronal ischemic preconditioning. Proc Natl Acad Sci USA 97: 436-441
114. Han BH, Holtzman DM (2000) BDNF protects the neonatal brain from hypoxic-ischemic injury in vivo via the ERK pathway. J Neurosci 20: 5775-5781
115. Maiese K, Boniece I, DeMeo D, Wagner JA (1993) Peptide growth factors protect against ischemia in culture by preventing nitric oxide toxicity. J Neurosci 13: 3034-3040
116. Jin KL, Mao XO, Greenberg DA (2000) Vascular endothelial growth factor: direct neuroprotective effect in in vitro ischemia. Proc Natl Acad Sci USA 97: 10242-10247
117. Siren AL, Fratelli M, Brines M, Goemans C, Casagrande S, Lewczuk P, Keenan S, Gleiter C, Pasquali C, Capobianco A, Mennini T, Heumann R, Cerami A, Ehrenreich H, Ghezzi P (2001) Erythropoietin prevents neuronal apoptosis after cerebral ischemia and metabolic stress. Proc Natl Acad Sci USA 98: 4044-4049
118. Yano S, Morioka M, Fukunaga K, Kawano T, Hara T, Kai Y, Hamada J, Miyamoto E, Ushio Y (2001) Activation of Akt/protein kinase B contributes to induction of ischemic tolerance in the CA1 subfield of gerbil hippocampus. J Cereb Blood Flow Metab 21: 351-360
119. Sakurai M, Hayashi T, Abe K, Itoyuama Y, Tabayashi K (2001) Induction of phosphatidylinositol 3-kinase and serine-threonine kinase- like immunoreactivity in rabbit spinal cord after transient ischemia. Neurosci Lett 302: 17-20
120. Ouyang YB, Tan Y, Comb M, Liu CL, Martone ME, Siesjo BK, Hu BR (1999) Survival- and death-promoting events after transient cerebral ischemia: phosphorylation of Akt, release of cytochrome C and Activation of caspase-like proteases. J Cereb Blood Flow Metab 19: 1126-1135
121. Chalecka-Franaszek E, Chuang DM (1999) Lithium activates the serine/threonine kinase Akt-1 and suppresses glutamate-induced inhibition of Akt-1 activity in neurons. Proc Natl Acad Sci USA 96: 8745-8750

122. Noshita N, Lewen A, Sugawara T, Chan PH (2001) Evidence of phosphorylation of Akt and neuronal survival after transient focal cerebral ischemia in mice. J Cereb Blood Flow Metab 21: 1442-1450
123. Kawano T, Fukunaga K, Takeuchi Y, Morioka M, Yano S, Hamada J, Ushio Y, Miyamoto E (2001) Neuroprotective effect of sodium orthovanadate on delayed neuronal death after transient forebrain ischemia in gerbil hippocampus. J Cereb Blood Flow Metab 21: 1268-1280

Gene expression and manipulation in injured neurons

Hiroshi Kiyama, Sumiko Kiryu-Seo, and Kazuhiko Namikawa

Department of Anatomy & Neuroscience, Graduate School of Medicine, Osaka City University, 1-4-3 Asahimachi, Abeno-ku, Osaka 545-8585, Japan

Summary: Neuronal cells subjected to injuries such as trauma and hypoxia are destined to die. Using the motor nerve injury model, we collected and screened several genes associated with nerve injury. This gene screening suggested some molecular mechanisms that might contribute to nerve survival and regeneration after injury. Some of these molecular mechanisms are not seen in the central nervous system. This might be a reason why central nervous system neurons are particularly fragile. To compensate for the lack of gene expression in the injured neuron, use of an adenovirus vector is effective. Adenovirus mediated gene expression prevented injury-induced neuronal death and accelerated neurite elongation *in vivo*.

Key words: Neuronal regeneration, Nerve injury, Adenovirus, Gene expression

Introduction

There are significant differences between the peripheral nervous system (PNS) and the central nervous system (CNS). One of the major differences is susceptibility to nerve injury. PNS neurons are rather resistant to injury, whereas CNS neurons are fragile. This difference could be key to exploring the molecular mechanism underlying neuronal death or survival. What sort of mechanism is essential for the survive and regeneration of PNS neurons? In the PNS motor neuron system, there is an intriguing phenomenon called axotomy-induced neuronal death. When we injure adult rat hypoglossal or sciatic nerve, for instance, the hypoglossal or spinal motor neurons can survive and regenerate, whereas in neonates most of the injured motor neurons eventually die [1,2]. This is intriguing because along with maturation, these motor neurons somehow gain resistance against injury. This might be a consequence of their gaining some molecular mechanisms along with maturation. Thus we attempted to establish a system to isolate genes whose expressions are upregulated in the surviving motor neurons, but are downregulated in dying motor neurons of neonates. We attempted to identify molecules associated with nerve regeneration using PNS motor neurons such as hypoglossal motor neurons. With this strategy several molecules involved in the regeneration process, and their possible underlying molecular mechanisms are gradually being explored. The lack of some molecule or a failure of gene expression causes neuronal death, which is often seen in CNS. Therefore, compensation for the lack or the failure, by manipulating gene expression in the injured neurons, is crucial for therapy of injured brain and degenerative diseases. In this chapter we will present a possible molecular mechanism underlying nerve regeneration, and also demonstrate that manipulation of gene expression rescues injured neurons, at least in an animal model.

Identification of nerve injury associated molecules

To identify molecules associated with neuronal injury, we took a molecular biological approachwith a rat hypoglossal motor neuron injury model. For the last few years, we have attempted to identify molecules involved in this process using a technique known as differential display-PCR (DD-PCR) and random cloning with a specific cDNA library derived from nerve-injured hypoglossal nuclei [3-7].

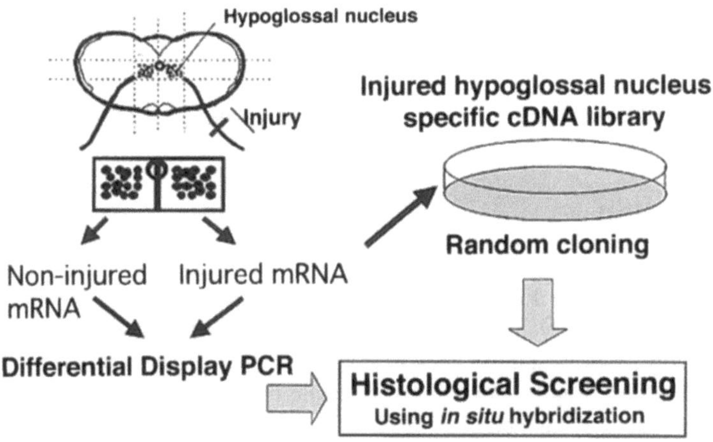

Fig. 1. Gene screening using hypoglossal nerve injury model. The hypoglossal nerve was transected unilaterally, and both the nerve-injured and control hypoglossal nuclei were excised. The RNAs from these tissues were purified, and DD-PCR was carried out. Alternatively, the injured hypoglossal nucleus specific cDNA library was made with nerve injured hypoglossal nucleus, and clones were picked up. All the gene fragments obtained by these methods were processed with histological screening using in situ hybridization histochemistry.

As shown in Fig. 1 the hypoglossal nerve was injured unilaterally. Then the hypoglossal nucleus was dissected under a microscope and collected from several animals. mRNAs from non-injured and injured sides were precipitated, respectively. We then utilized DD-PCR (Fig. 1 and 2) or made a cDNA library using mRNA from injured hypoglossal nuclei. In the case of the cDNA library, clones were randomly picked up, sequenced, and processed for histological screening, such as in situ hybridization. Through these methods we obtained a substantial number of candidate molecules, which are upregulated in adult injured motor neurons and downregulated in neonates. Subsequently, histological screening using a neonatal nerve injury model was performed.

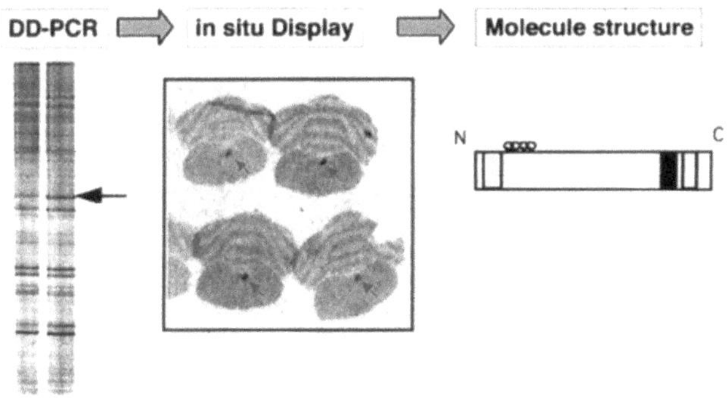

Fig. 2. Gene screening. Gene fragment obtained by DD-PCR (arrow) was used as a probe for the in situ Display screening. The in situ Display confirms whether the candidate gene is actually induced in injured motor neurons (arrows). If in situ Display showed a positive result, molecular structure was presumed according to the information of the nucleic acids sequence.

Gene responses for survival

Gene screening identifies many known and unknown molecules. A number of repeatedly hit molecules could be categorized into groups; Fig. 3 summarizes the major results. The major toxic events for the injured motor neurons would be glutamate and free radicals. In order to reduce these toxicities some molecule sets are induced. To reduce glutamate toxicity, glutamate transporters (EAAT3) and glutamine synthetase (GS) are upregulated in the injured motor neurons. In addition, glial glutamate transporter such as GLAST is also upregulated in the astrocytes. All these molecules function to reduce the extracellular glutamate level, which leads to a reduction of glutamate-induced hyper-excitation. For free radical scavenging, the super oxide dismutase (SOD), glutathion peroxidase (GPx), catalase are upregulated. Similarly oxidized protein by an oxidative stress seems to be repaired by the activation of thioredoxin (TRX) and glutathion (GSH) systems. The expression of TRH, TRH reductase (TRX-Red), and GSH-reductase (GSH-Red) is induced in the motor neurons after injury. In addition, our gene screening displayed a significant number of growth factor receptors and their downstream signaling molecules. In injured motor neurons, glial cell line-derived neurotrophic factor (GDNF) receptors (GFRalpha-1 and c-Ret), brain derived neurotrophic factor (BDNF) receptor (TrkB), and LIF receptor were upregulated (Table 1).

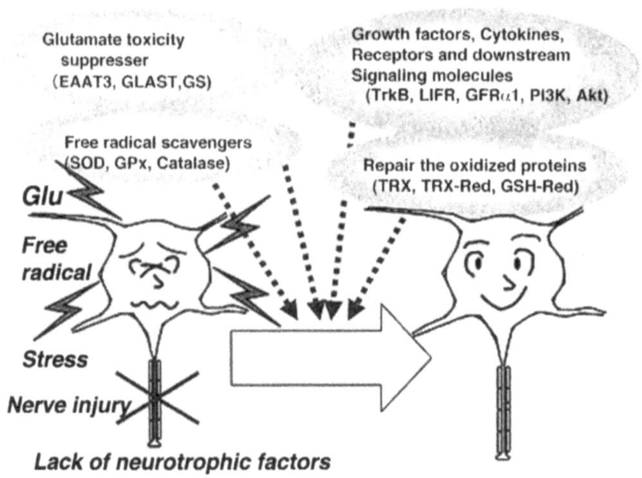

Fig. 3. Genes expressed after nerve injury.

Table 1. Growth factor receptor expression in injured motor neurons.

	Rescue activity	Receptor complex		Adult	Neonate
GDNF	++++	GFRa-1/c-Ret	c-Ret	↑	↑
			GFRa-1	↑	↓
BDNF	+++	TrkB	TrkB	↑	↓
CNTF	++	CNTFRa/LIFR/gp130	LIFR	↑	↓
NGF	-	TrkA	TrkA	n.d.	n.d.
NT-3	++(+)	TrkC	TrkC	↓	↓

n.d.; not detected

In addition, many intracellular signaling molecules, which locate downstream of these receptors, are expressed in response to nerve injury. Two major known signaling pathways located downstream of the growth factor receptors are Ras-ERK and PI3K-Akt. Strikingly, Shc, MEK, ERK, 14-3-3, PI3K, and Akt were all upregulated in expression and activated after nerve injury (Fig. 4). Similar upregulations were not found in PKC and PKA related molecules. It may be concluded therefore, that growth factor receptor signaling would be the most crucial signaling among intracellular signaling pathways after nerve injury.

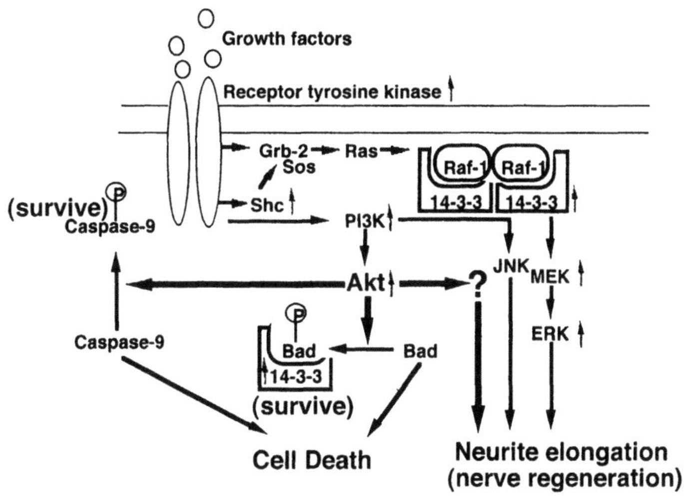

Fig. 4. Intracellular signaling molecules that responded to motor neuron injury. Molecules belonging to Ras-ERK and PI3K-Akt pathways are induced (arrows).

Gene transfer succeeded in rescuing dying neurons

Adenovirus mediated gene transfer

Among the vectors we examined, the adenovirus vector demonstrated relatively good results in expressing exogenous genes in neuronal cells [8]. Although the adenovirus as a gene transfer vector has disadvantages, such as short-term expression and slight toxicity, it is very easy to handle and achieves a high level of expression in neuronal cells. In addition, attempts to express a gene in certain types of cells are easily accomplishes using *Cre-loxP* system (Fig. 5). Namely, the switching unit in the vector contains a stuffer sequence encoding Neo, for instance, with a functional polyadenylation signal between the promoter and the inserted cDNA fragment, thereby blocking its expression during viral amplification in HEK293 cells. The stuffer is flanked by a pair of *loxP* sites, allowing for its excision by *Cre,* leading to expression of the inserted cDNA sequence. To obtain expression of the target gene (for instance lacZ in Fig. 5), we performed co-infection of the nuclear localization signal (NLS) tagged *Cre* recombinase expressing virus (AxCANCre) plus *Cre*-mediated NLS-LacZ virus (AxCALNLNZ). Using this *Cre-loxP* system, a cell type specific gene transfer was plausible. When astrocyte specific promoter such as GFAP is used instead of a general promoter such as CAG promoter (CA) for *Cre* expression, a target gene, which locates downstream of the second *loxP*, could be expressed only in astrocytes but not in neuronal and the other types of cells.

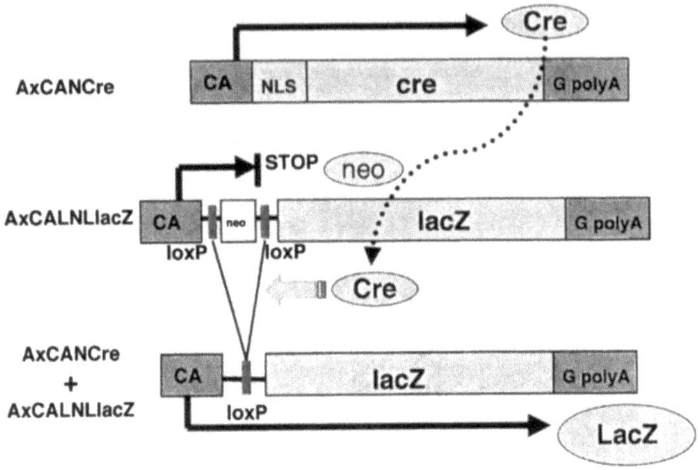

Fig. 5. *Cre-loxP* mediated gene expression system.

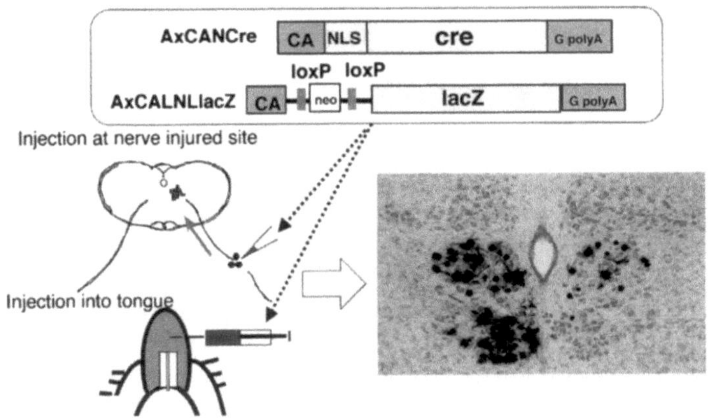

Fig. 6. Adenovirus is injected into tongue or nerve injured site. The photography demonstrated *LacZ* expressing hypoglossal motor neurons. The adenovirus was injected into the left–hand side of tongue.

There are several possible methods for adenoviral gene transfer into neural cells. In the case of peripheral motor neurons, methods include direct injection into the target nucleus of the brain, injecting the injured peripheral nerve site, or injecting the target skeletal muscle. The adenovirus is somehow taken up at the nerve terminal or injured axon site, transported to cell body retrogradely, and expressed in the target protein.As an application of this system in vivo, we demonstrated a rescue of neonatal injured motor neurons by changing the expression level and activities of the intracellular signaling molecules [8]. Previous gene screening suggested that two downstream signaling pathways are potentially important for survival. We examined if activation of either of these two pathways could rescue injured neurons. Adenoviruses, the constitutively active MEK (da-MEK), which activates Ras-ERK pathway, or the constitutively active Akt (myr-Akt), which activates PI3K-Akt pathway, were infected with *Cre* expressing adenovirus (AxCANCre)

Akt, but not MEK, prevents axotomy-induced neuronal death

To further clarify the roles of PI3K-Akt and Ras-ERK pathways in the prevention of axtomy-induced neuronal death *in vivo*, these recombinant adenoviruses were injected into the tongues of neonate rats (1 day old) to allow for retrograde infection of hypoglossal motor neurons. The efficacy of this method was preliminarily verified in neonates using AxCANLacZ. When AxCANLacZ was injected unilaterally into neonate tongues, more than 20% of ipsilateral hypoglossal motor neurons were labeled β-Galactosidase (β-Gal) positive (Fig. 6). Two days after injection, ipsilateral hypoglossal nerve was axotomized (on postnatal day 3). Adenoviral expressions of myr-Akt and da-MEK in injured motor neurons were observed immunohistochemically by using their corresponding tag (HA and c-Myc) antibodies (Fig. 7).

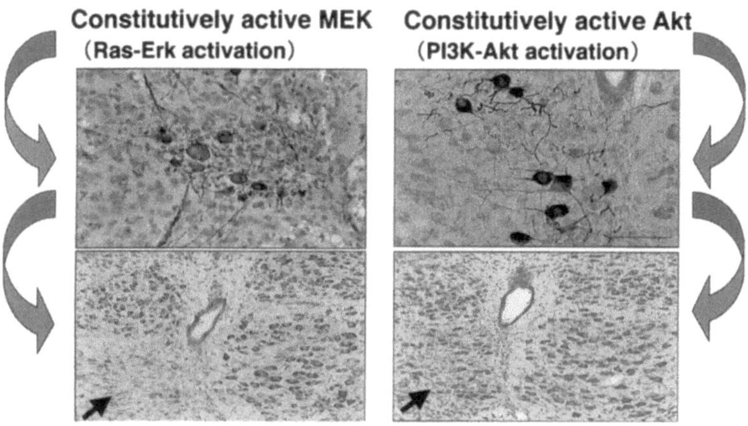

Fig. 7. Axotomy-induced neuronal death can be rescued by Akt, but not MEK.

Even though da-MEK was expressed in the surviving hypoglossal neurons on post-axotomy day 7, these cells clearly showed atrophic and degenerative changes. On the other hand, myr-Akt positive motor neurons seemed to be maintaining a healthy profile with large cell bodies and long processes even on post-axotomy day 12. Concomitantly, surviving neurons were counted on adjacent Nissle stained sections (Fig. 7). The surviving neurons were counted on both the injured and control sides and the survival ratio was obtained. The expression of myr-Akt significantly protected neonate motor neurons from axotomy-induced neuronal death with an efficacy similar to that observed with Bcl-2 overexpressing ones [8]. On the other hand, da-MEK failed to prevent axotomy-induced motor neuron death, even though it was expressed strongly (Fig. 7).

Gene transfer promotes nerve reprojection *in vivo*

Interestingly, myr-Akt promoted neurite elongation of the undifferentiated PC2 cells even without NGF application. We expected that the axon elongation activity might be enhanced in myr-Akt overexpressing motor neurons. In order to evaluate axon regeneration, we employed a retrograde tracer, Fluoro-Gold (FG), which, is taken up from axon terminals, and retrogradely transported into the cell bodies when injected into the tongue [9].

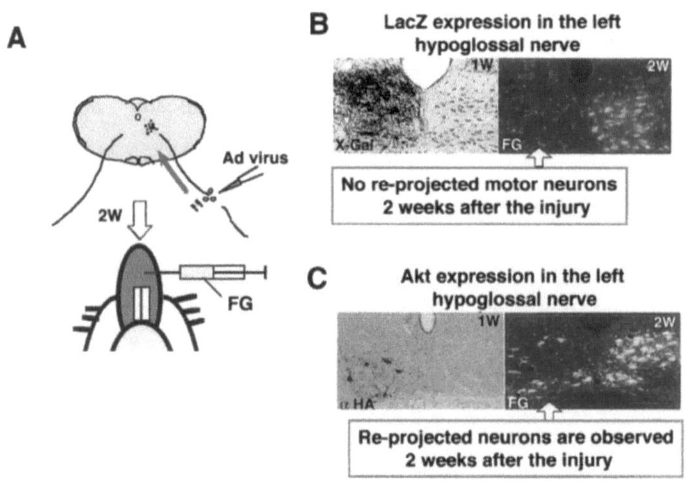

Fig. 8. Identification of neurite elongation activity. A Adenovrus (in this case either lacZ or Akt expressing virus) was injected into nerve injured site. Two weeks later, a retrograde tracer, Fluoro Gold (FG), was injected into tongue. If the regenerating nerve projects into the tongue at that time, FG labels the hypoglossal motor neurons (B and C).

FG was injected into both sides of the tongue two days before sacrifice to allow retrograde transport of the dye into the neuronal cell bodies. Animals were sacrificed at 2, 3, and 4 weeks after nerve transection and FG positive cells were counted on both injured and control sides. The axon reprojecting rate was evaluated by comparing FG positive cell number in the intact and the injured hypoglossal nuclei. By two weeks post-axotomy, approximately 20% of myr-Akt overexpressing motor neurons succeeded in reprojecting into the tongue, whereas the injured motor neurons overexpressing LacZ as control, failed to do so during the same period (Fig. 8). The number of successfully reprojecting cells increased with the passage of time. The reprojection ratios in the myr-Akt expressing neurons exceeded those in the LacZ overexpressing ones by more than 20 %. These results clearly indicate that Akt overexpression has a significant effect on enhancing axonal regeneration *in vivo* [8]. Not only Akt, but also some other gene expression with adenovirus succeeded in promoting the neurite elongation [10]. These results, therefore, suggest that the enhancement of neurite elongation by gene transfer is possible *in vivo*, and that a gene therapy to repair injured neural circuits might be achievable in the near future.

Conclusions

The hypoglossal nerve injury model proved that hundreds of gene expressions are implicated in the process of survival and regeneration after neuronal injury. Peripheral nerve regeneration orchestrates sequential changes in the expression of thousands of genes, which are necessary to protect damaged neurons from death, activate surrounding glial cells and accelerate neurite elongation. For neuronal survival, multiple defense lines are constructed in response to nerve injury. The primary defensive front would be the reduction of cell death initiators such as glutamate and the free radicals. For this purpose, scavengers such as glutamate transporters and SODs are induced. The second defense line could be the regulator of cytochrom C release from mitochondria on which Bax family and Bcl-2 family members are implicated in determining whether cytochrom C should be released or not. The final defense line could be neurotrophic factor-PI3K-Akt mediated signaling, which blocks the late process of the cell death cascade in addition to some upper part of the cascade. In the case of adult motor neurons all the defense lines are strong enough to protect the cell from death, however in the motor neurons of neonates these defense lines are not strong enough and motor neurons die. This would be the case for CNS neurons as well. The failure in constructing the defense lines (or mechanisms) in response to neuronal injury would be the major cause of cell death. Gene transfer could compensate for the weak points of defense lines, and in fact some gene expression protected injured neurons and also enhanced neurite regeneration. Therefore, the present approach using adenovirus mediated gene manipulation may provide a potential therapeutic intervention aimed at functional recovery in a number of clinical conditions like brain trauma, ischemia, or neurodegenerative diseases like amyotrophic lateral sclerosis (ALS).

References

1. Pollin MM, McHanwell S, Slater CR (1991) The effect of age on motor neurone death following axotomy in the mouse. Development 112:83-89
2. Snider WD, Elliott JL, Yan Q (1992) Axotomy-induced neuronal death during development. J Neurobiol 23:1231-1246
3. Kiryu S, Yao GL, Morita N, et al (1995) Nerve injury enhances rat neuronal glutamate transporter expression: identification by differential display PCR. J Neurosci 15:7872-7878
4. Morita N, Kiryu S, Kiyama H (1996) p53 independent cyclin G expression in a group of mature neurons and its enhanced expression during nerve regeneration. J Neurosci 16:5961-5966
5. Nakagomi S, Kiryu-Seo S, Kimoto M, et al (1999) Dimethylarginine dimethylaminohydrolase (DDAH) as a nerve injury associated molecule: The mRNA localization in the rat brain and its coincident up-regulation with neuronal NO synthase (nNOS) in axotomized motor neurons. Eur J Neurosci 11:2160-2166
6. Tanabe K, Nakagomi S, Kiryu-Seo S, et al (1999) Expressed-sequence-tag approach to identify differentially expressed genes following peripheral nerve axotomy. Mol Brain Res 64:34-40
7. Kiryu-Seo S, Sasaki M, Yokohama H, et al (2000) Damage induced neuronal endopeptidase (DINE) is a unique metallopeptidase expressed in response to neuronal damage and activates superoxide scavengers. Proc Natl Acad Sci USA 97: 4345-4350
8. Namikawa K, Honma M, Abe K, et al (2000) Akt / Protein kinase B prevents injury-induced motor neuron death and accelerates axonal regeneration. J Neurosci 20: 2875-2886
9. Hirota H, Kiyama H, Kishimoto T, et al (1996) Accelelated nerve regeneration in mice by upregulated expression of IL-6 and IL-6 receptor after trauma. J Exp Med 183:2627-2634
10. Tanabe K, Tachibana T, Yamashita T, et al (2000) The small GTP-binding protein TC10 promotes growth cone-like formation and nerve elongation in neuronal cells, and its expression is induced during nerve regeneration in rats. J Neurosci 20:4138-4144

4. Strategies for and from cortical spreading depression

Brain ischemia and spreading depression in a primate model

Chiaki Yokota[1], Yuji Kuge[2], Masafumi Tagaya[3], Yasuhiro Hasegawa[3], Takeo Abumiya[4], Go Kito[5], Takenori Yamaguchi[3], Kazuo Minematsu[3]

[1] Cerebrovascular Laboratory, Research Institute, and [3] Cerebrovascular Division, Department of Medicine, NATIONAL CARDIO-VASCULAR CENTER, 5-7-1 Fujishiro-dai, Suita, Osaka 565-8565, Japan
[2] Department of Tracer Kinetics, Graduate School of Medicine, Hokkaido University, Kita 15 Nishi 7, Kita-ku, Sapporo 060-8638, Japan
[4] Hokkaido Ebetu Hospital, 81-6 Yoyogi-cho, Nopporo, Ebetsu, Hokkaido 069-0817, Japan
[5] Shin Nippon Biomedical Laboratories, Ltd., 2438 Miyanoura, Yoshida, Kagoshima 891-1394, Japan

Summary: In order to investigate the pathophysiology of ischemic stroke, we developed a primate thromboembolic stroke model and examined serial changes in cerebral blood flow (CBF) and cerebral metabolic rate of glucose (CMRglc) using positron emission tomography (PET). In addition, we attempted to elicit spreading depression (SD), which is essential in the evolution of infarcts in small animal models, by chemical stimulation in primates.

In our thromboembolic stroke model (n=4), CBF in the temporal cortex and the basal ganglia decreased to < 40% of the contralateral values when measured at 1 hour following embolization. In these regions (ischemic core), CBF decreased further with time and CMRglc was found to be decreased at 24 h. In the parietal cortex and several regions surrounding the ischemic core, CBF was > 40% of that in the contralateral region at 1 h following embolization, and increased gradually thereafter. CMRglc at 24 h after embolization in these regions was increased compared with that in the contralateral. Thus, flow thresholds for the infarct development were considered to be 12-15 ml $100g^{-1}$ min^{-1} (40% of contralateral values) in this model.

We successfully elicited SD in 9 monkeys, and monitored the CBF by PET in 5 animals. The propagation of SD was limited to areas near the site of stimulation. Immediately after the first SD, focal cortical hyperemia was detected. However, this condition was not followed by spreading hypoperfusion or persistent hypoperfusion in the hemisphere ipsilateral to the site of stimulation. These unique features of SD in primates suggest that the role of SD in nonprimate animals may not be similar to that in stroke and migraine in humans.

Key words: Primate, PET, Focal brain ischemia, Spreading depression

Introduction

In 1998, stroke was the third leading cause of death in Japan, after cancer and heart disease. Although stroke mortality in Japan has markedly declined since 1960 [1], the incidence of stroke may be increasing as the elderly population increases. Acute stroke events and disability among stroke survivors places a great burden on the social and health care systems [2], therefore, the prevention and improved treatment of ischemic stroke have considerable public health significance [3]. From an analysis of trends in acute ischemic stroke trials through the 20th century, Kidwell et al. [4] have emphasized the emerging understanding of the pathophysiology of cerebral ischemia.

Although many animal studies have examined the pathophysiology of focal brain ischemia, only a small portion of this work has translated into effective treatment modalities for stroke [5]. Cortical spreading depression (SD), which is characterized by reversible depression of cortical electrical activity in the brain that spreads like a wave at a speed of 2-5 mm per minute [6], has been suggested as a target of pharmacological intervention because repetitive pathologic SDs in the peri-infarct border zone contributes to the evolution of infarcts in rat and cat models [7-14]. Although most neuroprotective agents known to block the occurrence of SDs in rodents [7,9,10] work well during brain ischemia in small animals [15], most of potential neuroprotective therapies modifying ischemic cell death cascades have not proven as beneficial in stroke patients. Moreover, peri-infarct depolarizations were not observed in human stroke patients on repetitive magnetic resonance diffusion imaging [12]. Further, eliciting an SD in the primate model has not been successful, and the participation of SD in ischemic stroke is a matter of speculation.

As proposed by the Stroke Therapy Academic Industry Roundtable, nonhuman primate studies are required to clarify the pathophysiology of ischemic stroke, and to verify the safety and efficacy of newly developed drugs that show promising results in rodents [16]. We have developed a primate thromboembolic stroke model [17], and determined serial changes in CBF and CMRglc using a high-resolution PET to characterize the primate model [18]. In addition, we sought to elicit SD by chemical stimulation in a non-ischemic primate model. Further, we examined the attendant changes in CBF using PET during the provocation of SD.

All procedures in this study were approved by our Institutional Animal Research Committee and were performed in accordance with the standards published by the National Research Council (Guide for the Care and Use of Laboratory Animals). In compliance with these standards, every effort was made to ensure that the animals were free from pain or discomfort.

Serial changes in cerebral blood flow and flow-metabolism uncoupling in primates with acute thromboembolic stroke

Material and methods

Animal preparation

In this study, we used 5 male cynomolgus monkeys weighing 3.5 to 3.8 kg.

The procedure for inducing thromboembolic stroke was previously described [17]. Briefly, animals were anesthetized by sevoflurane inhalation (0.5% to 2.0% sevoflurane delivered in a N_2O/O_2 (70%/30%) gas mixture) and artificially ventilated. They were implanted with an indwelling catheter filled with a heparin solution in their left internal carotid artery. Following their recovery from anesthesia, all animals were examined and were found free of neurological deficits. Two days after the operation, a single autologous blood clot was injected into the left internal carotid artery through the catheter under light sevoflurane anesthesia.

PET studies

The PET studies were performed using a multislice PET scanner (ECAT EXACT HR/47, Siemens/CTI, Knoxville, TN, USA) [19]. The spatial resolution at the center of the field of view (FOV) was 3.7 mm in-plane at full-width at half-maximum and 4.1 mm axially.

Each monkey was anesthetized by sevoflurane inhalation and artificially ventilated. The anesthetized animal was mounted on a custom-made stereotaxic instrument in a supine position, and the head was restrained. Body temperature was monitored and maintained at around 37 °C with heating pads. The arterial catheter was used for continuous blood pressure monitoring, and blood gas analyses were performed prior to each PET scan.

CBF and CMRglc were determined using ^{15}O-labeled water (^{15}O-H_2O) and 2-[^{18}F] fluoro-2-deoxy-D-glucose (^{18}F-FDG), respectively, according to the methods described in detail previously [20].

Study protocol and TTC staining

The CBF was measured in each monkey prior to the clot injection (baseline CBF) and at five timepoints following the injection. The baseline CBF was determined following carotid catheter implantation. After the PET scans were performed, the animals were allowed to recover from their anesthesia and were placed back into their cages. Two days after the baseline CBF measurement, embolization was performed as described above. The animals were allowed to recover from anesthesia, and any induced neurological deficits were confirmed. One monkey that showed no neurological deficits was excluded from the study. The other monkeys were anesthetized again by sevoflurane inhalation and prepared for the PET measurements. CBF was determined at 1, 2, 4 and 6 h following the embolization. After the procedure, the animals were allowed to recover from anesthesia and were placed in their home cages. Twenty-four hours following the embolization, each monkey was anesthetized again and the CBF was determined.

Immediately following the last CBF measurement at 24 h, ^{18}F-FDG was injected and CMRglc was measured. After completion of the CMRglc measurement, the brain was perfused with ice-cold saline and the animal was sacrificed by exsanguination under pentobarbital anesthesia. The brain was quickly removed and the blood clot located in the M1 portion of the left middle cerebral artery (MCA) was confirmed by inspection. The brain was sectioned coronally at 3-mm intervals and incubated in a 1% solution of 2,3,5-triphenyltetrazolium chloride (TTC) at 37°C for vital staining [17].

Data analysis

The PET images were reconstructed according to a standard filtered back-projection procedure using a Hanning filter. CBF images were calculated based on a diffusible autoradiographic method [21]. The CMRglc images were calculated according to an autoradiographic method [22] adapting the values of 0.102 ml g^{-1} min^{-1}, 0.130, 0.062, and 0.0068 min^{-1} for K_1, k_2, k_3, and k_4, respectively, and the value of 0.42 for the lumped constant.

A total of 18 circular regions of interest (ROIs, 10 mm in diameter) were determined for three coronal brain slices of baseline CBF images from the striatum to the thalamus level (Fig.1). The ROIs were superimposed on the CBF and CMRglc images obtained following embolization. An asymmetry index (AI) was defined as the ratio of the value for an ROI in the ipsilateral (to the arterial occlusion) hemisphere to that of the contralateral homologous ROI.

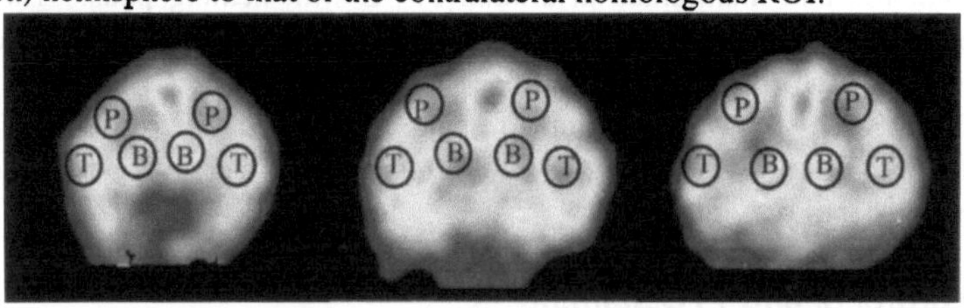

Slice 1 **Slice 2** **Slice 3**

P: Parietal Cortex T: Temporal Cortex B: Basal Ganglia

Fig. 1. An example of regions of interest (ROIs, 10 mm in diameter) placed on three coronal images from the striatum to the thalamus level. The slices are approximately 23 (slice 1), 32 (slice 2) and 41 mm (slice 3) from the frontal pole.

Multiple comparisons were analyzed using the one-way analysis of variance (ANOVA) and the Fisher's PLSD post hoc test. A two-way ANOVA was used to assess the significance of differences in the baseline CBF values, in the CMRglc values, and in the AIs at 24 h following embolization. A two-tailed probability value less than 0.05 was considered significant.

Results

During the experimental period, the physiological parameters examined did not change significantly.

Serial changes in CBF during focal ischemia in a primate model

Before the clot injection, no significant side-to-side differences were observed in the CBF images (Fig. 2).

Following the clot injection, a marked hypoperfusion developed throughout the MCA territory. Figure 3 shows serial changes in the AIs for CBF. At one hour after the clot injection, the AIs in the temporal cortex decreased significantly compared with those for baseline CBF. Subsequently, the AIs in these regions decreased gradually for 24 h following the clot injection. In the basal ganglia, CBF was significantly reduced after embolization. The AIs in these regions at 1-6 h were found to be decreased further at 24 h after embolization. The AIs in the parietal cortex at 1 h after embolization were significantly lower than those for baseline CBF. Subsequently, the AIs in the parietal cortex increased gradually for 24 h following the clot injection.

CMRglc at 24 h-ischemia in a primate model

Twenty-four hours after the ischemic insult, CMRglc was significantly reduced in most of the ipsilateral temporal cortex and the basal ganglia compared with the contralateral regions (Figs. 4, 5). In the ipsilateral parietal cortex, CMRglc significantly increased compared with that in the contralateral regions (Figs. 4, 5).

CBF-CMRglc relationship at 24 h-ischemia in a primate model

Twenty-four hours after the ischemic insult, CMRglc was significantly reduced in most of the ipsilateral temporal cortex and the basal ganglia compared with that in the contralateral regions (Figs. 4, 5). In the ipsilateral parietal cortex, CMRglc was significantly increased compared with that in the contralateral regions (Figs. 4, 5).

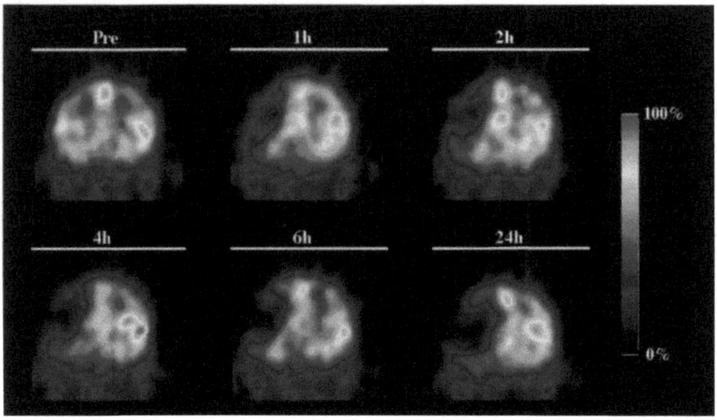

Fig. 2. Representative images of the time-courses of CBF changes for a coronal slice at the striatum level (approximately 32 mm from the frontal pole). CBF was measured before (Pre) and at 1, 2, 4, 6 and 24 h following embolization. The maximum CBF value in each PET measurement is indicated as 100%.

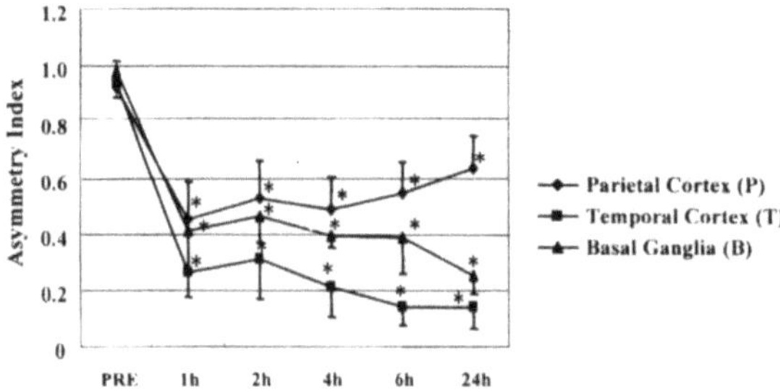

Fig. 3. The time-course of AIs for CBF in various ROIs. Data are the mean ± S.D. of 4 animals. The AIs for baseline CBF are shown as PRE values. * Significantly different from the AI for the baseline CBF.

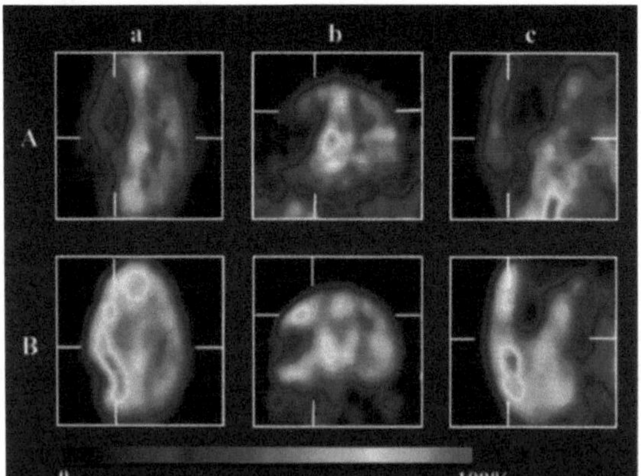

Fig. 4. Representative images of CBF and CMRglc at 24 h following embolization. A: CBF, B: CMRglc, a: transaxial slice, b: coronal slice, c: sagittal slice.

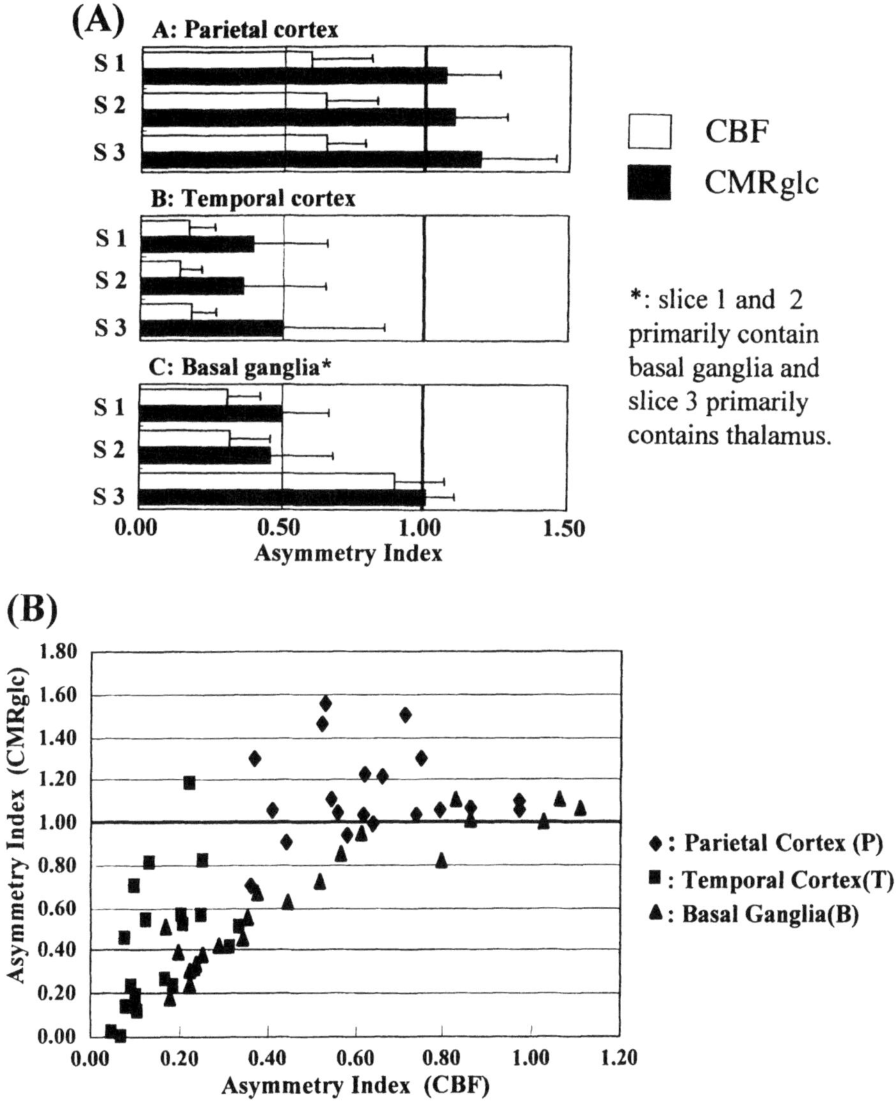

Fig. 5. (A): The AIs for CBF and CMRglc at 24 h after embolization. (B): The relationship between CBF and CMRglc in ROIs at 24 h after embolization.

Ischemic injury 24 h after ischemia by TTC staining

Lesions were detected predominantly in the temporal cortex and the basal ganglia. No obvious lesions were observed in the parietal cortex.

Spreading depression in a primate model

Material and methods

Animal preparation

Nine adult, male cynomolgus monkeys (#1-#9) were anesthetized with pentobarbital (50 mg/kg, i.p.), followed by tracheal intubation. Then, the animals were anesthetized with N_2O/O_2 (70%:30%) gas mixture inhalation under artificial ventilation. The rectal temperature was monitored continuously with a rectal probe and maintained at approximately 36 °C with a heating pad. An arterial catheter was used for continuous monitoring of heart rate and arterial pressure.

Electrophysiological measurement

The anesthetized animal was mounted on a custom-made stereotaxic instrument in a prone position, and the head was restrained. Three to four small burr holes were made in the left parietal bone and the dura was carefully excised. One burr hole was used for potassium chloride (KCl) application, and two to three were used for direct current (DC) potential recordings. Of the latter, two burr holes were made rostral to the hole for KCl application in all animals, for recording the DC potential through microelectrodes inserted into the cortical surface. Another hole for recording the DC potential was made caudal to the hole for KCl application in 2 animals (#4, #5). These burr holes were made along a line at 7-mm intervals. We also recorded the DC-shift in the right parietal cortex in one monkey (#4), although it has been reported that SD waves do not spread to the contralateral hemisphere [23,24].

The DC potential was monitored with an amplifier (Iso-DAM8, World Precision Instruments, Sarasota, FL, USA) using microelectrodes that had been inserted into the cortex to a depth of 1mm.

A sagittal slice through the insertion sites of the two microelectrodes was obtained from one monkey (#7) after the animal was sacrificed by exsanguination under pentobarbital anesthesia. The length of the cortical surface was measured between the two microelectrodes.

PET study

PET was performed using a multi-slice PET scanner (ECAT EXACT HR/47, Siemens/CTI, Knoxville, TN, USA) as described above [19].

Five of the nine animals (#1 to #5) underwent the PET study. Each animal was placed in the field of view in the prone position. The CBF was measured by PET with an intravenous bolus injection of ^{15}O-labeled water. Dynamic PET scanning (0-2 min) was initiated at the time of the ^{15}O-H_2O injection. A baseline CBF measurement was made prior to the topical application of 3.3 M of KCl solution in all animals. In animals where SD was observed, the CBF was measured within 10 minutes after the first SD was elicited (CBF1), followed by 3 to 5 PET scans at intervals of approximately 10-20 minutes.

Data analysis

The PET images were reconstructed according to a standard filtered back-projection procedure using a Hanning filter. Each activity image was globally normalized by relative ratio to regional counts of the cerebellar cortex ipsilateral to the site of KCl application. A total of 14 circular ROIs (10 mm in diameter each) were positioned in each hemisphere symmetrically on three transaxial brain slices as shown in Figure 6. We examined the data using the AI as defined previously.

The significance of differences in the sequential change of each physiological parameter was assessed using repeated-measures one-way analysis of variance (ANOVA) and Fischer's PLSD post hoc test. A two-tailed p-value less than 0.05 was considered to be significant.

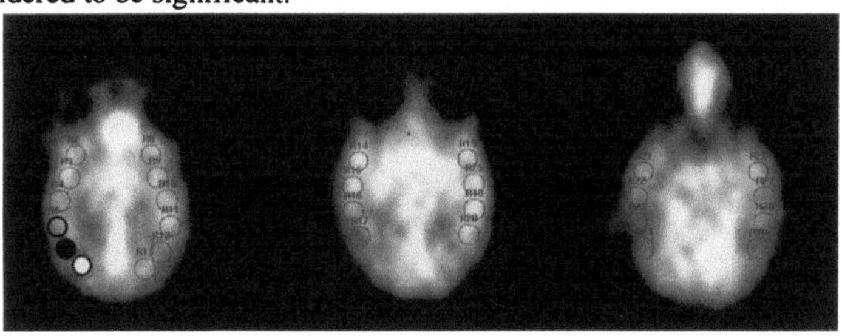

Fig. 6. Examples of ROIs (10 mm in diameter each) placed on three transaxial images. The slices are approximately 2.5 cm, 3.2 cm, and 4.2 cm, respectively, from the top of the precentral gyrus in the field of view. The ROI rostrally adjacent to the site of KCl application is indicated with a bold circle; the ROI caudally adjacent to the KCl application site is shown in white; and the KCl application site is indicated with a solid circle.

Results

Electrophysiological study

During the experimental period, physiological parameters of the monkeys did not change significantly.

The number and location of DC-shifts elicited by the KCl are listed in Table 1.

Table 1. The Number of DC-shifts Detected by Microelectrodes in each Site

Animal	Rostral site	Caudal site	Contralateral site	PET study
#1	0	-	-	+
#2	2	-	-	+
#3	1	-	-	+
#4	2	6	0	+
#5	0	8	-	+
#6	1	-	-	-
#7	1	-	-	-
#8	0	-	-	-
#9	6	-	-	-

-, not measured

A propagated DC shift was found on the recordings of DC potentials in two neighboring microelectrodes 7 mm apart in only one animal (#7). In this monkey, the length of the cortical convolution between the 2 microelectrodes was 48 mm. The DC-shift spread between the two microelectrodes in 12 minutes (Fig. 7), resulting in a propagation speed of 4 mm per minute. The amplitude was 20 mV. These values are consistent with the SD findings reported in previous studies [6,24].

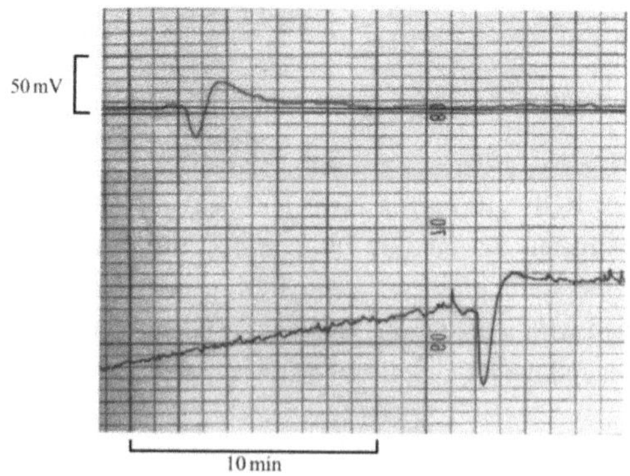

Fig. 7. Propagation of a spreading depression wave. Recordings of the DC potential obtained from the rostral holes close to (top line) and distant from (bottom line) the site of KCl application in animal #7 are shown.

PET study

Representative, multi-slice PET images in animal #2 in which SD was recorded

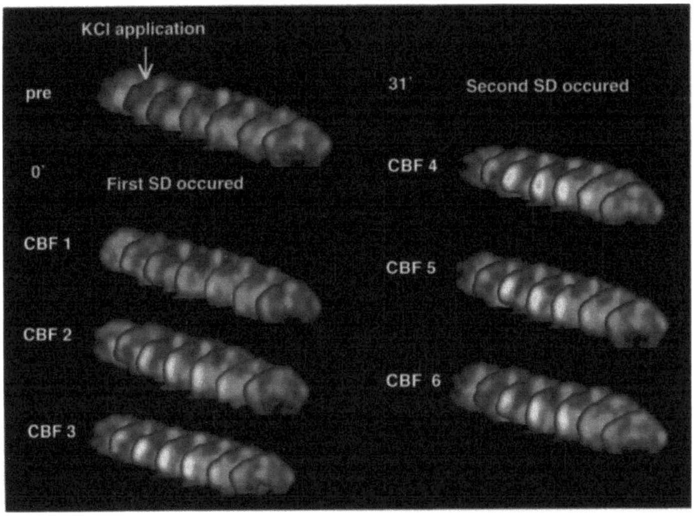

Fig. 8. Representative PET images (animal #2) showing the time course of CBF changes. The multi-slice PET images shows focal hyperemia in the temporal cortex ipsilateral to the site of KCl application.

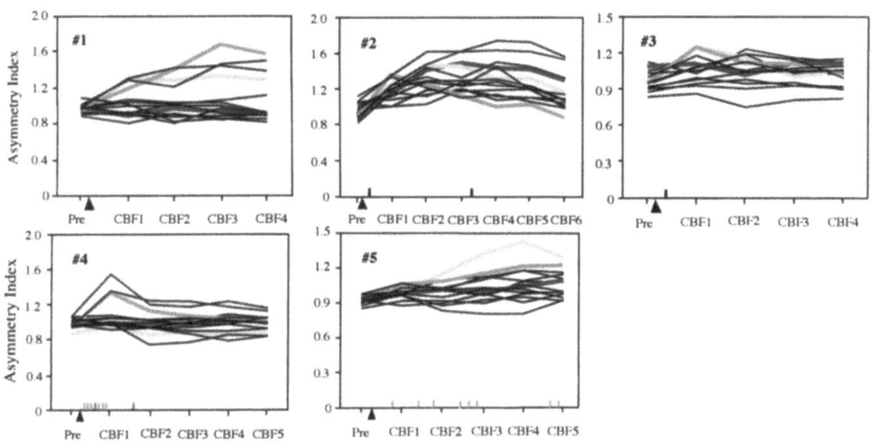

Fig. 9. Course of the AIs of CBF in the 14 ROIs in each of the 5 animals that underwent the PET study. The blue line shows the changes in the AIs in the ROIs rostrally adjacent to the site of KCl application; the pink line shows in the AIs caudally adjacent to the KCl application, and yellow line shows the KCl application site. The arrow-head indicates the time point of KCl application for eliciting SDs. The time points at which each SD was detected are indicated with vertical short lines above the x-axis: a blue line indicates SD in the rostral direction, and a pink line indicates SD in the caudal direction.

twice at the rostral site are shown in Figure 8. One episode was detected immediately after KCl application, and another episode occurred between the measurement of CBF3 and CBF4. The PET images obtained after the occurrence of SD demonstrated transient focal hyperemia in the ipsilateral temporal cortex to the site of KCl application. In the contralateral hemisphere, there were no obvious changes in regional CBF throughout the PET study in any of the animals.

Figure 9 shows the change in the AIs of CBF in the 14 ROIs during the experiment in each of the 5 animals. Focal increases in regional CBF were observed in accordance with the occurrence of SD. In animal #1 in which no SD episodes had been detected at the rostral sites, focal hyperemia was observed after the chemical stimulation. On the other hand, none of the animals had persistent hypoperfusion.

Discussion

Focal brain ischemia in a primate model

In this study, we have examined serial changes in the CBF and CMRglc in a primate thromboembolic stroke model by using PET.

In the temporal cortex and the basal ganglia, the CBF was reduced to less than approximately 40% of the contralateral values at 1 h after embolization. Most of these regions became infarcted at 24 h after embolization, suggesting that these regions represent the ischemic core. In the parietal cortex, the CBF was relatively preserved with no obvious TTC-unstained lesions at 24 h. Thus, the flow thresholds for infarct development were considered to be approximately 12-15 ml $100g^{-1}$ min^{-1} (approximately 40% of contralateral values) in our primate model of permanent occlusion, which are consistent with those in the previous reports [25,26]. In several studies of permanent [27-30] and temporary [30-32] occlusions of the MCA in nonhuman primates, acute changes in hemodynamics and oxygen metabolism were observed by PET. Differences in the reduction of the CBF following the occlusion were reported in those studies, which may be partly attributed to the differences in the species, anesthesia, occlusion method, and ROIs used in each study.

In this study, an elevated glucose metabolism and an uncoupling of flow and glucose metabolism were demonstrated in several regions surrounding the ischemic core. In other studies using rodent or cat models, the flow-metabolism uncoupling was observed in the arterial borderzone during several hours of acute ischemia [33-36] and were regarded as factors contributing to infarct development [34,36]. In primates, the relationship between CBF and CMRglc and its contribution to infarct development remain unclear. In this study, the elevated glucose metabolism and uncoupling of flow and metabolism were observed at 24 h following the embolization. The uncoupling of flow and metabolism may indicate the relatively long time window for the eventual recovery of tissue in the primates [29,37]. It is also notable that the CBF was relatively preserved, and recovered gradually during the course of the experiment in the regions where the uncoupling was observed. Therapeutic strategies affecting pathological biochemical mechanisms in the process of ischemic cell damage are necessary after the CBF has been, at least, partially restored by collateral perfusion, spontaneous reperfusion, or therapeutic intervention [37].

Spreading depression in a primate model

In our primate model of SD, SD waves were recorded infrequently at the rostral site, and neither spreading hypoperfusion nor persistent hypoperfusion was observed.

SD waves are known to propagate predominantly towards the caudal direction [6]. In a rat model, SD waves propagated throughout a hemisphere [23]. In the present study, however, SD waves were infrequently detected at the rostral site close to the source of stimulation. Only a single SD was detected at the site distant from the stimulation. Therefore, SD waves may propagate within a narrow range in primates. Differences in the cytoarchitecture among species, which are considered to reflect differences in the number and length of dendritic and axonal ramifications [38], may influence the propagation of SD.

The CBF pattern obtained in the present study differs from those obtained in rat- and cat-SD models [20,39,40]. Transient cortical hyperemia followed by persistent hypoperfusion was reported to be an epiphenomenon of SD in those models [20,39,40]. An increased extracellular potassium concentration *per se* may increase blood flow. However, the pattern of the serial change in CBF after KCl application varied, depending on the SD profile in the 5 animals that underwent the PET study. Although animal #1 did not show SD in the rostral direction, the pattern of the serial CBF change in this animal was similar to that in animal #5 that had 8 SD episodes in the caudal direction, but no episodes to the rostral direction. The dynamics of the CBF after chemical stimulation appear to be determined by the timing, as well as the number of SD episodes.

Previously, we demonstrated that a long-lasting CBF reduction followed a transient increase in the CBF after a single SD in the cortex ipsilateral to the site of KCl application in cats [20]. These findings are consistent with a rat-SD model [39]. Flow-metabolism uncoupling with persistent hypoperfusion in the cortex of cats with SD indicated that the cerebrovascular reactivity was impaired in association with SD [20]. In this study, persistent hypoperfusion was not seen in any ROIs in the 5 animals. Wahl et al. [41] demonstrated that the vascular responses to SD differed between cats and rats. Based on our study, the vascular responses to SD in primates may also differ from those in cats.

The changes in CBF during an SD phenomenon in primates were also distinct from those in patients with migraine [42-46]. Spreading hypoperfusion is regarded as an attendant change in CBF upon SD in patients with migraine attacks. However, the hypothesis that aura accompanied by SD phenomenon might be the trigger for migraine, particularly being pivotal to pain, was indicated to be implausible statement from the clinical point of view [47]. Recently, Ebersberger et al. [48] was unable to confirm the occurrence of inflammation as a cause of migraine headache. Because a pain stimulus results in a reduction in the global CBF in humans [49], the migraine headache itself may influence the dynamics of CBF in patients with a migraine attack. Furthermore, SD in the human brain, if present, would propagate much more slowly than observed in a previous migraine study [45], because SD waves propagate on the cortical convolution.

Conclusions

The present studies suggest that PET investigations of focal brain ischemia in the primate model provide a better understanding of the pathophysiology of human ischemic stroke than did studies with stroke models in small animals. Moreover, applying the experimental results of obtained from nonprimate animals to the pathogenesis of brain diseases in humans must be done with great care. Consideration of species' differences is crucial from the standpoint of the large series of failures in clinical trials of neuroprotective drugs.

To establish new therapeutic strategies for acute ischemic stroke, further interdisciplinary research using a nonhuman primate model is needed.

References

1. Liu L, Ikeda K, Yamori Y (2001) Changes in stroke mortality rates for 1950 to 1997: a great slowdown of decline trend in Japan. Stroke 32:1745-1749
2. Caro JJ, Huybrechts KF, Duchesne MS, et al (2000) Management patterns and costs of acute ischemic stroke: an international study. Stroke 31:582-590
3. Gorelick PB, Sacco RL, Smith DB, et al (1999) Prevention of a first stroke: a review of guidelines and a multidisciplinary consensus statement from the National Stroke Association. JAMA 281:1112-1120
4. Kidwell CS, Liebeskin DS, Starkman S, et al (2001) Trends in acute ischemic stroke trials through the 20th centry. Stroke 32:1349-1359
5. Kristian T, Siesjo BK (1998) Calcium in ischemic cell death. Stroke 29:705-718
6. Leao AAP (1944) Spreading depression of activity in the cerebral cortex. J Neurophysiol 7:359-390
7. Iijima T, Mies G, Hossmann KA (1992) Repeated negative DC deflections in rat cortex following middle cerebral artery occlusion are abolished by MK-801: Effect on volume of ischemic injury. J Cereb Blood Flow Metab 12:727-733
8. Takano K, Latour LL, Formato JE, et al (1996) The role of spreading depression in focal ischemia evaluated by diffusion mapping. Ann Neurol 39:308-318
9. Gill R, Andine P, Hillered L, et al (1992) The effect of MK-801 on cortical spreading depression in the penumbral zone following focal ischemia in the rat. J Cereb Blood Flow Metab 12:371-379
10. Chen Q, Chopp M, Bodzin G, et al (1993) Temperature modulation of cerebral depolarization during focal cerebral ischemia in rats: correlation with ischemic injury. J Cereb Blood Flow Metab 13:389-394
11. Nedergaad M, Hansen AJ (1993) Characterization of cortical depolarizations evoked in focal cerebral ischemia. J Cereb Blood Flow Metab 13:568-574
12. Back T, Kohno K, Hossmann KA (1994) Cortical negative DC deflections following middle cerebral artery occlusion and KCl-induced spreading depression: effect on blood flow, tissue oxygenation, and electroencephalogram. J Cereb Blood Flow Metab 14:12-19
13. Hossmann KA (1994) Viability thresholds and the penumbra of focal ischemia. Ann Neurol 36:557-565
14. Ohta K, Graf R, Rosner G, et al (2001) Calcium ion transients in peri-infarct depolarizations may deteriorate ion homeostasis and expand infarction in focal cerebral ischemia in cats. Stroke 32:535-543
15. del Zoppo GJ, Wagner S, Tagaya M (1997) Trends and future developments in the pharmacological treatment of acute ischemic stroke. Drugs 54:9-38
16. Stroke Therapy Academic Industry Roundtable (1999) Recommendations for standards regarding preclinical neuroprotective and restorative drug development. Stroke 30:2752-2758

17. Kito G, Nishimura A, Susumu T, et al (2001) Experimental thromboembolic stroke in cynomolgus monkey. J Neurosci Meth 105:45-53
18. Kuge Y, Yokota C, Tagaya M, et al (2001) Serial changes in cerebral blood flow and flow-metabolism uncoupling in primates with acute thromboembolic stroke. J Cereb Blood Flow Metab 21: 202-210
19. Wienhard K, Dahlbom M, Eriksson L, et al (1994) The ECAT EXACT HR: Performance of a new high resolution positron scanner. J Comput Assist Tomogr 18:110-118
20. Kuge Y, Hasegawa Y, Yokota C, et al (2000) Effects of single and repetitive spreading depression on cerebral blood flow and glucose metabolism in cats: a PET study. J Neurol Sci 176:114-123
21. Sakurada O, Kennedy C, Jehle J, et al (1978) Measurement of local cerebral blood flow with iodo [14C] antipyrine. Am J Physiol 234:H59-H66
22. Phelps ME, Hung SC, Hoffman EJ, et al (1979) Tomographic measurement of local cerebral glucose metabolic rate in humans with [18F]2-fluoro-2-deoxy-D-glucose: validation of method. Ann Neurol 6:371-388
23. Hasegawa Y, Latour LL, Formato JE, et al (1995) Spreading waves of a reduced diffusion coefficient of water in normal and ischemic rat brain. J Cereb Blood Flow Metab 15:179-187
24. Marshall WH (1959) Spreading cortical depression of Leao. Physiol Rev 39:239-279
25. Jones TH, Morawetz RB, Crowell RM, et al (1981) Thresholds of focal cerebral ischemia in awake monkeys. J Neurosurg 54:773-782
26. Yonas H, Gur D, Claassen D, et al (1988) Stable xenon-enhanced CT measurement of cerebral blood flow in reversible focal ischemia in baboons. J Neurosurg 19:228-238
27. Tenjin H, Ueda S, Mizukawa N, et al (1992) Positron emission tomographic measurement of acute hemodynamic changes in primate middle cerebral artery occlusion. Neurol Med Chir, Tokyo, pp 805-810
28. Pappata S, Fiorelli M, Rommel T, et al (1993) PET study of changes in local brain hemodynamics and oxygen metabolism after unilateral middle cerebral artery occlusion in baboons. J Cereb Blood Flow Metab 13:416-424
29. Touzani O, Young AR, Derlon JM, et al (1995) Sequential studies of severely hypometabolic tissue volumes after permanent middle cerebral artery occlusion. A positron emission tomographic investigation in anesthetized baboons. Stroke 26:2112-2119
30. Takamatsu H, Tsukada H, Kakiuchi T, et al (2000) Detection of reperfusion injury using PET in a monkey model of cerebral ischemia. J Nucl Med 41:1409-1416
31. Young AR, Sette G, Touzani O, et al (1996) Relationships between high oxygen extraction fraction in the acute stage and final infarction in reversible middle cerebral artery occlusion: an investigation in anesthetized baboons with positron emission tomography. J Cereb Blood Flow Metab 16:1176-1188
32. Touzani O, Young AR, Derlon JM, et al (1997) Progressive impairment of brain oxidative metabolism reversed by reperfusion following middle cerebral artery occlusion in anaesthetized baboons. Brain Res 767:17-25

33. Ginsberg MD, Reivich M, Giandomenico A, et al (1977) Local glucose utilization in acute focal cerebral ischemia: Local dysmetabolism and diaschisis. Neurology 27:1042-1048
34. Tanaka K, Greenberg JH, Gonatas NK, et al (1985) Regional flow-metabolism couple following middle cerebral artery occlusion in cats. J Cereb Blood Flow Metab 5:241-252
35. Hasegawa Y, Choki J, Yamaguchi T (1990) Cerebral blood flow, glucose utilization, and electrocorticograms following common carotid artery occlusion in gerbils. Stroke 21:112-118
36. Back T, Zhao W, Ginsberg MD (1995) Three-dimensional image analysis of brain glucose metabolism-blood flow uncoupling and its electrophysiological correlates in the acute ischemic penumbra following middle cerebral artery occlusion. J Cereb Blood Flow Metab 15:566-577
37. Heiss W-D, Graf R (1997) Therapeutic window in ischaemic stroke: Experimental concepts, neuroimaging studies, and implications for pharmacological treatment. CNS Drugs 8:474-491
38. Rockel AJ, Hiorns RW, Powell TPS (1980) The basic uniformity in structure of the neocortex. Brain 103:221-244
39. Lauritzen M, Jorgensen MB, Diemer NH, et al (1982) Persistent oligemia of rat cerebral cortex in the wake of spreading depression. Ann Neurol 12:469-474
40. Piper RD, Lambert GA, Duckworth JW (1991) Cortical blood flow changes during spreading depression in cats. Am J Physiol 261:H96-H102
41. Wahl M, Lauritzen M, Schilling L (1987) Change of cerebrovascular reactivity after cortical spreading depression in cats and rats. Brain Res 411:72-80
42. Olesen J, Larsen B, Lauritzen M (1981) Focal hyperemia followed by spreading oligemia and impaired activation of rCBF in classic migraine. Ann Neurol 9:344-352
43. Lauritzen M, Olsen TS, Lassen NA, et al (1983) Changes in regional cerebral blood flow during the course of classic migraine attacks. Ann Neurol 13:633-641
44. Lauritzen M, Olesen J (1984) Regional cerebral blood flow during migraine attacks by Xenon-133 inhalation and emission tomography. Brain 107:447-461
45. Woods RP, Iacoboni M, Mazziotta JC (1994) Bilateral spreading cerebral hypoperfusion during spontaneous migraine headache. New Engl J Med 331:1689-1692
46. Hadjikhani N, del Rio MS, Wu O, et al (2001) Mechanisms of migraine aura revealed by functional MRI in human visual cortex. Proc Natl Acad Sci USA 95:811-817
47. Goadsby PJ (2001) Migraine, aura, and cortical spreading depression: why are we still talking about it? Ann Neurol 49:4-6
48. Ebersberger A, Schaible HG, Averbeck B, et al (2001) Is there a correlation between spreading depression, neurogenic inflammation, and nociception that might cause migraine headache? Ann Neurol 49:7-13

49. Coghill RC, Sang CN, Berman KF, et al (1998) Global cerebral blood flow decreases during pain. J Cereb Blood Flow Metab 18:141-147

Infarct tolerance induced by repetitive cortical spreading depression is reproduced by prolonged intracerebral infusion of recombinant brain-derived neurotrophic factor

Hiroji Yanamoto[1,2], Jing-Hui Xue[1], Izumi Nagata[2], Nobuo Hashimoto[4], Masahiro Sakata[1], Ikuko Mizuta[1], Norimitsu Tohnai[1], and Haruhiko Kikuchi[3]

[1]Laboratory for Cerebrovascular Disorders, Research Institute of the NATIONAL CARDIO-VASCULAR CENTER, Suita, Osaka 565-8565, Japan
[2]Department of Cerebrovascular Surgery, Hospital of the [3]NATIONAL CARDIO-VASCULAR CENTER, Suita, Osaka 565-8565, Japan
[4]Department of Neurosurgery, Kyoto University Graduate School of Medicine, Kyoto 606-8507, Japan

Summary: Molecular mechanisms in infarct tolerance, the consistently increased cerebral resistance to ischemic stroke within 12 days following repetitive cortical spreading depression (CSD), were analyzed by measuring brain derived neurotrophic factor (BDNF)-content in the neocortex in rats. The levels of total BDNF protein were significantly elevated from day 0 to 12, peaking on days 0 and 6 following CSD. In contrast, the BDNF-like immunoreactivity in neuronal nuclei observed by confocal laser-scanning microscopy linearly increased until day 12. This indicated that the upregulation of BDNF and subsequent intranuclear translocation of BDNF-like protein was a key feature in infarct tolerance. Furthermore, it was confirmed that continuous and prolonged intracerebral infusion of exogenous recombinant BDNF induced infarct tolerance with similar histological findings of enhanced nuclear immunoreactivity for BDNF following CSD.

Key words: Infarct tolerance, Focal ischemia, Cortical spreading depression, Brain-derived neurotrophic factor, Review

Introduction

Tolerance of the brain against relatively mild stress, global ischemia, was induced by several types of preconditioning including hyperthermia, sublethal ischemia, or cortical spreading depression (CSD) in rodents [1-3]. However, induced resistance to ischemia, ischemic tolerance, was primarily limited to the most vulnerable hippocampus CA1, and the potential for neuroprotection was limited to a brief period of global ischemia of less than 8 min [4]. In our previous study aimed at enhancing cerebral tolerance to overcome focal ischemia, a repetitive CSD for 48 h was introduced as preconditioning. The prolonged CSD could be utilized in the trial to enhance ischemic tolerance since CSD itself was known to be safe in the normal brain, which is in contrast to sublethal ischemia [6-8]. After the repetitive CSD, the resistance to severe stress, focal ischemia, was enhanced up to 12 days, i.e. the lowest level cerebral infarction was observed after 12 to 15 days [8] (Fig. 1). The optimal interval between preconditioning and the peak of infarct tolerance was much longer than that previously reported, which had ranged from 1 to 4 days following a brief period of CSD [1,4,9-11]. Knowledge of the molecular mechanisms behind the tolerance to cerebral ischemia may lead to new neuroprotective interventions against cerebral damage caused by stroke. This article reviews our recent studies that examined the production-levels of brain-derived neurotrophic factor (BDNF) following prolonged CSD in the development of an enhanced ischemic tolerance; infarct tolerance, and the role of upregulated BDNF in cerebral resistance to ischemic stroke.

Methods

Repetitive CSD-preconditioning

Cortical spreading depression (CSD) was generated by a continuous infusion of 4 M potassium chloride (KCl) (1.0μl/h) for 48 h via an osmotic pump. The infusion needle was implanted at 1 mm posterior to the bregma and 4 mm left lateral to the sagittal suture in the neocortex (SSp, Fig. 2) at 2 mm depth from the cranial surface [8,12].

Quantitative measurement of BDNF-protein content

Ipsilateral cortex samples were collected on day 0 (the day of pump removal), day 6, 12, 18 or 24 after KCl- or vehicle (saline)- preconditioning and without pump implantation (normal control) (n=6, each). The homogenized samples were used for ELISA assay.

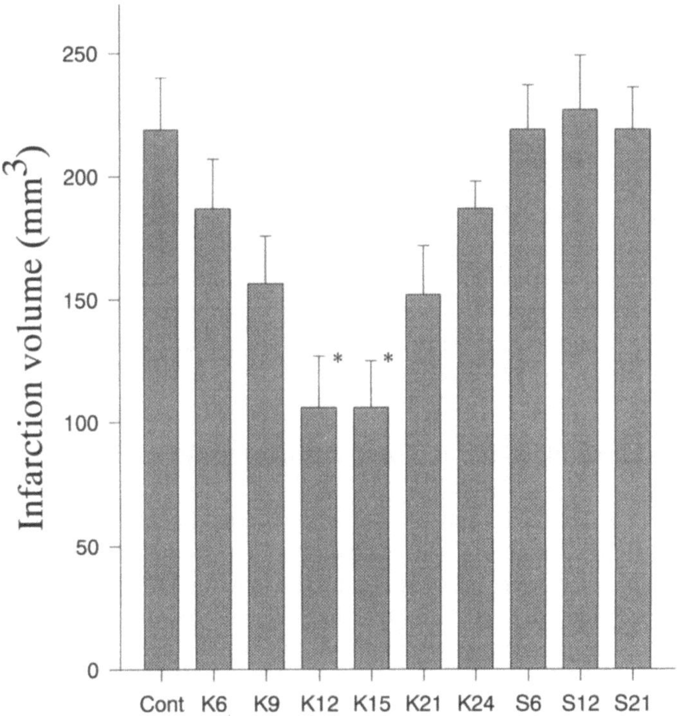

Fig. 1. The infarct tolerance phenomenon following repetitive CSD in rats. Abbreviations: 6(K6)-24(K24), 6(S6)-21(S21), days after KCl or saline-pump removal (from reference [8], with permission).

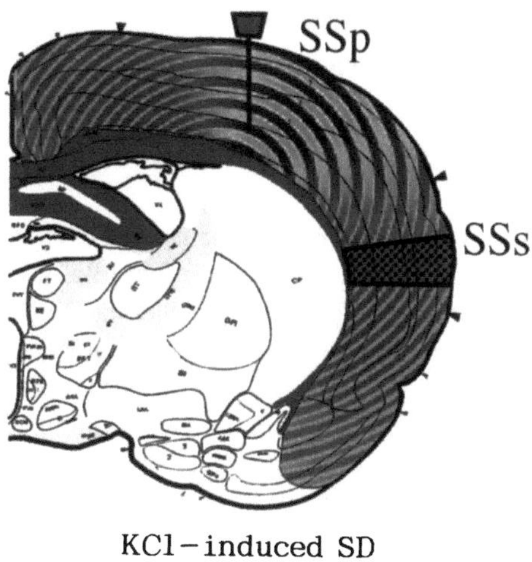

Fig. 2. The location of the needle insertion to induce CSD, the region of densitometric analysis (dotted area), the primary somatosensory area (SSp), and the supplementary somatosensory area (SSs) are all indicated on the brain map [12].

Protocols for temporary focal ischemia

The surgical procedures of this model are described elsewhere [13]. Briefly, both common carotid arteries (CCAs) and the left middle cerebral artery (MCA) were occluded for 2 h. After 2 hs of three-vessel occlusion, the microclip was removed and the neck snares released. Rectal and temporal muscle temperature, mean arterial blood pressure, blood gases (PO_2, PCO_2, pH) and the concentration of blood sugar were monitored pre, during and after ischemia. The infarction volumes were analyzed using 2,3,7-triphenyltetrazolium chloride (TTC) staining of the brain slices 2 days after ischemia. The infarction area and hemispheric areas of each section were traced using the image analysis system, and the infarction volume in each rat was calculated.

Immunohistochemical and regional densitometric analysis of BDNF

On days 0, 1, 3, 6, 12, 18 and 24 after the preconditioning, or without pump implantation (normal control) (n=6 each), rat brains were removed under deep anesthesia. The brains were immersed and fixed in methyl Carnoy's solution. The regional expression of BDNF was investigated by immunohistochemical techniques. A coronal section from each rat, 2 μm thick, taken at the SSs (Fig. 2), 1 mm posterior to the bregma, the region of interest, was employed for the densitometric analysis.

BDNF-immunoreactivity in the same brain sections was also analyzed with a laser-scanning confocal imaging system. Densitometric analyses of FITC-labeled BDNF-like immunoreactivity in the neuronal nuclei were carried out with the image from each rat taken at the SSs (Fig. 2).

After continuous infusion of rBDNF for 14 days as described below, the brains were removed and prepared for immunohistochemical analysis [14].

Intracerebral infusion of recombinant BDNF

The same amount (8 μg) of human recombinant (r)BDNF or saline for the vehicle was infused into the left neocortex using a different total infusion-period from 2.5 day to 14 days preischemia plus 2 days postischemia (Fig. 3), and the effect of temporary focal ischemia on the infarcted lesion sizes were compared (n=6, each).

In the first group, focal temporary ischemia was induced as described. In the remaining groups, a cerebral infusion cannulae was implanted at the same location as the KCl-injection in Fig. 2. In the second to the fifth group, rBDNF dissolved in 200 μl of saline with 0.2% rat albumin, set in the pump under the skin, was continuously infused for various periods. In group 2, rBDNF was infused for 2.5 days preischemia plus 2 days postischemia (injection rate, 1.92 μg /day). In group 3, rBDNF was infused for 7 days preischemia plus 2 days postischemia (injection rate, 0.96 μg /day). In group 4, rBDNF was infused for 10 days preischemia plus

2 days postischemia (injection rate, 0.72 μg /day). In group 5, rBDNF was infused for 14 days preischemia plus 2 days postischemia (injection rate, 0.54 μg /day). Focal ischemia was induced on day 2, 5, 7, 10 or 14 (day 0: the day of pump implantation), respectively. In group 6, rBDNF was infused for 14 days (injection rate, 0.54 μg /day) and focal ischemia was induced 7 days after pump removal in group 6. In groups 7 and 8, saline with 0.2% rat albumin was infused for 7 or 14 days plus 2 days postischemia, respectively. Temporary focal ischemia was induced 7 days (in group 7) or 14 days (in group 8) after pump implantation (Fig. 3).

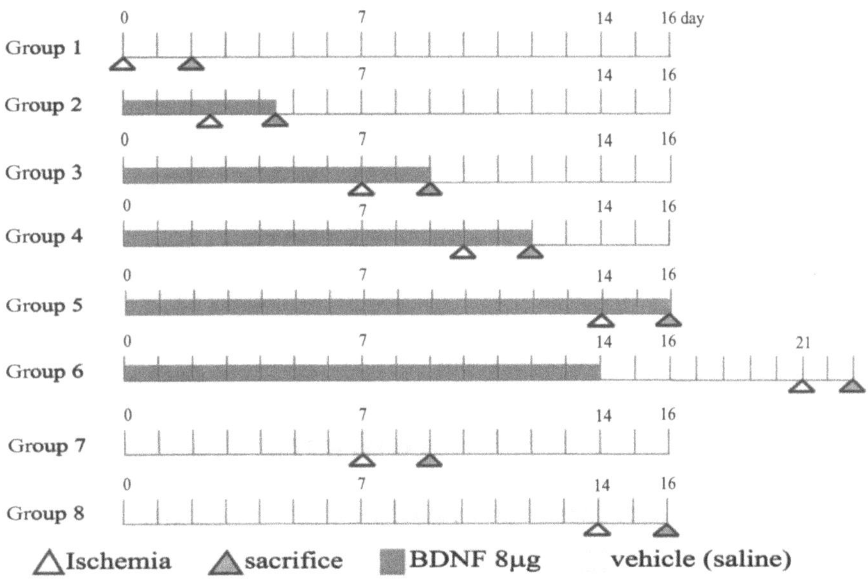

Fig. 3. The diagram shows the BDNF-treatment protocol. The volume of the neocortical infarct was assessed 2 days after the induction of focal ischemia. The osmotic mini-pump with rBDNF or vehicle remained implanted until the time of sacrifice.

Measurement of regional cerebral blood flow

The absolute rCBF values before ischemia following continuous intracerebral 8 μg BDNF or saline-injection for 14 days were monitored using a hydrogen clearance flow meter (n=5, each) [14]. In a separate set of animals on day 14 following 8 μg rBDNF or saline-infusion (n=5, each), rCBF at the point for the hydrogen clearance method was monitored before and during focal ischemia with a laser-Doppler flowmetry system. The $rCBF_{LDF}$ values during ischemia were calibrated by the preischemic $rCBF_{HC}$ value [14]. The data were analyzed by ANOVA. If multiple comparisons were indicated, the Student-Newman Keuls test was applied. The results are presented in the text as the mean ± SEM. A value of $p < 0.05$ was considered significant.

Results

Quantitative measurement of BDNF-protein content following CSD

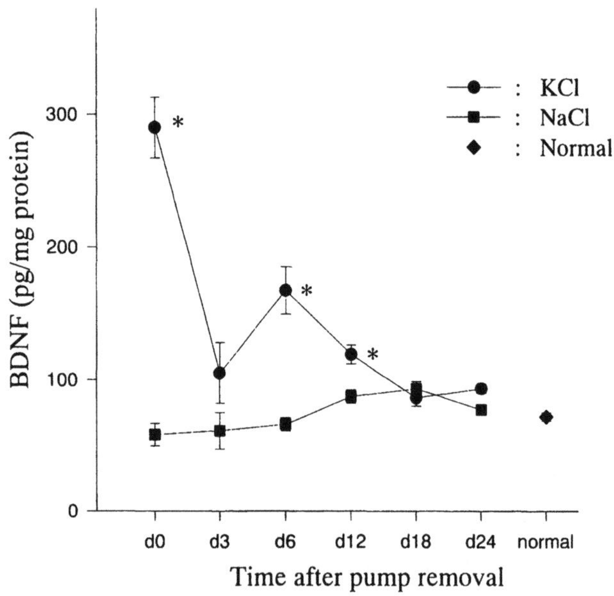

Fig. 4. The levels of BDNF protein in the rat neocortex preconditioned with saline or KCl for repetitive CSD, analyzed by ELISA. There were significant elevations in protein levels on days 0, 6 and 12 after the end of CSD compared to those in normal brain. (from reference [15], with permission).

The BDNF protein-level was significantly elevated from day 0 to 12, peaking on day 0 and 6 (Fig. 4). There was a biphasic elevation pattern consistent with that seen in the densitometric analysis (Fig. 5). However, the elevated level of BDNF protein at the acute phase analyzed by ELISA rapidly decreased following the second peak.

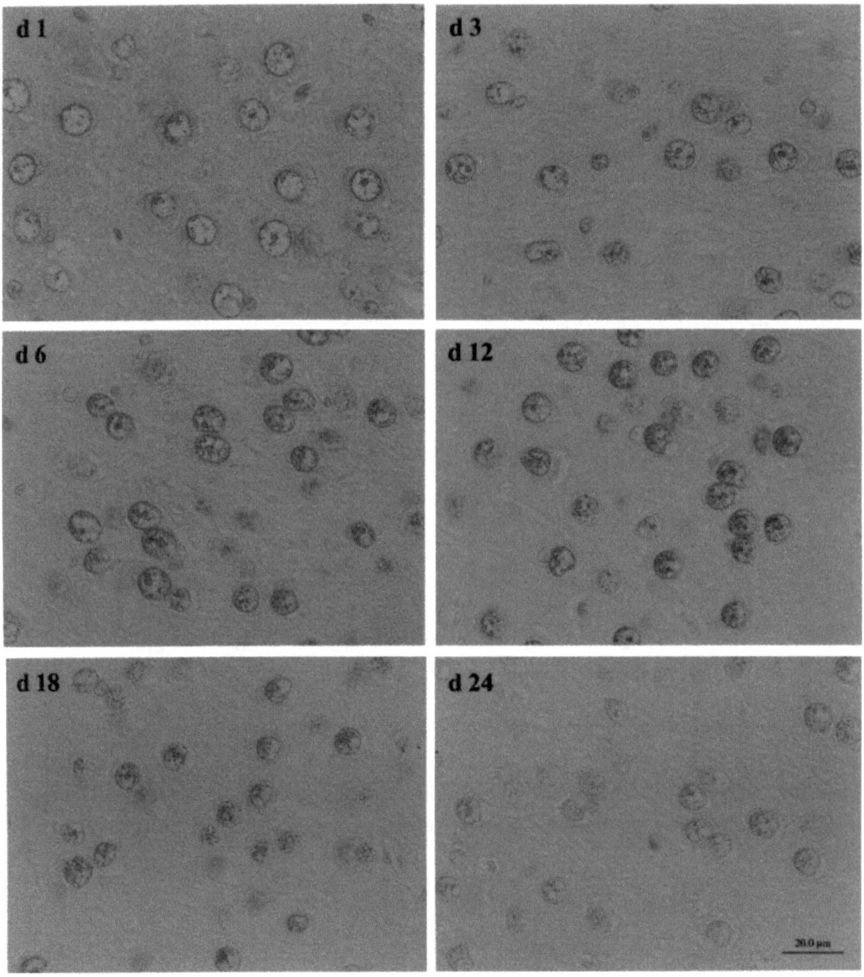

Fig. 5. The immunoreactivity for BDNF appeared strongly positive in widespread areas in the neocortex from day 1 to 18 following repetitive CSD analyzed by the indirect immunoperoxidase technique. Nuclear and background immunoreactivity was observed from day 1 to day 18, but was faint on day 24. Furthermore, the nuclear BDNF-like immunoreactivity was enhanced gradually until day 12 (from reference [15], with permission).

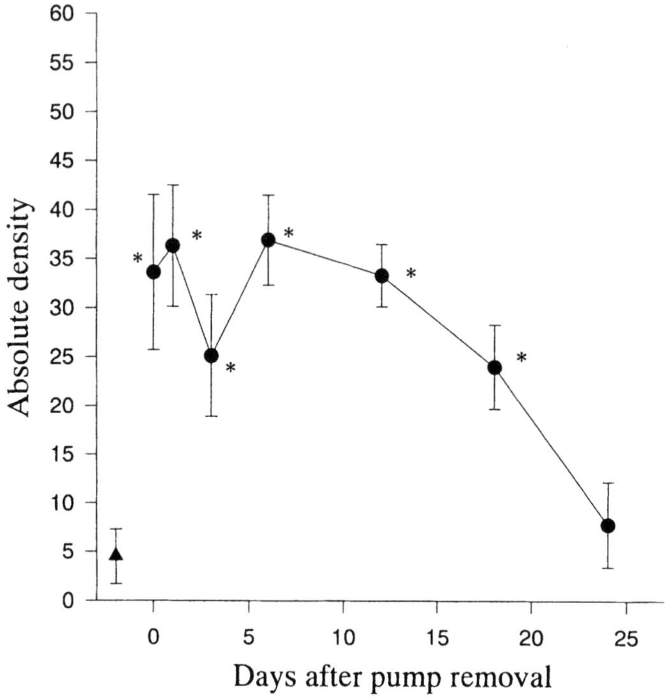

Fig. 6. The densitometric analyses of BDNF-like immunoreactivity in the neocortex in the normal cortex and neocortex following repetitive CSD at the SSs. The mean density expressing BDNF-like immunoreactivity following CSD (circle) was significantly higher from day 0 to 18 than the values of the normal neocortex (triangle) (from reference [15], with permission).

Immunohistochemical and regional densitometric analysis for BDNF following CSD

BDNF-immunoreactivity was detected primarily in neurons in a wide area of the left neocortex using indirect immunoperoxidase (Fig. 5). The elevations in the density for BDNF-like immunoreactivity were significant from days 0 to 18, peaking on day 3 and 6 following CSD (Fig. 6).

Thin slicing-images for FITC-labeled BDNF following CSD are shown in Fig. 7. There was an obvious increase in the nuclear BDNF-like immunoreactivity during the initial 12 day-period following CSD. The absolute density for BDNF-like immunoreactivity in the nuclei measured in the SSs area is shown in Fig. 8. There was a linear increase peaking on day 12 with a subsequent slight decline thereafter. The intranuclear condensation of the BDNF-like immunoreactivity correlated well with the time course of the development and enhancement of the infarct tolerance (Fig. 1) [8,15].

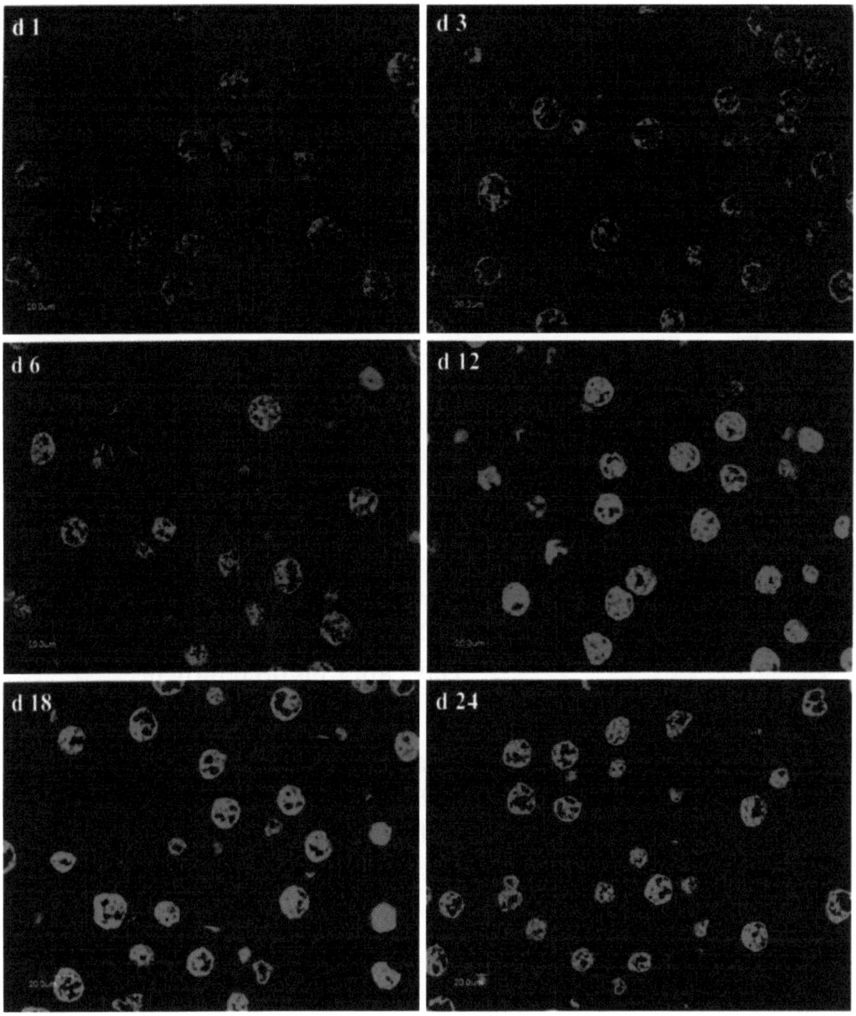

Fig. 7. The results of FITC-labeled immunostaining following repetitive CSD in the neocortex detected by laser scanning confocal imaging, on days 1, 3, 6, 12, 18 and 24. In the spatial expression of the BDNF-like immunoreactivity, only intranuclear density was observed in the thin slicing scan-images. There was a tendency for the nuclear FITC-BDNF density to increase from day 1 to day 12 (×600 originally, from reference [15], with permission).

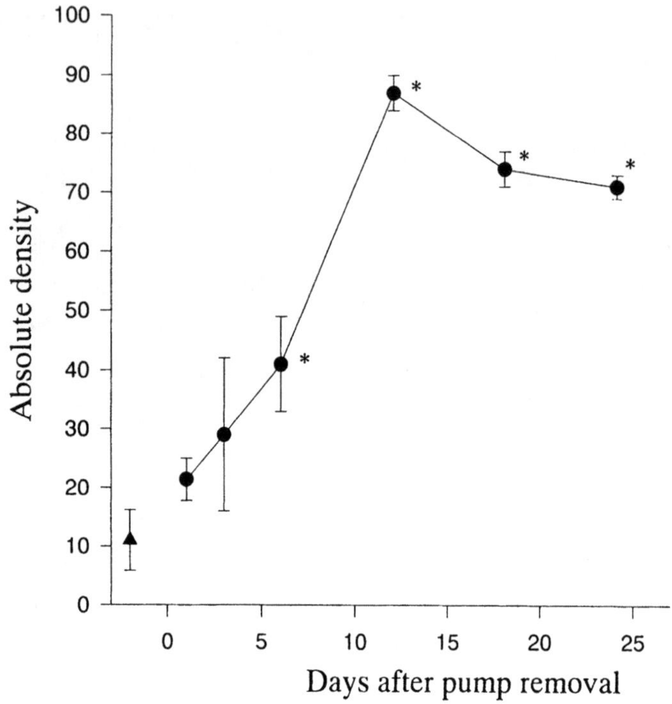

Fig. 8. The absolute density for intranuclear BDNF-like immunoreactivity visualized by FITC-labeling and laser scanning confocal imaging at the SSs. The density was constantly elevated for 12 days following repetitive CSD. There were significant differences on days 6, 12, 18, and 24 following CSD (circle) compared to the values in normal brain (triangle) (from reference [15], with permission).

Infarction volumes after temporary focal ischemia following rBDNF infusion

The values of total infarcted volume in the neocortex for all the groups following intracerebral rBDNF or vehicle infusion are shown in Fig. 9. The volume tended to decrease as the duration of intracerebral rBDNF-infusion of 8 μg of BDNF was extended. A significant tolerance to the development of cerebral infarct following focal ischemia was induced by the rBDNF-infusion only when the period of infusion was extended beyond 7 days. In contrast, there were no reductions in infarct volume in the vehicle control-group or in the group infused with 8 μg of rBDNF for 14 days in which focal ischemia was induced 7 days later (Fig. 9).

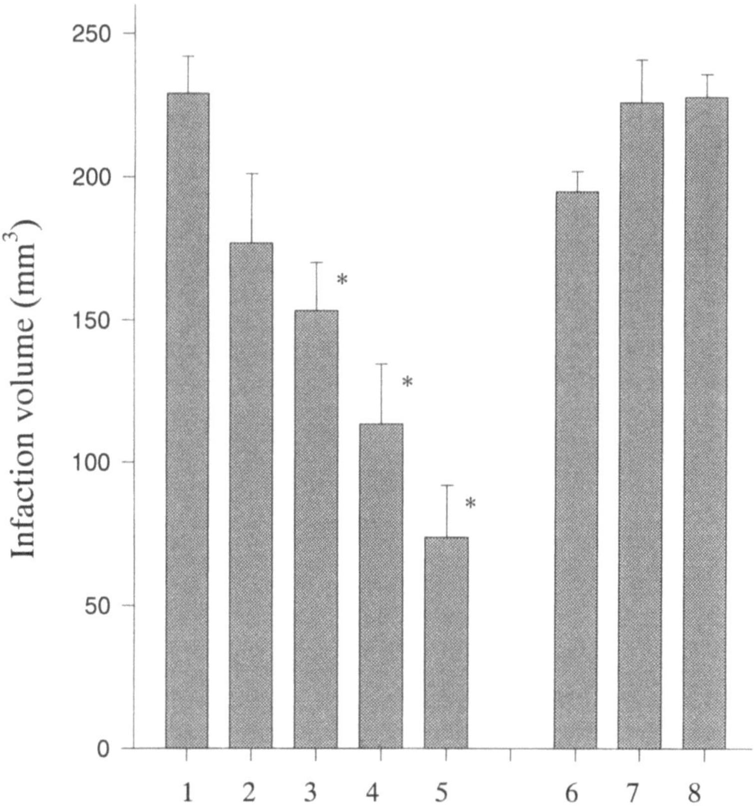

Fig. 9. The average infarction volumes. There was a tendency for the infarction volume to decrease when the duration of treatment (8 μm of rBDNF) was extended (groups 3, 4, and 5). After a 7 day-interval between the termination of intracerebral infusion for 14 days and the induction of ischemia (group 6), there was no significant reduction in infarct volume compared to that of the control or vehicle groups (from reference [14], with permission).

Measurement of regional cerebral blood flow following rBDNF infusion

The results of the rCBF values pre- and during ischemia following intracerebral 8 μg of BDNF or saline-infusion for 14 days are shown in Fig. 10. It was confirmed that the severity of ischemia was not affected, i.e. that the alteration in rCBF was not the reason for the reduction of cerebral infarction volume.

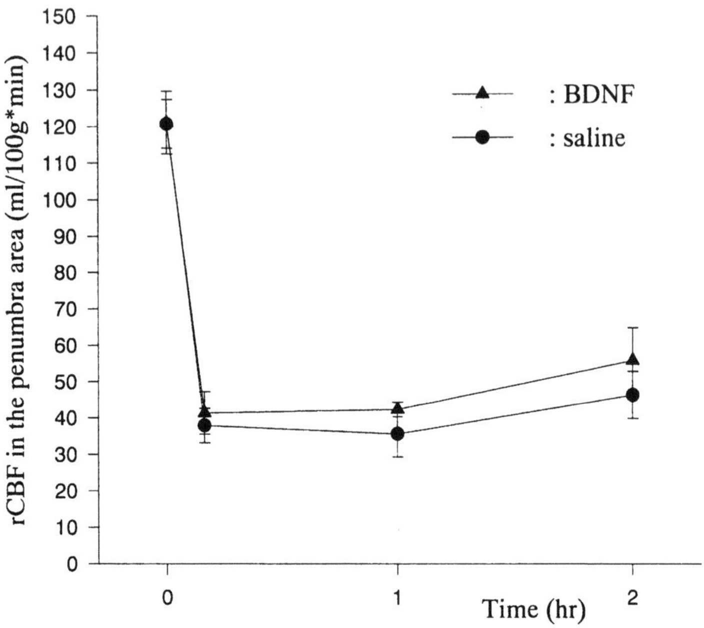

Fig. 10. Regional cerebral blood flow (rCBF) values at the left piriform cortex (penumbra area in this model) after 8 μg of rBDNF or vehicle (saline)-injection for 14 days. There was no significant difference in rCBF values during either the ischemic or postischemic period among the groups (from reference [14], with permission).

Immunohistochemical analysis of BDNF following prolonged rBDNF infusion

In the new paradigm of infarct tolerance induced by a continuous and prolonged intracerebral infusion of exogenous rBDNF, strong BDNF-like immunoreactivity was observed in the neuronal cytoplasm as well as in the background area close to the infusion-needle (Fig. 11 upper). Distant from the infusion needle, the nuclei of cortical neurons expressed intense BDNF-like immunoreactivity with a faint background density (Fig. 11 middle). The intensity of the nuclear BDNF was enhanced similar to that in the areas close to and distant from the needle after 14-day infusion (Fig. 11 upper and middle). In contrast, there was only faint staining for rBDNF in the contralateral neocortex (Fig. 11 lower). By FITC-labeled-immunostaining observed using a laser-scanning confocal microscope system, neuronal nuclear condensation was demonstrated (Fig. 12 middle and lower). In contrast, there was only weak immunostaining in the normal brain (Fig. 12 upper). In the paradigm of infarct tolerance following prolonged exposure to intrinsic, or exogenous BDNF, intranuclear condensation of the immunoreactivity for BDNF-like substance was a common feature.

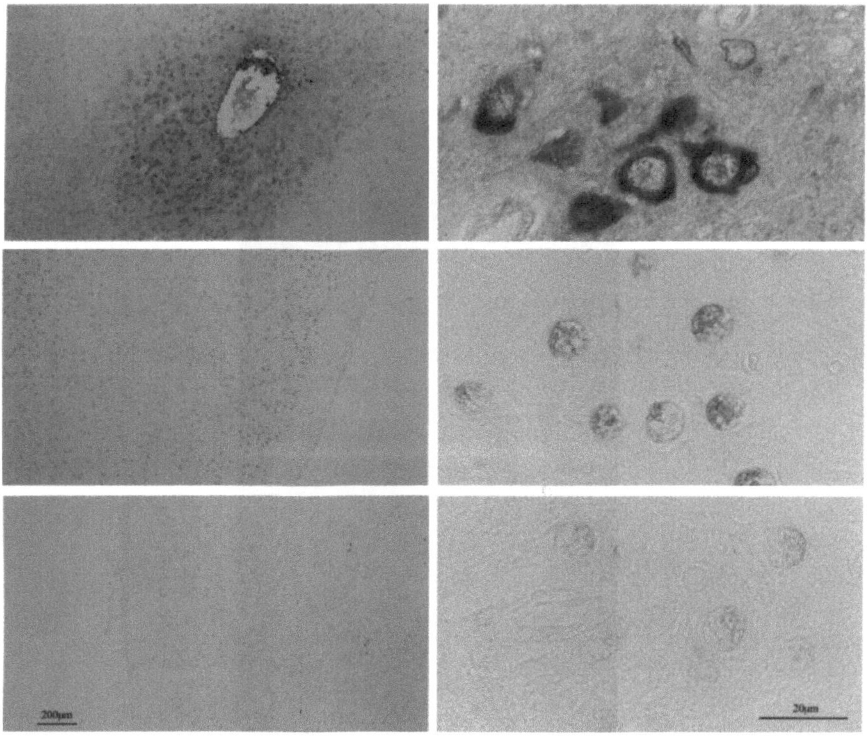

Fig. 11. The immunoreactivity for rBDNF in brain sections after a 14-day intracortical infusion (8μg in total) at the time when the ipsilateral neocortex achieved infarct tolerance. Strong immunoreactivity was demonstrated in the brain tissue limited to around the tip of the infusion needle (upper left). The neurons contained immunoreactivity both in the perikarya and the nuclei (upper right). In the area distant from the needle, enhanced immunoreactivity was detected in nuclei (middle panels). Faint immunoreactivity for rBDNF was detected in the nuclei of the contralateral neocortex (lower panels) (Left: ×40; Right: ×600 originally, from reference [14], with permission).

Discussions

The "ischemic tolerance" phenomenon was first reported by Kitagawa et al. in gerbils in 1990 [1]. Sublethal ischemia was used as an ischemic preconditioning, which induced neuronal resistance in the most vulnerable neurons against subsequent forebrain ischemia. Using the ischemic tolerance model, the molecular mechanisms in intrinsic resistance to ischemia have been studied to determine the neuronal survival-promoting mechanisms involved. The production of heat-shock proteins (hsps), especially hsp70 (72), had been considered a key feature for generating ischemic tolerance [9,10,16-18]. A brief period of sublethal global ischemia increased the synthesis of hsp70 in the hippocampus, which accompanied ischemic tolerance following sublethal ischemia [1].

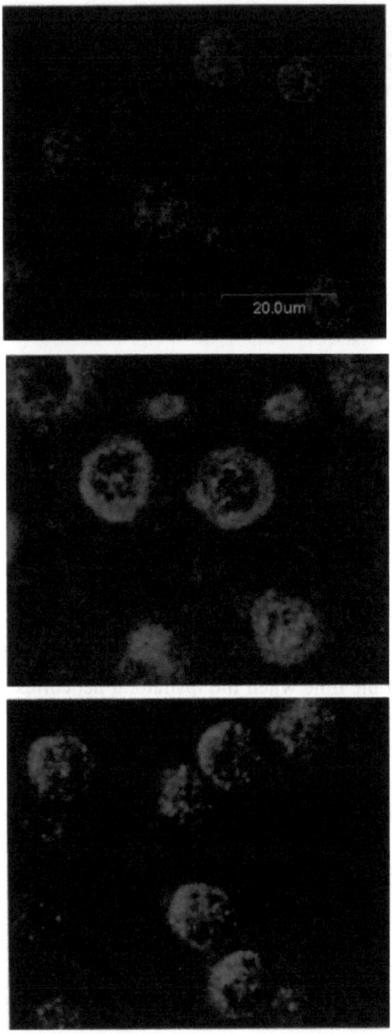

Fig. 12. The immunoreactivity for FITC-labeled BDNF. There was a weak staining for BDNF in the nuclei in the neocortex of the normal rat (upper panel). After continuous intracerebral infusion of rBDNF for 14 days (8μg in total), at the time when the ipsilateral neocortex was resistant to temporary focal ischemia, strong immunoreactivity for BDNF was detected in the perikarya as well as in the nuclei of neurons in the neocortex in the area close to the infusion site (middle panel). Enhanced immunoreactivity for rBDNF was also detected in the neuronal nuclei at the remote area of the infusion needle (lower panel) (×600 originally) (from reference [14], with permission).

However, a limitation in the neuroprotective effect of hsp70 was also demonstrated [4]. Later, it was found that CSD evoked by KCl application over the dura without ischemia similarly induced a resistance in hippocampus CA1 neurons against brief global ischemia with a 3-day interval [19]. In general, sublethal ischemia is linked to neuronal depolarization (anoxic depolarization), which creates CSD involving the surrounding brain tissues [20-22]. Therefore, CSD is part of the components of ischemic stress that induce anoxic depolarization. It had been reported that the expression of hsp70 mRNA was not elevated following KCl-induced CSD [23]. In 1995, induction of ischemic tolerance was confirmed to occur without any significant induction of hsp70 protein in rat neocortex [5]. We also confirmed that hsp70 immunoreactivity was not detected in the brain during the achievement of infarct tolerance [15]. The report that the duration of postischemic depolarization necessary for the induction of the ischemic tolerance was much shorter than that necessary for upregulation of hsp70 explains the lack of hsp70 expression following CSD [24]. Given the available evidence, the induction of hsp70 is not an essential factor in the induction of ischemic/infarct tolerance, although the postulated neuroprotective effects of hsp70 are not denied [25].

CSD has been known to induce c-fos RNA, c-fos-like immunoreactivity encoding transcription factors, nerve growth factor (NGF) mRNA, BDNF mRNA and BDNF in neurons through the activation of voltage-sensitive calcium channels [5,26-31]. BDNF was found at extremely low levels in the nervous system in 1982 [32-34], which has consequently been shown to be neuroprotective *in vivo* [35-39]. In a recent study designed to elucidate the mechanism of ischemic tolerance in the hippocampus, BDNF mRNA was upregulated in the ipsilateral cortex 0 to 4 h after a brief period of CSD (2 h), but not in the ipsilateral hippocampus for 7 days [40,41]. The result did not explain the phenomenon of ischemic tolerance by the local BDNF-expression, since the tolerance was observed in the hippocampus peaking at 3 days after the CSD. In the case of ischemic preconditioning, BDNF mRNA was not upregulated in the hippocampus CA1 either [42-43]. Although, the CA1 sector does not induce BDNF mRNA after CSD, it is possible that upregulated BDNF in the cortex after CSD is transferred to the hippocampus within 3 days (through retrograde axonal transport and following intranuclear translocation) and may contribute to the ischemic tolerance in the CA1, given that BDNF could be transported within the brain via the neurons [44]. However, it is probably difficult to detect the "BDNF transported to CA1", if any, by means of the two-site ELISA assay [40], since the intranuclear BDNF-like (in which the structure is possibly modified from the native form) protein visualized in the neocortex by immunohistochemical analysis was not detected by the ELISA assay (Fig. 3 and 5). The intranuclear BDNF-like protein may have undergone molecular processing to become lucent for ELISA assay-detection.

In 1991, Wetmore et al. reported that BDNF-like immunoreactivity was observed in the cytoplasm, dendrites, and nuclei in neurons of adult rat brain [45].

The immunoreactivity was detected in BDNF mRNA-expressing and non-expressing neurons. It was speculated that "one form" of the BDNF protein enters the neuronal nucleus following dendro-axonic interneuronal transfer, internalization, and retrograde axonal transport, and influences transcription in postmitotic neurons in the brain. The active transport mechanism of BDNF inside the neurons following the receptor-ligand-initiated signal transduction and rapid (8-16 μm/sec) retrograde signal transduction was later reported [46-48]. Exogenous rBDNF enters neurons by phosphorylated TrkB-internalization, moves in axons toward cell bodies and enters the nuclei in mature neurons [49]. The enhanced immunoreactivity for rBDNF in the neurons around the infusion-needle observed in our study may represent rapid internalization combined with the TrkB receptor in the cortical neurons and the subsequent intracellular retrograde transport to neuronal perikarya [50-52]. In contrast, the possible transport from the neuronal perikarya to the intra-nuclei observed in the whole cortical areas was a delayed phenomenon.

An autocrine or paracrine role for central BDNF has been also postulated. [53-56]. The observation that a subpopulation of CA1 hippocampal neurons coexpressing the high-affinity tyrosine kinase receptor for BDNF, TrkB and BDNF were resistant to transient forebrain ischemia suggests that a BDNF/TrkB-autocrine loop is regulating autologous cell survival in these neurons [54]. The expression of TrkB is primarily restricted to the nervous system and TrkB mRNA has been detected at high levels in hippocampal pyramidal neurons [55,56]. In addition, TrkB immunoreactivity was widespread in the adult rat, including in the cerebral cortex, and on the surface of neuronal cell bodies, axons and dendrites [49].

Following global ischemia, the levels of BDNF mRNA and protein were increased in the rat hippocampus dentate gyrus, which is known to be resistant to a brief global ischemia [42-43]. The stress of temporary focal ischemia also elevated the expression of BDNF mRNA, TrkB mRNA, and TrkB protein in the cortex [57-59]. The BDNF and TrkB mRNA upregulation followed by the increase in protein synthesis triggered by ischemic stress suggests that intrinsic defense mechanisms against ischemic stress exist in neurons. Possible intracellular (outside of nuclei) cascades in the downstream of TrkB receptor-tyrosine kinase could be related to phospholipase C (PLC)-γ, sucassociated neurotrophic factor-induced tyrosine-phosphorylated target (SNT), Shc, Ras, Raf, MAP kinase and PI-3 kinase [60-66]. Recently, clathrin-mediated signal-transduction of neurotrophin was postulated from axon terminals to cell bodies with internalized activated receptors and Erk1/2 attached to the vesicles leading to the activation of Elk (signaling endosome hypothesis) [67,68]. However, the signal transductions are considered to proceed within hours after the cell-contact of BDNF. To clarify the mechanisms of "extremely slowly progressive and prolonged signal-transduction from cytoplasm to the nucleus" requires further investigation.

In hippocampal slice cultures exposed to the stress of oxygen and glucose deprivation, pre but not post-ischemic addition of rBDNF reduced neuronal damage [69]. Furthermore, in global ischemia, exogenously administered intraventricular rBDNF (pre and post-treatment, infusion rate: 0.3 μg /day, or 1.44 μg /day post-treatment) reportedly prevented ischemic neuronal death in the hippocampus CA1 *in vivo* [37,70]. In addition, in focal ischemia, intraventricular infusion of rBDNF (infusion rate, 2.1 μg /day, started 24 h before ischemia and continued for 7 days postischemia) significantly reduced the infarct volume of the neocortex assessed 7 days after permanent focal ischemia in rats [71]. Following these results, we also tried the intraventricular infusion of rBDNF (infusion rate, 1.92 μg /day) for 2.5 days prior to, during, and for 2 days after temporary focal ischemia. However, the treatment did not reduce the volume of neocortical infarct as assessed 2 days after ischemia (data not shown). Concerning the distribution of BDNF following intraventricular administration, it has been reported that intraventricularly administered radio-labeled rBDNF did not penetrate the brain parenchyma, but remained on the ventricular walls 20 h after ventricular injection, and only intraparenchymal injections of rBDNF resulted in transport throughout the CNS [46,72]. In our previous study using intracerebral infusion of another growth factor, platelet-derived growth factor-BB (PDGF-BB) to induce infarct tolerance, continuous infusions for more than 7 days were necessary to achieve significant reductions of infarcted lesion following focal ischemia [73]. The precise effects of the intraventricular or intracerebral administration of BDNF on the brain damage following temporary focal ischemia and the histological evidence in terms of the distribution of exogenous rBDNF requires further clarification.

More rapid and effective neuroprotection has been reported using intravenous administration of rBDNF against focal ischemia in rats [74]. Despite the results, we could not reproduce positive protective effects by intravenous administration of rBDNF (a gift from Regeneron Pharmaceuticals, Inc, NY, through Sumitomo Pharmaceuticals Co Ltd. Research Center, Osaka) in our focal ischemia model, since systemically delivered BDNF, which is not transported across the blood-brain barrier (BBB), did not reduce the infarction size, although BDNF should enter the brain after the breakdown of the BBB during or after ischemia [74]. Considering the timing of the BBB-destruction after temporary focal ischemia, it may be too late to protect the brain at risk *in vivo* [75,76]. We have yet to find an effective protocol for demonstrating neuroprotection by a simple systemic or local administration of BDNF "after" the onset of focal ischemia. Hopefully, any positive results of reduced infarction sizes should be confirmed in other laboratories before clinical trials, since many positive data on drug-treatments for experimental cerebral infarction cannot be reproduced (personal communication). Recently, it was reported that intravenous administration of BDNF conjugated to a drug designed to pass through the BBB reduced the size of cortical infarction [77].

In search of downstream cascades of the repetitive CSD, we have performed a microarray analysis for the brain to detect inducible gene products that may enhance the endogenous defense system against, or which may accelerate recovery function following ischemic stress by using the brain that is in the process of achieving infarct tolerance [78, 79]. From the microarray analysis, genes related to DNA damage and repair, GADD45 and PCNA [80-84] were upregulated in the neocortex following CSD. Since ischemia and reperfusion are known to induce oxidative stress, free radicals [85-90], and subsequent oxidative DNA damage before neuronal cell death [91-94], the defense mechanism for the ischemic DNA damage may be altered following CSD to a level designed to protect the brain from focal ischemia.

The repetitive CSD upregulated BDNF in the neocortex during the process to infarct tolerance. Prolonged exposure to exogenous rBDNF to the normal brain triggered survival-promoting signals against focal ischemia, developing infarct tolerance. In both cases, the brain with infarct tolerance expressed enhanced immunoreactivity for BDNF in the nuclei. The key mechanisms behind the potent survival promoting cascades in neurons after prolonged exposure to BDNF should be elucidated to provide new strategies for protecting or rescuing the brain from ischemic stroke.

Acknowledgment: These studies were supported by Special Coordination Funds for the Promotion of Science and Technology, a Grant-in-Aid for Scientific Research, from the Ministry of Education, Culture, Sports, Science and Technology (MEXT) of Japan, and by a grant from The Japan Health Sciences Foundation. We acknowledge the valuable assistance of Yasuda T, Okuno A, Kurimoto M, and Nishimori K.

References

1. Kitagawa K, Matsumoto M, Tagaya M, et al (1990) 'Ischemic tolerance' phenomenon found in the brain. Brain Res 528:21-24
2. Kitagawa K, Matsumoto M, Tagaya M, et al (1991) Hyperthermia-induced neuroprotection against ischemic injury in gerbils. J Cereb Blood Flow Metab 11:449-452
3. Chopp M, Chen H, Ho K-L, et al (1989) Transient hyperthermia protects against subsequent forebrain ischemic cell damage in the rat. Neurology 39:1396-1398
4. Liu Y, Kato H, Nakata N, et al (1992) Protection of rat hippocampus against ischemic neuronal damage by pretreatment with sublethal ischemia. Brain Res 586:121-124
5. Kobayashi S, Harris VA, Welsh FA (1995) Spreading depression induces tolerance of cortical neurons to ischemia in rat brain. J Cereb Blood Flow Metab 15:721-727
6. Nedergaard M, Hansen AJ (1988) Spreading depression is not associated with neuronal injury in the normal brain. Brain Res 449:395-398
7. Gehrmann J, Mies G, Bonnekoh P, et al (1993) Microglial reaction in the rat cerebral cortex induced by cortical spreading depression. Brain Path 3:11-17
8. Yanamoto H, Hashimoto N, Nagata I, et al (1998) Infarct tolerance against temporary focal ischemia following spreading depression in rat brain. Brain Res 784:239-249

9. Kitagawa K, Matsumoto M, Kuwabara K, et al (1991) 'Ischemic tolerance' phenomenon detected in various brain regions. Brain Res 561:203-211
10. Kirino T, Tsujita Y, Tamura A (1991) Induced tolerance to ischemia in gerbil hippocampal neurons. J Cereb Blood Flow Metab 11:299-307
11. Kato H, Liu Y, Araki T, et al (1991) Temporal profile of the effects of pretreatment with brief cerebral ischemia on the neuronal damage following secondary ischemic insult in the gerbil: cumulative damage and protective effects. Brain Res 553:238-242
12. Swanson LW (1992) Brain maps. Structure of the rat brain. Elsevier, New York, pp 102-103
13. Yanamoto H, Nagata I, Hashimoto N, et al (1998) Three-vessel occlusion using a micro-clip for the proximal left middle cerebral artery produces a reliable neocortical infarct in rats. Brain Res Protoc 3:209-220
14. Yanamoto H, Nagata I, Sakata M, et al (2000) Infarct tolerance induced by intra-cerebral infusion of recombinant brain-derived neurotrophic factor. Brain Res 3:240-248
15. Yanamoto H, Mizuta I, Nagata I, et al (2000) Infarct tolerance accompanied enhanced BDNF-like immunoreactivity in neuronal nuclei. Brain Res 877:331-344
16. Nishi S, Taki W, Uemura Y, et al (1993) Ischemic tolerance due to the induction of HSP70 in a rat ischemic recirculation model. Brain Res 615:281-288
17. Glazier SS, O'Rourke DM, Graham DI, et al (1994) Induction of ischemic tolerance following brief focal ischemia in rat brain. J Cereb Blood Flow Metab 14:545-553
18. Liu Y, Kato H, Nakata N, et al (1993) Temporal profile of heat shock protein 70 synthesis in ischemic tolerance induced by preconditioning ischemia in rat hippocampus. Neuroscience 56:921-927
19. Kawahara N, Ruetzler CA, Klatzo I (1995) Protective effect of spreading depression against neuronal damage following cardiac arrest cerebral ischemia. Neurol Res 17:9-16
20. Back T, Kohno K, Hossmann K-A (1994) Cortical negative DC deflections following middle cerebral artery occlusion and KCl-induced spreading depression: Effect on blood flow, tissue oxygenation, and electroencephalogram. J Cereb Blood Flow Metab 14:12-19
21. Nedergaard M, Hansen AJ (1993) Characterization of cortical depolarizations evoked in focal cerebral ischemia. J Cereb Blood Flow Metab 13:568-574
22. Iijima T, Mies G, Hossmann K-A (1992) Repeated negative DC deflections in rat cortex following middle cerebral artery occlusion are abolished by MK-801: Effect on volume of ischemic injury. J Cereb Blood Flow Metab 12:727-733
23. Nowak TSJr, Osborne OC, Mies G (1991) Cortical spreading depression induces the proto-oncogene, c-fos, but not the stress protein, hsp70. J Cereb Blood Flow Metab 11:S215
24. Abe H., Xue Z-C, Nowak TSJr (1995) Threshold depolarization intervals for ischemic tolerance vs. expression of HSP72 and other ischemia-induced mRNAs. J Cereb Blood Flow Metab 15:S67
25. Rajdev S, Hara K, Kokubo Y, et al (2000) Mice overexpressing rat heat shock protein 70 are protected against cerebral infarction. Ann Neurol 47:782-791
26. Herdegen T, Sandkuhler J, Gass P, et al (1993) JUN, FOS, KROX, and CREB transcription factor proteins in the rat cortex: basal expression and induction by spreading depression and epileptic seizures. J Comp Neurol 333:271-288

27. Herrera DG, Robertson HA (1990) Application of potassium chloride to the brain surface induces the c-fos protooncogene: reversal by MK-801: effect on volume of ischemic injury. Brain Res 510:166-170
28. Herrera DG, Maysinger D, Gadient R, et al (1993) Spreading depression induces c-fos-like immunoreactivity and NGF mRNA in the rat cerebral cortex. Brain Res 602:99-103
29. Kokaia Z, Gido G, Ringstedt T, et al (1993) Rapid increase of BDNF mRNA levels in cortical neurons following spreading depression: regulation by glutamatergic mechanisms independent of seizure activity. Mol Brain Res 19:277-286
30. Takahashi M, Hayashi S, Kakita A, et al (1999) Patients with temporal lobe epilepsy show an increase in brain-derived neurotrophic factor protein and its correlation with neuropeptide Y. Brain Res 13:579-582
31. Ghosh A, Carnahan J, Greenberg ME (1994) Requirement of BDNF in activity-dependent survival of cortical neurons. Science 263:1618-1623
32. Barde Y-A, Rdgar D, Thoenen H (1982) Purification of a new neurotrophic factor from mammalian brain. EMBO J 1:549-553
33. Leibrock J, Lottspeich F, Hohn A, et al (1989) Molecular cloning and expression of brain-derived neurotrophic factor. Nature 341:149-152
34. McDonald NQ, Lapatto R, Murray-Rust J, et al (1991) New protein fold revealed by a 2.3-A resolution crystal structure of nerve growth factor. Nature 354:411-414
35. Barde Y-A (1989) Trophic factors and neuronal survival. Neuron 2:1525-1534
36. Beck T, Lindholm D, Castren E, et al (1994) Brain-derived neurotrophic factor protects against ischemic cell damage in rat hippocampus. J Cereb Blood Flow Metab 14:689-692
37. Acheson A, Conover JC, Fandl JP, et al (1995) A BDNF autocrine loop in adult sensory neurons prevents cell death. Nature 374:450-453
38. Hofer MM, Barde Y-A (1988) Brain-derived neurotrophic factor prevents neuronal death *in vivo*. Nature 331:261-262
39. Endres M, Fan G, Hirt L, et al (2000) Ischemic brain damage in mice after selectively modifying BDNF or NT4 gene expression. J Cereb Blood Flow Metab 20:139-144
40. Kawahara N, Croll SD, Wiegand SJ, et al (1997) Cortical spreading depression induces long-term alterations of BDNF levels in cortex and hippocampus distinct from lesion effects: implications for ischemic tolerance. Neurosci Res 29:37-47
41. Kariko K, Harris VA, Rangel Y, et al (1998) Effect of cortical spreading depression on the levels of mRNA coding for putative neuroprotective proteins in rat brain. J Cereb Blood Flow Metab 18:1308-1315
42. Lindvall O, Ernfors P, Bengzon J, et al (1992) Differential regulation of mRNAs for nerve growth factor, brain-derived neurotrophic factor, and neurotrophin 3 in the adult rat brain following cerebral ischemia and hypoglycemic coma. Proc Natl Acad Sci U.S.A. 89:648-652
43. Kokaia Z, Nawa H, Uchino H, et al (1996) Regional brain-derived neurotrophic factor mRNA and protein levels following transient forebrain ischemia in the rat. Mol Brain Res 38:139-144
44. Mafson EJ, Kroin JS, Sendera TJ, et al (1999) Distribution and retrograde transport of trophic factors in the central nervous system: functional implications for the treatment of neurodegenerative diseases. Prog Neurobiol 57:451-484

45. Wetmore C, Cao YH, Pettersson RF, et al (1991) Brain-derived neurotrophic factor: subcellular compartmentalization and interneuronal transfer as visualized with anti-peptide antibodies. Proc Natl Acad Sci U.S.A. 88:9843-9847
46. Bhattacharyya A, Watspm FA, Bradlee TA, et al (1997) Trk receptors function as rapid retrograde signal carriers in the adult nervous system. J Neurosci 17:7007-7016
47. Bhattacharyya A., Watson FL, Zhang Y, et al (1998) Immunolocalization of the neurotrophin signaling complex within sciatic nerve axons. Soc Neurosci Abst 24:705.2
48. Watson FL, Bhattacharyya A, Moheban D, et al (1998) Retrograde signaling in dorsal root ganglia neurons by target-derived neurotrophins. Soc Neurosci Abst 24:705.3
49. Yan Q, Radeke MJ, Matheson CR, et al (1997) Immunocytochemical localization of TrkB in the central nervous system of the adult rat. J Comp Neurol 378:135-157
50. Middlemas DS, Lindberg RA, Hunter T (1991) trkB, a neural receptor protein-tyrosine kinase: evidence for a full-length and two truncated receptors. Mol Cell Biol 11:143-153
51. Soppet D, Escandon E, Maragos J, et al (1991) The neurotrophic factors brain-derived neurotrophic factor and neurotrophin-3 are ligands for the trkB tyrosine kinase receptor. Cell 65:895-903
52. Squinto SP, Stitt TN, Aldrich TH, et al (1991) trkB encodes a functional receptor for brain-derived neurotrophic factor and neurotrophin-3 but not nerve growth factor. Cell 65:885-893
53. Bothwell M (1991) Keeping track of neurotrophin receptors. Cell 65:915-918
54. Ferrer I, Ballabriga J, Marti E, et al (1997) BDNF and TrkB co-localize in CA1 neurons resistant to transient forebrain ischemia in the adult gerbil. J Neuropathol Exp Neurol 56:790-797
55. Klein R, Martin-Zanca D, Barbacid M, et al (1990) Expression of the tyrosine kinase receptor gene trkB is confined to the murine embryonic and adult nervous system. Development 109:845-850
56. Klein R, Parada LF, Coulier F, et al (1989) trkB, a novel tyrosine protein kinase receptor expressed during mouse neural development. EMBO 8:3701-3709
57. Kokaia Z, Zhao Q, Kokaia M, et al (1995) Regulation of brain-derived neurotrophic factor gene expression after transient middle cerebral artery occlusion with and without brain damage. Exp Neurol 136:73-88
58. Arai S, Kinouchi H, Akabane A, et al (1996) Induction of brain-derived neurotrophic factor (BDNF) and the receptor trk B mRNA following middle cerebral artery occlusion in rat. Neurosci Lett 211:57-60
59. Merlio J-P, Ernfors P, Kokaia Z, et al (1993) Increased production of the trkB protein tyrosine kinase receptor after brain insults. Neuron 10:151-164
60. Atwal JK, Massie B, Miller FD, et al (1998) Analysis of trk signal transduction pathways in the growth and survival of sympathetic neurons. Soc Neurosci Abst 24:514.4
61. Rabin SJ, Cleghon V, Kaplan DR (1993) SNT, a differentiation-specific target of neurotrophic factor-induced tyrosine activity in neurons and PC12 cells. Mol Cell Biol 13:2203-2213
62. Ginty DD, Bonni A, Greenberg ME (1994) Nerve growth factor activates a Ras-dependent protein kinase that stimulates c-fos transcription via phosphorylation of CREB. Cell 77:713-725

63. Kaplan DR, Stephens RM (1994) Neurotrophin signal transduction by the Trk receptor. J Neurobiol 25:1404-1417
64. Stephens RM, Loeb DM, Copeland TD, et al (1994) Trk receptors use redundant signal transduction pathways involving SHC and PLC-gamma 1 to mediate NGF responses. Neuron 12:691-705
65. van der Geer P, Wiley S, Lai VK, et al (1995) A conserved amino-terminal Shc domain binds to phosphotyrosine motifs in activated receptors and phosphopeptides. Curr Biol 1:404-412
66. Mazzoni IE, Paquet L, Miller FD, et al (1998) Multiple Ras signal transduction pathways differentially affect neuronal cell survival. Soc Neurosci Abst 24:514.6
67. Howe CL, Valletta JS, Rusnak AS, et al (2001) NGF signaling from clathrin-coated vesicles: evidence that endosomes serve as a platform for the Ras-MAPK pathway. Neuron 32:801-814
68. Beattie EC, Howe CL, Wilde A, et al (2000) NGF signals through TrkA to increase clathrin at the plasma membrane and enhance clathrin-mediated membrane traffic. J Neurosci 20:7325-7333
69. Pringle AK, Sundstrom LE, Wilde GJC, et al (1996) Brain-derived neurotrophic factor, but not neurotrophin-3, prevents ischaemia-induced neuronal cell death in organotypic rat hippocampal slice cultures. Neurosci Lett 211:203-206
70. Kiprianova I, Freiman TM, Desiderato S, et al (1999) Brain-derived neurotrophic factor prevents neuronal death and glial activation after global ischemia in the rat. J Neurosci Res 1:21-27
71. Schabitz WR, Schwab S, Spranger M, et al (1997) Intraventricular brain-derived neurotrophic factor reduces infarct size after focal cerebral ischemia in rats. J Cereb Blood Flow Metab 17:500-506
72. Yan Q, Matheson C, Sun J, et al (1994) Distribution of intracerebral ventricularly administered neurotrophins in rat brain and its correlation with Trk receptor expression. Exp Neurol 127:23-36
73. Sakata M, Yanamoto H, Hashimoto N, et al (1998) Induction of infarct tolerance by pletelet-derived growth factor against temporary focal ischemia. Brain Res 784:250-255
74. Schabitz WR, Sommer C, Zoder W, et al (1999) Effect of intravenous brain-derived neurotrophic factor in infarct size and apoptosis after focal cerebral ischemia. J.Cereb.Blood Flow Metab 19:S134
75. Pardridge WM, Kang YS, Buciak JL (1994) Transport of human recombinant brain-derived neurotrophic factor (BDNF) through the rat blood-brain barrier *in vivo* using vector-mediated peptide drug delivery. Cell 65:915-918
76. Yanamoto H, Hashimoto N, Kassell NF, et al (1996) Disruption of blood brain barrier triggered by reperfusion following transient focal ischemia in rats. Soc Neurosci Abst 838.3
77. Zhang Y, Pardridge WM (2001) Neuroprotection in transient focal brain ischemia after delayed intravenous administration of brain-derived neurotrophic factor conjugated to a blood-brain barrier drug targeting system. Stroke 32:1378-1384
78. Xue J-H, Tohnai N, Nagata I, et al (2001) Cortical spreading depression up-regulates DNA damage-inducible gene gadd45 and proliferating cell nuclear antigen (PCNA) in rat brain. Soc Neurosci Abst 27:205.12

79. Xue J-H, Yanamoto H, Nagata I, et al (2001) Cortical spreading depression up-regulates the growth arrest and DNA damage-inducible gene (GADD45) in rata brain. J Cereb Blood Flow Metab 21:S240
80. Nichols AF, Sancar A (1992) Purification of PCNA as a nucleotide excision repair protein. Nucleic Acids Res 20:2441-2446
81. Hollander MC, Alamo I, Jackman J, et al (1993) Analysis of the mammalian *gadd45* gene and its response to DNA damage. J Biol Chem 268:24385-24393
82. Hall PA, Kearsey JM, Coates PJ, et al (1995) Characterization of the interaction between PCNA and Gadd45. Oncogene 10:2427-2433
83. Fornace AJJr, Nebert DW, Hollander MC, et al (1989) Mammalian genes coordinately regulated by growth arrest signals and DNA-damaging agents. Mol Cell Biol 9:4196-4203
84. Fornace AJJr, Alamo IJr, Hollander MC (1988) DNA damage-inducible transcripts in mammalian cells. Proc Natl Acad Sci U.S.A. 85:8800-8804
85. Kil HY, Zhang J, Piantadosi CA (1996) Brain temperature alters hydroxyl radical production during cerebral ischemia/reperfusion in rats. J Cereb Blood Flow Metab 16:100-106
86. Piantadosi CA, Zhang J (1996) Mitochondrial generation of reactive oxygen species after brain ischemia in the rat. Stroke 27:327-332
87. Solenski N, Kwan A-L, Yanamoto H, et al (1997) Differential hydroxylation of salicylate in core and penumbra regions during focal reversible cerebral ischemia. Stroke 28:2545-2552
88. Morimoto T, Globus M, Busto R, et al (1996) Simultaneous measurement of salicylate hydroxylation and glutamate release in the penumbral cortex following transient middle cerebral artery occlusion rats. J Cereb Blood Flow Metab 16:92-99
89. Globus MYT, Busto R, Lin B, et al (1995) Detection of free radical activity during transient global ischemia and recirculation: effects of intraischemic brain temperature modulation. J Neurochem 65:1250-1256
90. Lancelot E, Callebert J, Revaud M-L, et al (1995) Detection of hydroxyl radicals in rat striatum during transient focal cerebral ischemia: possible implication in tissue damage. Neurosci Lett 197:85-88
91. Liu PK, Hsu CY, Dizdaroglu M, et al (1996) Damage, repair, and mutagenesis in nuclear genes after mouse forebrain ischemia-reperfusion. J Neurosci 16:6795-6806
92. Chopp M, Chan PH, Hsu CY, et al (1996) DNA damage and repair in central nervous system injury: national institute of neurological disorders and stroke workshop summary. Stroke 27:363-369
93. Huang D, Shenoy A, Cui J, et al (2000) *In situ* detection of AP sites and DNA strand breaks bearing *3'*-phosphate termini in ischemic mouse brain. FASEB J 14:407-417
94. Cui J, Holmes EH, Greene TG, et al (2000) Oxidative DNA damage precedes DNA fragmentation after experimental stroke in rat brain. FASEB J 14:955-967

5. Strategies using hypothermia

The importance of thermal changes in the pathophysiology of stroke: post-stroke fever and hypothermia therapy

Hiroaki Naritomi, Kazuyuki Nagatsuka, Kotaro Miyashita, Hiroshi Oe, Hiroshi Moriwaki, Zhen He, and Takemori Yamawaki

Department of Cerebrovascular Medicine, NATIONAL CARDIO-VASCULAR CENTER, 5-7-1 Fujishiro-dai, Suita, Osaka 565-8565, Japan

Summary: In order to elucidate the significance of thermal changes in the pathophysiology of stroke, experimental and clinical studies were performed in rats and stroke patients, respectively. In rats, small infarction restricted to the hypothalamus was produced with intraluminal methods occluding hypothalamic artery selectively. The body temperature increased significantly by 0.6-1.1 ℃ for 72 hours. Changes in body temperature were retrospectively studied in 45 patients with cardio-embolic stroke admitted within 24 hours after stroke. Body temperature was found to increase significantly during the first 4 days of stroke correlating with the size of infarction. Mild hypothermia (32.5-33.5 ℃ for 3-5 days) was induced within 6 hours after stroke in 13 patients with embolic occlusion of major cerebral artery. The frequency of good functional outcome as defined by Barthel Index (BI) 75 or more at 3 months after stroke (50%) was significantly larger as compared with that in patients with the similar stroke severity who were admitted at 6-24 hours after stroke and underwent no hypothermic or antipyretic therapy (10%). Antipyretic therapy with oral administration of non-steroidal antipyretic drug (loxoprofen 180 mg/day) was induced within 12 hours after stroke and continued for 5 days in 17 patients with embolic occlusion of major cerebral artery. Good functional outcome at 3 months after stroke (41%) was significantly larger as compared with that in patients without hypothermic or antipyretic therapy (12%). The results of the present study suggest that post-stroke fever is developed commonly following large infarction and aggravates clinical outcome. The management of temperature may bring about better clinical outcome and is considered important for the treatment of severe stroke.

Key words: Stroke, Hypothermia, Fever, Antipyretics, Hypothalamus

Introduction

It has been repeatedly demonstrated by experimental studies in animals during the last decade that even a moderate increase or decrease in brain temperature significantly aggravates or ameliorates ischemic cerebral injury (1, 2). In stroke patients, body temperature increases rather commonly during the acute phase of stroke, and the elevation of body temperature is closely correlated with poor clinical outcome (3, 4). It, thus, seems that body temperature in the acute phase of stroke is a significant determinating factor of ischemic cerebral injury and clinical outcome. Respiratory tract or urinary tract infection may be the main cause of post-stroke fever. Several workers, however, have assumed that post-stroke fever may be developed partly mediating central mechanisms, since the fever may be observed even in patients without infectious signs or symptoms (4).

In spite of the accumulation of experimental data concerning excellent protective effects of hypothermia on ischemic brain, little has yet been known as to effects of body temperature manipulation on clinical outcome of stroke patients. The present experimental and clinical studies were, therefore, performed to elucidate mechanisms of post-stroke fever and effects of temperature manipulation on clinical outcome of ischemic stroke.

Experimental study: mechanisms of post-ischemic fever

Experimental study was performed to elucidate whether ischemic damage to the unilateral hypothalamus causes increase of body temperature (5, 6). Forty-seven 10-week-old rats purchased from Oriental Yeast Co (Kyoto, Japan) were used in the study. Rats were anesthetized with 2% isoflurane in a mixture of 30% oxygen and 70% nitrous oxide delivered by a face mask. During the operation, rats were warmed by a heating pad set at 37.0 °C. An intraluminal occluder was introduced from the common carotid artery (CCA) into the internal carotid artery (ICA) in order to obstruct the hypothalamic artery (HTA) arising from the distal ICA proximal to the middle cerebral artery (MCA) bifurcation selectively and to produce an isolated hypothalamic infarction. The operation was initiated within 25 minutes after anesthetic induction. After the operation, the rats were kept in a separate cage and allowed to recover from anesthesia at room temperature (21± 1°C).

Rats were divided into two groups, such as a group for hypothalamic infarction and a sham-operated control group. In the group for hypothalamic infarction (n=36), an occluder , a 3-0 nylon suture coated with 0.1% poll-L-lysine, was introduced through the right common carotid artery (CCA) into the right internal carotid artery (ICA) and advanced intracranially until resistance was encountered. When the advanced distance from the CCA bifurcation was shorter than 18 mm, the occluder tip was presumed to have reached the MCA bifurcation. The occluder was then withdrawn 2 mm to allow the MCA origin to remain unobstructed and to obstruct the deep penetrating arteries free to receive blood retrograde from the anterior cerebral artery (ACA). If the occluder could be advanced more than 18 mm from the CCA bifurcation without feeling resistance, it was assumed that the tip had crossed beyond the MCA origin and was now within the ACA. The occluder was then withdrawn to a position 15-16 mm from the CCA bifurcation. In the sham-operated control group (n=11), the occluder was advanced 13 mm from the CCA bifurcation, thereby avoiding the obstruction of HTA, MCA or other branches of ICA supplying the brain.

Body temperature was measured by a probe temporarily inserted 2 cm into the rectum. Measurements were recorded before and 1, 3, 24, 48, and 72 hours after the operation in hand-handled non-anesthetic rats. The resting level temperature before operation was measured at 3:00-3:30 PM in all animals. Seventy-two hours after obstructive surgery, each animal was reanesthetized with pentobarbital (50 mg/kg) and killed by decapitation. The brain was removed for histological analysis with TTC, hematoxylin and eosin and TUNEL staining method.

Following the histological examinations, 13 rats were found to have a small infarction restricted to the ipsilateral hypothalamus. The absolute success rate for production of isolated hypothalamic infarction was 36%. Changes in body temperature after obstructive surgery are illustrated in Fig 1. Average body temperature prior to the occluder introduction was the same in hypothalamic infarction group and sham-operated control group (37.6 ℃ vs 37.8 ℃). Following the obstructive surgery, the temperature remained unaltered for 72 hours in the control group. In the hypothalamic infarction group, the temperature increased significantly at 1 hour after ischemia and kept showing 0.6-1.1 ℃ higher values as compared with the control group until 72 hours after ischemia. The differences in body temperature between the two groups were significant throughout 72-hour period ($p<0.05$).

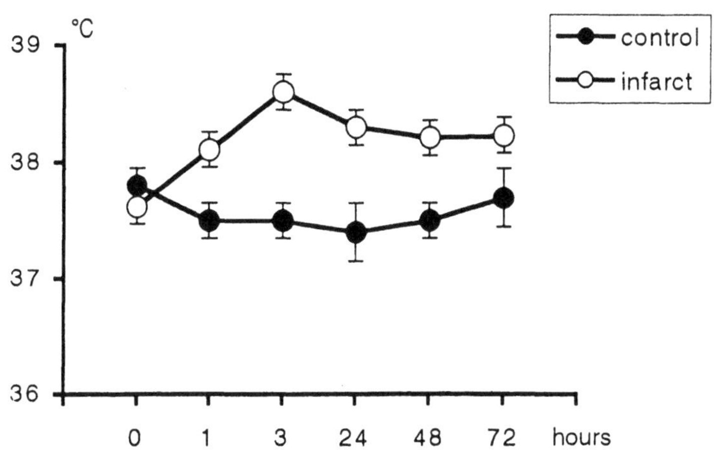

Fig. 1. Changes in body temperature after hypothalamic infarction.

Post-stroke fever and infarction size

Retrospective study was performed in 45 patients with cardio-embolic stroke in ICA territory who were admitted within 24 hours after stroke to clarify whether the development of post-stroke fever is related with the size of ischemia. Patients with definitive evidence of pneumonia or urinary tract infection were excluded from the study. The patients were divided into 3 groups according to the size of infarction on computed tomography (CT) obtained more than 3 weeks after onset, such as a large infarction group with hypodensity area exceeding the size of whole MCA territory , a small infarction group with hypodensity area restricted to the basal ganglia area and a medium-size group with hypodensity area smaller than the whole MCA territory but not restricted to the basal ganglia area. In each patient, body temperature values were averaged for the first day of stroke, the second to forth days of stroke and the fifth to seventh days of stroke. The temperature values in each period were compared between the groups.

As shown in Table 1, body temperature in the small infarction group was normal throughout the 1-week period ranging from 36.4 to 36.6 ℃. The temperature was somewhat higher in the medium-size infarction group than in the small infarction group, although the difference was not significant. Body temperature in the large infarction group was significantly higher than that in the small infarction group at the first day and the second to fourth days of stroke ($p<0.05$).

Table 1. Post-stroke body temperature in 3 different sizes of infarction

size of infarction		1st day	2nd-4th days	5th-7th days
small	n=25	36.5 ± 0.7 ℃	36.4 ± 0.7 ℃	36.6±0..6 ℃
medium	n=11	37.0 ± 0.8	37.1 ± 0.5	37.1±0.5
large	n=9	37.7 ± 0.8 *	37.5 ± 0.8 *	37.1±0.7

* p<0.05 as compared with small infarction.
Values are expressed in mean and standard deviation.

Effects of mild hypothermia on hyperacute stroke

In order to clarify effects of mild hypothermia on ischemic stroke, mild hypothermia was induced in 13 patients with malignant cerebral infarction, and neuroimaging findings and clinical outcome were studied (7, 8). Entry criteria for the induction of hypothermia included ages below 75 years, admission within 4 hours after stroke, hemiparesis in association with consciousness disturbance grade more than 2 in Japan Come Scale (JCS), no hemorrhagic change on CT, neurological or ultrasonographic findings suggestive of embolic occlusion of ICA, MCA (M1 portion) or basilar artery (BA), no improvement of neurological symptoms for more than 30 min following administration of recombinant tissue plasminogen activator (rt-PA), if ever given, and no association of severe organ failure in the heart, liver or kidney.

Mild hypothermia therapy was undertaken in our stroke care unit. Age, gender, the site of occlusion and the initial severity of stroke in 13 patients undergoing hypothermia therapy are listed in Table 1. Conventional angiography was performed prior to the induction of hypothermia in 3 patients and following mild hypothermia in the remaining 9 patients. Prior to hypothermia therapy, thrombolytic therapy was performed intravenously in 7 patients and intraarterially in one patient within 4 hours after stroke. None of them showed a noticeable neurological recovery, so that they were subjected to hypothermia therapy. In another patient with BA top occlusion, intraarterial thrombolysis was performed following the induction of hypothermia at 7 hours after stroke resulting in the achievement of partial recanalization. The remaining 4 patients underwent no thrombolytic therapy.

Table 2. The initial clinical conditions in 13 patients with hypothermia therapy

case no	age/sex	occluded site	initial NIHSS	thrombolysis	time reaching 33 °C
1	60/M	lt-ICA	29	intraarterial	4.5 hours
2	68/M	rt-MCA	13	intravenous	4.3
3	43/F	lt-ICA	17	intravenous	5.9
4	36/F	rt-MCA	14	intravenous	5.7
5	71/M	lt-MCA	26	intravenous	5.8
6	64/F	rt-ICA	12	none	7.5
7	65/M	rt-ICA	26	intraarterial	4.7
8	57/F	lt-ICA	31	intravenous	7.8
9	63/M	BA	37	intraarterial	5.7
10	45/M	rt-MCA	16	intravenous	6.0
11	70/M	lt-ICA	28	none	2.7
12	61/M	lt-ICA	25	none	5.5
13	50/M	rt-MCA	22	none	6.5

age in years; M, male; F, female; lt, left; rt, right

The hypothermia therapy was induced under general anesthesia with fentanyl and midazolum. Prior to the induction of general anesthesia, 1,000 ml plasma expander was infused intravenously in order to avoid excessive blood pressure reduction accompanied by anesthesia. Following the anesthesia, the body was cooled using hypothermic blanket combined with an alcohol compress to reach the target brain temperature 33.0 ℃. The brain temperature was monitored at the internal jugular vulb, and the core temperature was monitored at the bladder. 1.6 ±0.7 hours were required to obtain the target brain temperature. Hypothermia at 32.5-33.5 ℃ was maintained for 3-6 days according to the following criteria: 3 days in cases of small or medium-sized lesion without mass effects on CT, 5 days in cases of large lesion without mass effects, and more than 5 days in cases of large lesion with mass effects. Following hypothermic treatment, the body was rewarmed with a speed of 1-2 ℃/day in brain temperature to return toward the normothermia. During the hypothermic and post-hypothermic period, carotid ultrasonographic examinations were performed serially in order to assess the state of recanalization.

As listed in Table 2, all the 13 patients undergoing hypothermia therapy had occlusion of major cerebral artery, such as ICA, proximal M1 portion or BA, and the grade of consciousness disturbance on admission ranged from 3 to 100 in JCS. Their initial stroke severity was 21.8 ±9.3 in National Institute of Health Stroke Scale (NIHSS). The body cooling started at 3.6±0.8 hours after stroke onset, and the target brain temperature was obtained at 5.6±1.3 hours. During and after the hypothermic period, none of the patients suffered from severe infectious diseases, such as sepsis, although 5 patients had pneumonia. 3 patients developed moderate congestive heart failure during the hypothermic period, and 2 patients exhibited a confusional state in association with involuntary movements during the rewarming period. All these complications were, however, treatable and did not disturb the continuation of therapy. Severe arrhythmia was observed in none of the patients.

Two patients with ICA occlusion (Cases 7 and 8) died during the acute phase. Case 7 with the initial NIHSS 26 received intraarterial thrombolysis prior to the induction of hypothermia. This patient developed massive hemorrhagic changes on CT at 2 days after stroke, which expanded further at 3 days after stroke leading to the fatal outcome. Case 8 with the initial NIHSS 31 underwent no thrombolytic therapy. She suffered from recurrent multiple emboli causing bilateral ICA occlusion with unilateral vertebral artery occlusion. , which led to the fatal outcome. Except for these 2 patients, none died in the acute or chronic phase. One patient (Case 10) undergoing intravenous thrombolysis prior to the induction of hypothermia developed large hemorrhagic transformation on CT during the hypothermic period and was subjected to a craniotomy. In this patient, the hypothermia was continued following the craniotomy. The total hypothermic duration in this patient became 4 days. Those 11 surviving patients showed a considerably good functional recovery. At 3 months after stroke, they showed mRS of 2.8±1.5 and BI of 69±35.

Table 3 compares clinical outcome in the 12 patients with hypothermia therapy and 30 embolic stroke patients who had the similar stroke severity due to major

Table 3. Clinical outcome in patients with hypothermia and without hypothermia

	hypothermia	no hypothermia
number of cases	12	30
ages	59±12 years	67±11 years
initial NIHSS	21.8 ± 9.3	21.5 ± 6.9
time of admission	less than 4 hours	6-12 hours
mortality	2/12 (17%)	9/30 (30%)
BI ≥75 at 3 months	6/12 (50%)	3/30 (10%)

BI, Barthel Index.
Case 10 with good outcome (BI 80) is not included into this analysis because of surgical intervention.

cerebral artery occlusion but underwent no hypothermia therapy because of late arrival at the hospital. Case 10 was excluded from this analysis because of

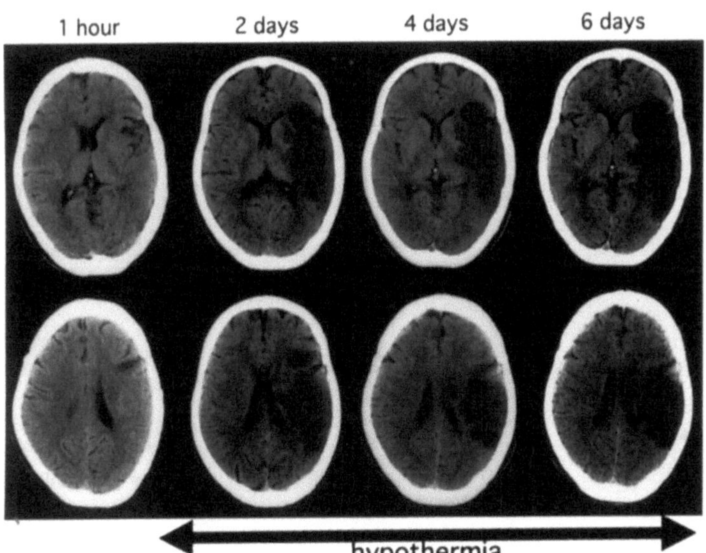

Fig. 2. Serial CT images in a case of left ICA occlusion. In spite of the development of large low density area, little mass effects are observed. Note that the ischemic lesion is sharply demarcated from the surrounding areas even at 2 days after stroke.

surgical intervention, although this case had good clinical outcome showing BI 80 at 3 months after stroke. 30 control patients arrived at our institue more than 6 hours after stroke and hence received neither thrombolytic nor hypothermia therapy. They were, however, admitted within 12 hours after stroke and underwent the same medical treatment as the hypothermic patients except for hypothermia or thrombolysis. Their initial NIHSS (21.5±6.9) was comparable with that in the hypothermic patients. As shown in Table 3, the mortality and good functional outcome at 3months after stroke are apparently better in the hypothermic patients than in the control patients.

In the 11 surviving patients, several interesting CT findings were observed during hypothermia therapy. First, definitive mass effects were obsevred in none of the patients except for Case 10 who developed a large hemorrhagic transformation and was treated with a craniotomy. As shown in Figure 2, the developmet of ischemic lesion was not accompanied by appreciable mass effects even in cases of large lesion occupying more than two third of MCA territory. This was true whether CT was obtained in the hypothermic period or post-hypothermic period. Second, ischemic lesions were sharply demarcated from the surrounding regions even in the early phase such as 2 days after stroke (Figure 2). Third, contrast CT demonstrated little parenchymal enhancement in ischemic lesions. Definitive contrast enhancement was observed only in 2 of 11 patients who had early recanalization within 3 days after stroke as confirmed by serial carotid ultrasonographic studies. One is Case 7 with a fatal hemorrhagic infarc-

Table 4. CT findings in hypothermic patients

case no	recanalization within 3 days	CT findings: hemorrhage	enhancement	mass effect	slow develop
1	+	-	-	±	-
2	+	+	±	-	-
3	-	-	-	±	-
4	+	+	±	±	-
5	+	+	-	-	-
6	-	-	-	-	+
7*	+	+++	+	+++	unknown
8*	-	-	not done	+++	unknown
9	+	-	-	-	-
10 **	+	++	not done	not evaluated	unknown
11	-	-	-	±	+
12	-	-	-	±	+
13	+	+	+	±	-

* Cases 7 and 8 were fatal. ** Case 10 underwent a craniotomy during hypothermia.

tion, and the other is case 13 with excellent functional recovery. Excluding these 2 patients, 6 others had early recanalization within 3 days after stroke. All of these patients with early recanalization showed no contrast enhancement, although contrast study was not performed in one of them (Table 4). Fourth, gradual expansion of ischemic lesion over 48 hours was observed in 3 cases (Cases 6, 11 and 12). All these cases had ICA occlusion. Arterial recanalization was not observed within 3 days in these patients (Table 4).

Effects of antipyretic therapy on acute stroke

Hypothermia therapy in the above mentioned fashion requires general anesthesia and body-cooling system, such as hypothermic blanket. Because of the requirement of such a special system and invasive nature, the use of hypothermia therapy may be restricted to a small number of patients who are untreatable with other therapies. Exploring more feasible and non-invasive therapy, we considered that the prevention of post-stroke fever by means of antipyretics may be useful for stroke treatment. After exploring several drugs , we decided to choose loxoprofen -Na (sodium 2-p-2-oxocyclopentylmethyl phenyl propionate dihydrate: Sankyo Co. Ltd., Japan) (8). Loxoprofen-Na is a relatively novel non-steroidal anti-inflammatory drug (NSAID), which is commercially available in Japan. Adverse effects of this drug on gastrointestinal system are known to be small. The use of loxoprofen-Na for stroke patients is, therefore, advantageous over other NSAIDs in this respect.

The anipyretic therapy was performed in 17 stroke patients (72±8 years of age). Inclusion criteria included ages below 80 years, admission within 6-12 hours after stroke, initial NIHSS 10 or more, neurological and ultrasonographic findings suggestive of ICA or MCA occlusion, no intracranial hemorrhage on CT, and no history of gastrointestinal ulcer. Loxoprofen-Na (180 mg/day) was administered orally for 5 days in association with 4-point ice cooling. 60 mg powdered form loxoprofen-Na diluted in 10 ml water was given via a stomach tube every 8 hours. In order to prevent gastrointestinal disorders, H2 receptor antagonists (famotidine 20 mg twice a day) were also administered. Axillary temperature was measured 3-4 times a day, and daily average temperatures were calculated. CT scans were obtained serially on admission, and 2 days, 4 days , 7 days and 30 days after stroke. Clinical outcome was evaluated at 3 months after stroke. The results were compared with 50 age-matched stroke patients (71± 11) who were admitted within 12 hours after stroke with initial NIHSS 10 or more and were not treated with antipyretic therapy, hypothermia therapy or thrombolytic therapy.

As shown in Fig 3, antipyretic therapy successfully prevented the elevation of axillary temperature. In the control group, axillary temperature exceeded 37.0 ℃ at 2-7 days after stroke. In the antipyretic group, axillary temperature at 2-7 days remained within the normal range showing values of approximately 36.5 ℃. There were significant differences in temperatures at 2-7 days between the two groups ($p<0.05$).

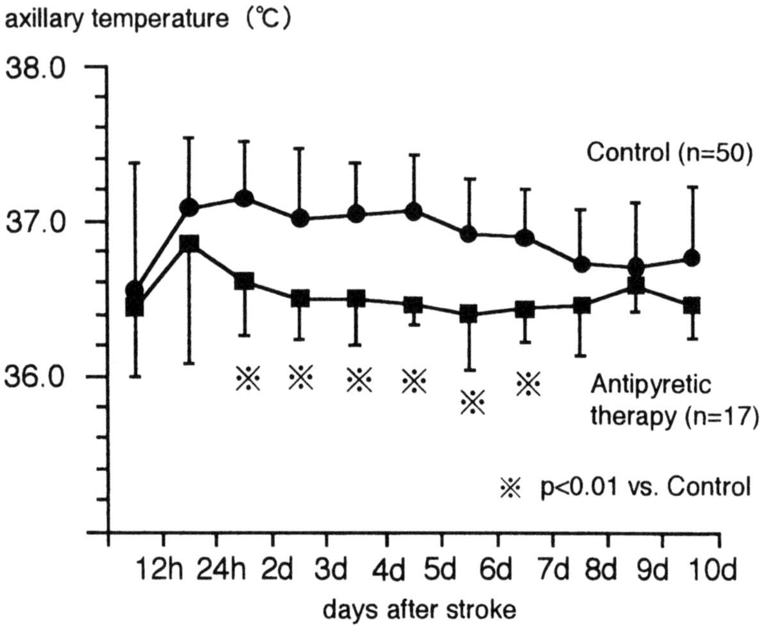

Fig. 3. Axillary temperature differences between the antipyretic and control groups.

NIHSS on the admission was almost the same in the antipyretic group (18.0±4.0) and control group (18.7±4.8). In serial CT examinations, hemorrhagic transformation in association with definitive mass effects occurred less frequently in the antipyretic group (3/17, 17.5%) than in the control group (19/50, 38.0%), although the difference was not significant. The shift of midline structure resulting from severe mass effects was observed in the majority patients in the both groups. However, the magnitude of maximum midline shift was significantly smaller in the antipyretic group (3.9±3.2 mm) than in the control group (9.2±6.7 mm)($p<0.005$). The mortality during the first 3 months of stroke was the same in the antipyretic group (2/17, 11.8%) and control group (7/50, 14.0%). However, good functional outcome at 3 months after stroke as difined by BI 75 or more was significantly more common in the antipyretic group (7/17, 41.2%) than in the control group (6/50, 12.0%)($p<0.05$).

Discussion

Mechnisms of post-stroke fever

In experimental studies of cerebral ischemia, body temperature is usually regulated under anesthetic condition. However, the fact that body temperature may increase transiently following forebrain ischemia has been recognized for years by workers obstructing both common carotid arteries in gerbils under a short-term anesthesia. The elevation of body temperature can be observed also in focal cerebral ischemia produced by intraluminal obstruction of MCA in rats (9). Zhao et al. assumed that such a post-ischemic body temperature elevation may be attributable to the damage of anterior hypothalamus and preoptic area (9). Our experimental study inducing isolated infarction in the hypothalamus has affirmed that ischemic damage of unilateral hypothalamus can cause elevation of body temperature.

The hypothalamus is known to play an important role in regulation of body temperature. This region senses changes in local brain temperature, integrates information of temperature from other parts of the body, and sends efferent signals to various regions. Mechanisms of body temperature elevation following hypothalamic ischemia can be explained as follows. Following hypothalamic ischemia, the ipsilateral hypothalamus senses reduction of body temperature erroneously, since hypothalamic blood flow reduction causes local hypothalamic temperature decrease. The hypothalamus, then, provokes a compensatory action to increase body temperature and sends erroneous efferent signals to various regions. Body temperature, thus, increases as a compensatory reaction of hypothalamic. It is, however, unclear as to whether local hypothermia in the unilateral hypothalamus can cause systemic body temperature changes. More detailed studies are needed to elucidate mechanisms of post-ischemic temperature elevation further.

Post-stroke fever and infarction size

In stroke patients, mild fever is observed rather commonly. Several reports indicated that the presence of fever in the acute phase of stroke was closely connected with poor clinical outcome (3, 4, 10). The frequency of post-stroke fever in previous reports largely differs ranging from 22% to 61% probably due to the difference in definition of fever (3, 4). The major cause of fever is undoubtedly the association of infectious diseases. The fever is, however, occasionally developed even in patients without signs or symptoms of infection (3, 10). Such a fact suggests that post-stroke fever may be developed mediating by central mechanisms. Przelmoski reported that post-stroke fever was observed commonly in embolic stroke but not in lacunar stroke (3). Rare occurrence of post-stroke fever is likely attributable to rare occurrence of infection or to rare involvement of central mechanisms in lacunar stroke because of small lesion size. Boysen and Christensen pointed out that post-stroke fever was developed more commonly in patients with severe stroke than in those with moderate stroke (10). Common occurrence of post-stroke fever in severe stroke patients is likely attributable either to common occurrence of infection or to common involvement of central mechanisms in severe stroke because of large lesion size

The results of our study have clearly indicated that the presence or absence of post-stroke fever is determinated largely by the size of infarction. In the patients with small lesions, body temperature did not increase significantly during the acute phase of stroke. To the contrary, in the patients with large lesions, body temperature increased definitively during the first 5 days of stroke. This increase of body temperature may be attributable partly to infectious diseases, since patients with large lesions commonly suffer from consciousness disturbance which accelerates infectious complications. The increase of body temperature may be also attributable partly to the involvement of central mechanisms. It was not clear from CT findings whether the hypothalamus was involved by ischemia in our patients with large lesions suffering from post-stroke fever. Even if the hypothalamus is not involved by ischemia, the decrease of local temperature in wide areas of cerebral hemisphere, which are adjacent to the hypothalamus, may be sensed by the hypothalamus as the reduction of whole body temperature erroneously. As a consequence, the hypothalamus may provoke a compensatory reaction and send efferent signals to various regions to increase body temperature.

Effects of mild hypothermia on hyperacute stroke

During the last decade, experimental studies have repeatedly demonstrated that protective effects of mild hypothermia on ischemic brain are excellent (11, 12). To the contrary, clinical results of multi-centered randomized trial of hypothermia in patients with severe head injury recently performed in USA were rather disappointing (13). In their study, mild hypothermia (33°C, 2 days) did not improve the mortality or functional outcome in patients with severe head injury (13). In their randomized trial, however, only 23% of patients had an extremely elevated intracranial pressure at the beginning of study. Previously, Shiozaki et al demonstrated that hypothermia was effective in patients with severe head injury associating with extremely high intracranial pressure (14) but not in those without high intracranial pressure (15). Hypothermic treatment under general anesthesia is accompanied by various side effects, such as infection (15). Because of such adverse effects, hypothermia may be rather harmful, provided it is applied for the treatment of mild or moderate cerebral injury. Beneficial effects of hypothermia may be obtained, only if it is applied for the treatment of life-threatening severe stroke caused by massive cerebral injury.

In our study, hypothermia therapy was indicated only for the hyperacute phase of severe embolic stroke due to ICA, MCA (M1) or BA occlusion. Other therapies can rarely improve clinical conditions in such patients with severe embolic stroke. Therefore, the use of hypothermia in such patients is considered permissible, even though it may carry with various adverse effects. In our study, body cooling was initiated within 6 hours after stroke in all the patients. Such an early start of therapy is considered necessary to obtain neuroprotective effects of hypothermia definitively, since the viability of brain is likely lost within 6 hours after stroke. In our study, good functional outcome was obtained in 50% of patients with hypothermia therapy. The results are considered excellent, although the number of patients is small. In a study of Schwab et al, the mortality of patients treated with hypothermia was high reaching 44%, since hypothermia was initiated late at 14 ± 7 hours after stroke (16). The time, 14 hours after stroke, is considered too late to protect the brain from ischemic insults.

In our imaging studies, 3 characteristic CT findings were observed in the hypothermic patients, such as little mass effects, sharp demarcation of lesions in the early phase, and rare enhancement of ischemic lesions. These CT findings suggest that hypothermia protects both neuronal and vascular cells in ischemic territory suppressing the development of severe edema and blood-brain barrier disruption. Peculiar CT observation found in 3 patients, a slow and gradual expansion of lesions over 48 hours, probably indicates that the process of ischemic neuronal death takes a longer time under hypothermia. This observation may indicate that the expansion of lesions can be prevented by blood flow recovery within 48 hours after stroke under normothermic condition. Thus, therapeutic time window for thrombolysis may be widened under hypothermic condition.

Effects of antipyretic therapy on acute stroke

As discussed above, post-stroke fever is developed rather commonly in patients with severe stroke. Kuroiwa et al clearly demonstrated in experimental studies that the prevention of post-ischemic fever can prevent the deterioration of ischemic neuronal injury (17). The prevention of post-stroke fever is, therefore, considered to exert protective effects on the ischemic brain, although the effects may not be so potent as hypothermia. The results of our study have suggested that oral administration of NSAID for the first 5 dyas of stroke can successfully prevent the development of post-stroke fever and bring about better clinical outcome.

NSAIDs are known to prevent prostaglandin synthesis by inhibiting cyclooxygenase activity. The inhibition of cyclooxygenase activity may provide suppression of inflammatory reaction in ischemic brain thereby reducing ischemic neuronal injury (18). It is, therefore, unclear as to whether good clinical outcome obtained by loxoprofen administration is attributable to its antipyretic action or anti-inflammatory action. Whichever the mechanism it is, the use of NSAID for the treatment of acute stroke is considered advantageous over hypothermia therapy in its feasibility and non-invasiveness. In our antipyretic therapy using loxoprofen, axillary temperature was maintained at approximately

36.5 °C. The temperature may be reduced to lower levels such as 35.5-36.0 °C, provided more potent antipyretics are used for the therapy. Such a potent antipyretic drug should be explored in order to improve neuroprotective therapy in acute stroke.

References

1. Busto R, Dietrich WD, Globus MY-T, et al (1987) Small differences in intraischemic brain temperature critically determine the extent of ischemic neuronal injury. J Cereb Blood Flow Metab 7:729-738
2. Dietrich WD, Busto R, Halley M, et al (1990) The importance of brain temperature in alterations of the blood-brain barrier following cerebral ischemia. J Neuropathol Exp neurol 49:486-497
3. Przelomski MM, Roth RR, Gleckman RA, et al (1986) Fever in the wake of stroke. Neurology 36:427-429
4. Castillo J, Davalos A, Marrugat J, et al (1998) Timing for fever-related brain damage in acute ischemic stroke. Stroke 29:2455-2460
5. He Z, Yang S-H, Naritomi H, et al (2000) Definition of the anterior choroidal artery territory in rats using intraluminal occluding technique. J Neurol Sci 182:16-28
6. He Z, Yamawaki T, Yang S (1999) Experimental model of small deep infarcts involving the hypothalamus in rats. Changes in body temperature and postural reflex. Stroke 30:2743-2751
7. Naritomi H, Nagatsuka K, Yamawaki T, et al (2000) Treatment of hyperacute embolic stroke with major cerebral artery occlusion by mild hypothermia. In: Hayashi N (ed) Brain Hypothermia, Springer-Verlag, Tokyo, pp169-174
8. Naritomi H, Nagatsuka K, Miyashita K, et al (2001) Effects of hyperthermia and hypothermia on ischemic vascular damages. In: Fukuuchi Y, Tomita M, Koto A (eds) Ischemic Blood Flow in the Brain, Springer-Verlag, Tokyo, pp448-454
9. Zhao Q, Memezawa H, Smith M-L, et al (1994) Hyperthermia complicates middle cerebral artery occlusion induced by an intraliminal filament. Brain Res 649:253-259
10. Boysen G, Christensen H (2001) Stroke severity determines body temperature in acute stroke. Stroke 32:413-417.
11. Morikawa T, Ginsberg MD, Dietrich WD, et al (1992) The significance of brain temperature in focal cerebral ischemia: histopathological consequences of middle cerebral artery occlusion in rats. J Cereb Blood Flow Metab 12:380-389
12. Yanamoto H, Hong S-C, Soleau S, et al (1996) Mild postischemic hypothermia limits cerebral injury following transient focal ischemia in rat neocortex. Brain Res 718:207- 211
13. Clifton GL, Miller ER, Choi SC, et al (2001) Lack of effect of induction of hypothermia after acute brain injury. N Engl J Med 344:556-563
14. Shiozaki T, Sugimoto H, Taneda M, et al (1993) Effect of mild hypothermia on uncontrollable intracranial hypertension after severe head injury. J Neurosurg 79:363-368
15. Shiozaki T, Hayakata T, Taneda M, et al (2001) A multicenter prospective randomized controlled trial of the efficacy of mild hypothermia for severely head injured patients with low intracranial pressure. J Neurosurg 94:50-54

16. Schwab S, Schwarz S, Spranger M, et al (1998) Moderate hypothermia in the treatment of patients with severe middle cerebral artery infarction. Stroke 29:2461-2466
17. Kuroiwa T, Bonnekoh P, Hossmann KA, et al (1990) Prevention of postischemic hyperthermia prevents ischemic injury of CA1 neurons in gerbils. J Cereb Blood Flow Metab 10:550-556
18. Yen MH, Lee SH (1987) Effect of cyclooxygenase and lipooxygenase inhibitors on cerebral oedema induced by freezing lesions in rats. Eur J Pharmacol 133:369-373

Cerebrovascular disease and hypothermia Part I: effects of mild hypothermia in the management of cerebrovascular disease

Nobuyuki Yasui[1], Shingo Kawamura[1], Akifumi Suzuki[1], Hiromu Hadeishi[1], and Jun Hatazawa[2]

Departments of Surgical Neurology[1] and Radiology and Nuclear Medicine[2], Research Institute for Brain and Blood Vessels–Akita, 6-10 Senshu-Kubota-machi, Akita 010-0874, Japan

Summary: Previous reports have established the effectiveness of hypothermia in preserving cerebral function and integrity after various insults. However, certain complications persist when hypothermic therapy is used in clinical settings such as head injury and stroke. While several clinical trials of hypothermic therapy have been performed, the efficacy of the hypothermia has not been definitively proven. The current paper describes the development and use of a hypothermia bed used in the treatment of patients with stroke and summarizes the pathophysiological data obtained from these trials.

Key words: Brain protection, Mild hypothermia, Stroke

Introduction

The effectiveness of hypothermia in protecting the brain from the adverse effects of cerebral ischemia has been well established [10,18]. Siebke has previously reported a case in which an individual survived 40 minutes' period of submersion without subsequent cerebral sequelae, an outcome thought to be a direct result of hypothermia [25]. The cerebral protective effect of deep hypothermia, in which the body temperature is lowered to less than 30°C, has also been applied to cardiac surgery and neurosurgery [2,4]. Experiments using deep hypothermia as a therapeutic approach to prevent brain injury were performed in the 1950's [12,17,23]. However, the maintenance of low body temperature and associated management proved difficult; serious complications arose as the duration of deep hypothermia increased. Thus, deep hypothermia was rarely utilized in the years following these experiments.

In 1987, Busto reported that a cerebral protective effect was also present with mild hypothermia, in which the brain temperature is lowered only by several degrees [5]. Since this study, other investigators have reassessed mild hypothermia as a method for preventing cerebral damage [19,20,22,24].

Beginning in 1997, we have utilized a new mobile bed system that functions to maintain hypothermia in patients with severe cases of cerebrovascular disease [15,16]. The current paper summarizes our findings and reviews the present knowledge regarding mild hypothermia and its use to prevent cerebral damage.

Hypothermia bed system for stroke patients

A mobile hypothermia bed was constructed for use during the treatment of cerebrovascular disease. The bed consists of a Servo Ventilator 900C (Siemens-Elema AB; Life Support System Division, Solna, Sweden), three gas cylinders (O_2, N_2O, and compressed air), a cooler with a water bed (Cool Bath NCB-3100; Tokyo Rikakikai, Tokyo), water-circulating blankets, a hand-held computer (PC-9821 Np®; NEC Corporation, Tokyo), a temperature monitor (Coretemp CTM-205®; Terumo, Tokyo), an electrocardiographic monitor for heart rate, arterial blood pressure, and percutaneous O_2 saturation (Dynascope DS-5100E®; Fukuda-Denshi, Tokyo), and a storage battery providing one hour of electrical supply for use during patient transfers. Two syringe pumps were placed under the bed for intravenous administration of medications.

The patient underwent surface cooling using water blankets, and hypothermia was maintained during radiological examination. Patients were anesthetized with an imidazo-benzodiazepine compound, midazolam (Dormicum®; F.Hoffmann-La Roche Co., Ltd., Basle, Switzerland), administered continuously (0.125 mg/kg/hr IV). Patients were paralyzed with pancuronium (0.05 mg/kg/hr IV) and artificially ventilated with air and supplementary oxygen. Arterial blood pressure was monitored through a catheter in the radial or dorsal pedis artery, and arterial blood was obtained from the catheter for blood-gas analysis. Swan-Ganz catheter and Vigilance® monitor (Baxter, Irvine, Calif., U.S.A.) were used to evaluate cardiac and hemodynamic function during hypothermia.

Core temperature was monitored continuously from the urinary bladder, pulmonary artery, and rectum. The water temperature in the blankets was maintained between 5-40°C based on the bladder temperature using a feedback computer program (Daikin Industries, Osaka). The core temperatures at the

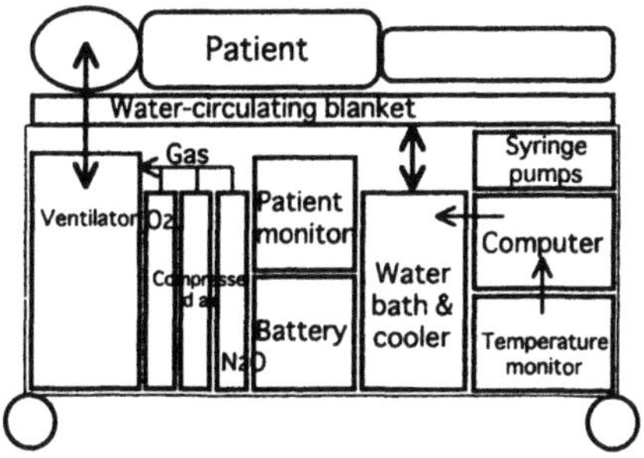

Fig. 1. Hypothermia bed system for patients with stroke. (from [15], with permission)

bladder and rectum did not significantly differ.

The core temperature was lowered to 33-34°C over the course of approximately 48 hours, and then increased over a subsequent 48 hours. The total duration of hypothermia was 4-5 days. At a bladder temperature of 36.5°C, the patient was moved from the hypothermia bed to a standard bed. Bladder temperature was maintained at <38.0°C using the Medi-Therm for 2 weeks following stroke onset.

Radiological examination performed during hypothermic therapy included x-ray computed tomography (CT), single photon emission CT, and measurements of regional cerebral blood flow (CBF) and O_2 metabolism using positron emission tomography (PET). CT was also performed simultaneous to PET studies, allowing accurate identification of the anatomical structures of the brain. The transfer time for radiological examination was approximately 5 minutes. During CT and PET examination, the core temperature was maintained within ±0.1°C of the target temperature. There were no remarkable complications during patient transfer or radiological examination.

Effect of hypothermia tharapy in severe cerebrovascular disease

Mild hypothermia is indicated in patients less than 70 years old with stroke and no history of ischemic heart disease (including myocardial infarction and angina pectoris). Further, patients must satisfy the following criteria: (1) patients with aneurysmal subarachnoid hemorrhage (SAH) must be admitted within 6 hours after onset of hemorrhage with spontaneous respiration and Stage IV or V consciousness level according to the World Federation of Neurological Surgeons (WFNS) scale [9]; (2) patients with intracerebral hemorrhage (ICH) must be admitted within 6 hours of onset of hemorrhage, with consciousness level of semicomatose or worse and clinical brain stem responses such as light reflex, cilio-spinal reflex, or Doll's eye phenomenon; (3) patients with embolic occlusion of the internal carotid or middle cerebral arteries must be admitted within 24 hours of stroke with cortical neurological signs and no spontaneous eye opening.

CT, magnetic resonance imaging (MRI), or both were performed upon admission. In addition, patients underwent conventional or CT angiography to determine the location of vascular lesions. Informed consent was obtained from the patient's closest relative (spouse, or family member), and surgery for aneurysm clipping in the case of SAH, or hematoma evacuation in the case of ICH, was performed. During surgery, hypothermia was induced using a cooling blanket (Medi-Therm®; Gaymer Industries, Inc., Orchard Park, N.Y., U.S.A.) until the temperature measured in the urinary bladder reached 35.0-35.5°C. Cerebrospinal fluid (CSF) was drained from the basal cisterns or the sylvian fissure to maintain intracranial pressure within normal range following surgery in patients with SAH. Hypothermia was maintained postoperatively in the intensive care unit. Patients with embolic stroke did not undergo thrombolytic therapy to evaluate the therapeutic effects of hypothermia alone.

From 1997, mild hypothermia was utilized in 11 cases of severe stroke, 7 cases of SAH, 3 cases with ICH and one case of embolic stroke; Table 1 summarizes the clinical data of these cases. Among the 7 SAH cases, 4 were attributed to middle cerebral aneurysm, 2 cases to internal carotid aneurysm, 1 case to distal anterior cerebral aneurysm and another to superior cerebellar basilar aneurysm. Among these, 5 cases had associated intracerebral hemorrhage. Two cases with ICH were secondary to hypertensive putaminal hemorrhage and one case was associated with right parietal subcortical hematoma caused by rupture of an arterio-venous malformation. Another case was the result of left internal carotid artery occlusion caused by emboli of cardiac origin. Most cases were admitted within 2 hours of onset and begun on hypothermia within 6 hours of onset, except for one case of ICH. Level of consciousness at the time of admission was worse than 8 evaluated by Glasgow Coma Scale (GCS). Three cases of SAH and 2 cases of ICH recovered to moderate disability based on Glasgow Outcome Scale (GOS) and greater than 55 points on the Bathel index.

Case presentation

Case 2: A 49-year-old man was admitted after 30 minutes' episode of sudden-onset loss of consciousness with subsequent right hemiparalysis, left anisocoria and diminished left light reflex with GCS 8. Massive subarachnoid hemorrhage was revealed on CT scan, especially at the left basal cistern (Fig. 2a). Vertebral angiogram demonstrated a left basilar superior cerebellar artery aneurysm (Fig. 2b).

Table 1. Case summary of the mild hypothermia

Case	Age/Sex	Diagnoss	Onset-Admission	GCS	GOS	Bathel index
1	37 / F	SAH	30 min	4	MD	85 (16 mo)
2	49 / M	SAH	30 min	8	GR	100 (10 mo)
3	54 / M	SAH	90 min	3	MD	60 (17 mo)
4	67 / F	SAH	4 hrs	7	SD	0 (12 mo)
5	43 / M	SAH	20 min	6	SD	0 (12 mo)
6	65 / F	SAH	0 min	4	SD	5 (12 mo)
7	47 / F	SAH	60 min	7	SD	0 (6 mo)
8	41 / M	ICH	6 hrs	4	MD	55 (12 mo)
9	59 / F	ICH	11 hrs	6	SD	5 (12 mo)
10	50 / M	ICH	40 min	4	MD	90 (14 mo)
11	63 / M	INF	60 min	8	D	/

GCS: Glasgow Coma Scale, GOS: Glasgow Outcome Scale, F: female, M: male, min: minute, hr: hour, mo: month, SAH: subarachnoid hemorrhage, ICH: intracerebral hemorrhage, INF: infarction, GR: good recovery, MD: moderate disability, SD: severe disability, D: dead

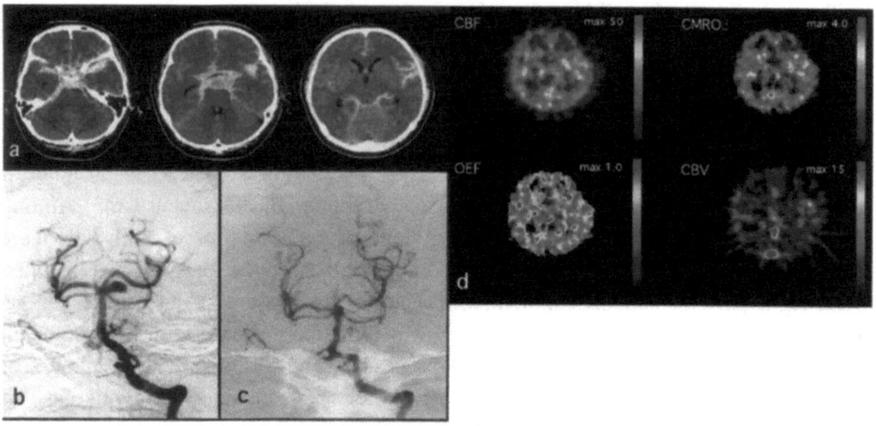

Fig. 2a,b,c,d. 49-year-old man admitted 3 hours after insult. **a** CT scan shows massive subarachnoid hemorrhage, especially in the left-basal cistern. **b** Pre-operative angiogram shows Lt-BA-SCA aneurysm. **c** Aneurysm was clipped; post-operative angiogram. **d** PET performed during hypothermia on day 2 demonstrated CBF and $CMRO_2$ approximately 50% of normal. Oxygen metabolism was maintained. The patient recovered well without residual neurological deficit.

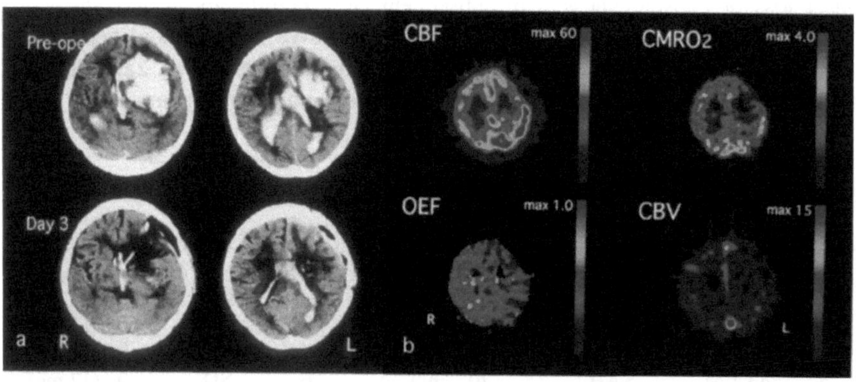

Fig. 3a,b. 59-year-old female admitted 3 hours after onset with GCS 6. **a** Pre-operative CT scan shows massive Lt-putaminal hemorrhage (upper); removed post-operatively. **b** PET scan performed during hypothermia on day 3 showed increased CBF in left parietal area and diffusely decreased $CMRO_2$. This patient began rehabilitation 40 days after the onset.

Emergency operation was performed at WFNS grade 4 and hypothermia was induced following surgery and continued for 48 hours at 34 centigrade before rewarming to 36 centigrade. PET was performed during hypothermia on day 2 (Fig. 2d), demonstrating that both CBF and cerebral metabolic rate of oxygen ($CMRO_2$) decreased to less than 50% of normal. $CMRO_2$, however, was relatively maintained. Post-operative angiogram showed complete neck obliteration with aneurysm clip (Fig. 2c). After rewarming, the patient gradually recovered to consciousness level GCS 14 with mild right hemiparesis on day 6. On day 7, aphasia and disorientation occurred secondary to vasospasm and resulted in left parietal infarction. Patient recovered gradually and was independent in activities of daily living approximately 1 year later.

Case 9: A 59-year-old female was admitted 3 hours after the onset with GCS 6, right hemiplegia and leftt-conjugate deviation. Massive hematoma was demonstrated in left putamen by CT scan (Fig. 3a). Following emergency evacuation of the hematoma, mild hypothermic treatment was initiated 3 days after admission. PET scan was performed during the hypothermia (Fig. 3b), demonstrating increased CBF in left parietal area and diffusely decreased $CMRO_2$. Four months after the onset, CBF decreased in the left hemisphere and $CMRO_2$ was maintained, except in the area of the hematoma. The patient began rehabilitation 40 days after the onset on the insult, but functional recovery was poor.

Table 2. Perfusion state in middle cerebral artery area during hypothermia

Case	ICH	Ipsilateral	Contralateral
2	-	misery	misery
3	+	luxury	coupling
4	+	luxury	coupling
5	-	luxury	coupling
6	+	mixed*	misery
7	+	luxury	misery
9	+	luxury	coupling
11	-	0	coupling

ICH: intracerebral hematoma,

* luxury around ICH and misery perfusion at superior temporal area

Effect of hypothermia therapy on cerebral blood flow and oxygen metabolism

We investigated the effects of hypothermia (33-34°C) on cerebral blood flow and oxygen metabolism using PET (Table 2). Briefly, CBF was 35.7±7.6 ml/100ml/min and $CMRO_2$ was 1.76±0.39 ml/100ml/min in areas of the middle cerebral artery ipsilateral to the ruptured aneurysms, whereas these values were 32.3±5.6 and 2.28±0.34 ml/100ml/min, respectively, on the contralateral side. This represents a decrease of 35.7±14.1% compared to normal CBF and 54.3±9.9% compared to normal $CMRO_2$ ($p<0.01$) in the ipsilateral areas, and decreases of 41.8±10.1% and 41.2±8.6%, respectively, on the contralateral side. These results provide evidence of decreased CBF and $CMRO_2$ during hypothermia in humans. Description of the perfusion state in the middle cerebral artery area during hypothermia in ICH and cerebral infarction (INF) are also summarized (Table 2). CBF and $CMRO_2$ decreased in these cases. In the case of INF, marked reduction of the CBF and $CMRO_2$ was present in the ischemic area and resulted in fatal infarction with brain swelling.

Discussion

The cerebral protective effect of hypothermia has been described in clinical cases and experimental study, but its usefulness in the treatment of clinical entities such as head injury and stroke remained unclear. Unaddressed issues included whether the severity of the cerebral insult would limit the effectiveness of hypothermic therapy and what systemic complications could be attributed to this therapy. Other investigators have suggested that hypothermic therapy results in higher incidence of suppression of immunity leading to infectious disease, hemodynamic instability due to systemic hypotension and cardiac arrhythmias, electrolyte imbalance (particularly hypokalemia), coagulopathy, and multi-organ failure [3,7,16,18]. Even with mild hypothermia, severe complications can occur with increased duration of hypothermia.

The mechanism by which hypothermia exerts its protective effects may include decreased cerebral metabolism, decreased excitatory neurotransmitter release [6,11,21], decreased accumulation of lipid peroxidation products and free radical generation [1]. Other possible protective mechanisms include prevention of postischemic hyper- and hypo-perfusion, decreased blood-brain barrier disruption, prevention of brain edema [8,13], and attenuation of brain acidosis and inflammatory responses.

A decrease in CBF and $CMRO_2$ during hypothermia in humans is demonstrated in the current paper through PET. During hypothermia, the mean decrease in $CMRO_2$ was approximately 1.5 times that of CBF in the middle cerevral artery areas ipsilateral to the lesion side. The present PET data obtained during hypothermia are consistent with those of previous PET studies in non-hypothermia cases, in which $CMRO_2$ decreased more than CBF in SAH patients with mild-to-moderate severity, a condition known as relative luxury perfusion [16,26]. Taken together, these data indicate that hypothermia may not alter the underlying perfusion state. Reduced $CMRO_2$ may result in a decrease in energy demand by the brain.

In the present study, hypothermic therapy was maintained 4-5 days postoperatively based on the belief that suppression of initial brain damage following stroke minimizes secondary brain damage. Patients did not develop hypothermia-related complications, likely secondary to the short duration of the therapy. The present data suggest some limitation of mild hypothermia for severe brain damage despite early induction of cooling. Out of a total 11 cases, hypothermia appears to have been relatively effective in 5 cases (3 of 7 cases with subarachnoid hemorrhage, 2 of 3 cases with intracerebral hemorrhage), leaving 6 cases with poor outcome. Because of the small sample size, we are unable to definitively conclude whether mild hypothermia is effective for severe stroke. Further investigation must be performed, with comparison to a control population.

This work was supported by Special Coordination Funds for Promoting Science and Technology from the Ministry of Education, Culture, Sports, Science and Technology of Japan, and from the Frontier Project of Stroke, Research Institute for Brain and Blood Vessels-Akita.

References

1. Baiping L, Xiujuan T, Hongwei C, et al (1994) Effect of moderate hypothermia on lipid peroxidation in canine brain tissue after cardiac arrest and resuscitation. Stroke 25:147-152
2. Bigelow WG, Callaghan JC, Hopps JA (1950) General hypothermia for experimental intracardiac surgery. Ann Surg 132:531-537
3. Bigger WD, Bohn D, Kent G (1983) Neutrophil circulation and release from bone marrow during hypothermia. Infect Immun 40:708-712
4. Botterell EH, Lougheed WM, Scott JW, et al (1956) Hypothermia, and interruption of carotid, or carotid and vertebral ciruculation, in the surgical management of intracranial aneurysms. J Neurosurg 13:1-42
5. Busto R (1987) Small defferences in intraischemic brain temperature crutically determine the extent of ischemic neuronal injury. J Cereb Blood flow Metab 7:729-738
6. Busto R, Globus MYT, Dietrich WD, et al (1989) Effect of mild hypothermia on ischemia-insduced release of neurotransmitter and free fatty acids in rat brain. Stroke 20:904-910
7. Clifton G (1992) Systemic hypothermia in treatment of brain injury. J Neurotrauma 9 (Suppl):S487-495
8. Dietrich WD, Busto R, Halley M, et al (1990) The importance of brain temperature in alterations of the blood-brain barrier following cerebral ischemia. J Neuropathol Exp Neurol 49:486-497
9. Drake CG (1988) Report of world federation on neurological surgeons committee on a universal subarachnoid hemorrhage grading scale. J Neurosurg 68:985-986
10. Ginsberg MD et al (1992) Therapeutic modulation of brain temperatuere: relevance to ischemic brain injury. Cerebrovasc Brain Metab Rev 4:189-225
11. Hagerdal M, Harp J, Siesjo BK (1975) The effect of induced hypothermia upon oxygen consumption in the rat brain. J Neurochem 24:311-316
12. Howell DA, Stratford JG, Posnikoff J (1956) Prolonged hypothermia in treatment of massive cerebral haemorrhage. Can Med Assoc J 75:388-394

13. Karibe H, Chen J, Zarow GJ, Graham SH, et al (1994) Delayed induction of mild hypothermia to reduce infarct volume after temporary middle cerebral artery occlusion in rats. J Neurosurg 80:112-119
14. Kawamura S, Suzuki A, Hadeishi H, et al (2000) Cerebral blood flow and oxygen metabolism during mild hypothermia in patients with subarachnoid haemorrhage. Acta Neurochir (Wien) 142:1117-1122
15. Kawamura S, Suzuki E, Yasui N, et al (1999) Hypothermia bed system for stroke patients – Technical note -. Neurol Med Chir (Tokyo) 39:466-470
16. Lawrence R (1990) Hypothermia and blood coagulation: dissociation between enzyme activity and clotting factor levels. Circulatory Shock 32:141-152
17. Lazorthes G, Campan L (1958) Hypothermia in the treatment of craniocerebral traumatism. J Neurosurg 15:162-167
18. Maher J, Hachinski V (1993) Hypothermia as a potential treatment for cerebral ischemia. Cerebrovasc Brain Metab Rev 5:277-300
19. Marion DW, Obrist WD, Carlier PM, et al (1993) The use of moderate therapeutic hypothermia for patients with severe head injuries: a preliminary report. J Neurosurg 79:354-362
20. Metz C, Holzschuh M, Bein T, et al (1996) Moderate hypothermia in patients with severe head injury: Cerebral and extracerebral effects. J Neurosurg 85:533-541
21. Mitani A, Kataoka K (1991) Critical levels of extracellular glutamete mediating gerbil hyppocampal delayed neuronal death during hypothermia. Neurosci 42:661-670
22. Naritomi H, Shimizu T, Oe H, et al (1996) Mild hypothermia therapy in acute embolic stroke: a pilot study. J Sttroke Cerebrovascl Dis 6: Suppl 1 pp193-196
23. Sedzimir CB (1959) Therapeutic hypothermia in cases of head injury. J Neurosurg 16:407-414
24. Shiozaki T, Sugimoto H, Taneda M, et al (1993) Effect of mild hypothermia on uncontrollable intracranial hypertension after severe head injury. J Neurosurge 79: 363-368
25. Siebke H, Rod T, Breivik H, et al (1975) Survival after 40 minutes' submersion without cerebral sequelae. Lancet 1:1275-1277
26. Voldby B, Enevoldsen EM, Jensen F (1985) Regional CBF, intraventricular pressure, and cerebral metabolism in patients with ruptured intracranial aneurysms. J Neurosurg 62:48-58
27. Yasui N, Kawamura S, Suzuki A, et al (2001) Role of hypothermia in the monagement of severe cases of subarachnoid hemorrhage. Acta Neurochirgica Suppl. (in press)

Cerebrovascular disease and hypothermia Part II: an experimental approach for ischemic neuronal death

Yasuji Yoshida[1], Octavio J Arroyo[2], Carlos A Arellanes[2], and Nobuyuki Yasui[2]

Departments of [1]Pathology and [2]Surgical Neurology, Research Institute for Brain and Blood Vessels-AKITA, 6-10 Senshu-Kubota-machi, Akita 010-0874, Japan

Summary: To evaluate the hypothermic effect on cerebral focal ischemia induced in rats, we carried out histological and immunohistochemical studies of mitochondrial pathways with or without energy dependency, and Fas (Apo-1/CD95) pathway in normothermic (NT; 37°C; n=44) and hypothermic (HT; 33°C; n=43) groups. Histologically, areas of cerebral ischemia and neuronal damage were significantly mitigated in the HT group. Bax, cytochrome c, Fas and caspase-3 immunoreactivities were suppressed, but Bcl-2 was increased in the HT group. Apoptosis-inducing factor (AIF) was not detected in either group. The large molecular DNA ladder of the hypothermic ischemia group was located at 20kbp. The results suggest that mild hypothermia protects both the energy dependent mitochondrial and Fas (Apo-1/CD95) pathways of apoptotic cell death, where the AIF is not involved.

Key words: Focal cerebral ischemia, Hypothermia, Cell protective effect, Apoptosis, Cytochrome c, Fas, AIF

Introduction

Apoptosis is one of the mechanisms contributing to neuronal degeneration in ischemic insult [1]. To achieve programmed cell death in ischemic apoptosis, three metabolic pathways have been proposed: mitochondrial pathways with or without energy dependency; and Fas (Apo-1/CD95) activated caspase-3 pathways [2-7]. Mitochondrial pathway with energy dependency acts by releasing cytochrome c into the cytoplasm, which subsequently forms a complex with caspase-9 and Apaf-1 and activates the procaspase-3. Mitochondrial pathway without energy dependency acts via apoptosis-inducing factor (AIF); the mitochondria releases AIF into cytoplasm where it translocates to the nucleus and causes nuclear fragmentation [8,9]. Fas (Apo-1/CD95) activated caspase-3 pathway is regarded as a member of the tumor necrosis factor superfamily that can transduce cell death signals via activated caspase-3.

Mild hypothermia has been previously shown to exert beneficial effects on cerebral focal ischemia induced in rats [10-13], and many studies suggest mechanistic approaches to this effect [14-16]. However, the influence of hypothermia on these pathways remains unclear. The present study evaluates the effects of hypothermia on apoptogenic pathways using histology and immunohistochemistry [17,18].

Materials and methods

Middle cerebral artery occlusion (MCAo) was achieved by inserting a nylon monofilament (#3-0) to the anterior cerebral artery via the external carotid artery of Sprague-Dawley rats (275±10g; n=87) as described earlier [19]. During surgery a thermistor probe was introduced into the rectum to monitor the core temperature, which was 37°C for the normothermic (NT) group and 33°C for the hypothermic (HT) group of rats. The HT group was maintained at 33°C for 1h on the pad. After 1h the monofilament was withdrawn to allow recirculation. The HT rats were gradually rewarmed to 37°C.

Rats subjected to MCAo were allowed to survive for either 1 (n=10), 3 (n=10), 5 (n=10), or 24h (n=20), 4 (n=10) or 10d (n=15). After anesthesia with pentobarbital (50mg/kg), they were sacrificed by perfusion fixation with 4% paraformaldehyde in 0.1M phosphate-buffer solution (PB). Brains were removed and fixed in the same fixative for 24h and were cut into four coronal blocks (3mm in thickness) using brain matrix. The blocks were embedded in paraffin wax and 3μm sections were prepared for histological and immunohistochemical evaluation.

A hematoxylin-eosin (H&E)-stained section through the optic chiasm, where the maximum lesion was detected, was used to observe the infarct area. In the section, striatal and cortical areas of infarction were measured using an image analyzer (Leica Q500: Leica Cambridge Ltd., UK). Infarcts were calculated by integrating the necrotic areas. Coronal sections were used for morphological evaluation of the lesions, as described by Garcia et al [20].

Immunostaining was performed with primary antibodies of anti Bcl-2 (Dako), anti Bax (Upsate), anti cytochrom c (Upsate), anti Fas (Dako), and anti caspace-3 (Dako). The reaction was visualized by the avidin-biotin complex method partly associated with the Catalysed Signal Amplification System (Dako) and diaminobenzidine.

In situ detection of DNA fragmentation was carried out using the TdT-mediated dUTP-biotin nick-end labeling (TUNEL) method according to Gavrieli et al [21]. The reaction was visualized by streptavidin-biotin-peroxidase complex (Apop Tag kid; Intergen, NY, USA) and diaminobenzidine.

The rats treated with 1h ischemia were decapitated after 2 and 24h and the brains were quickly removed (NT, n=6; HT, n=6). The ischemic portion of the brains was carefully isolated on an ice-cold platform. The contralateral side of the brain was used as negative controls. The DNA was extracted using a kit (Sepa

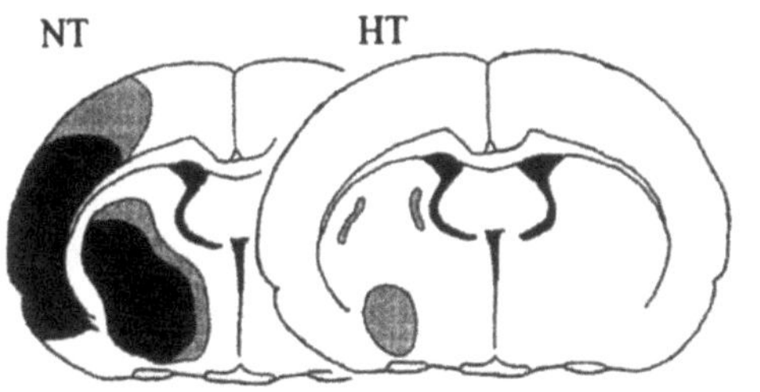

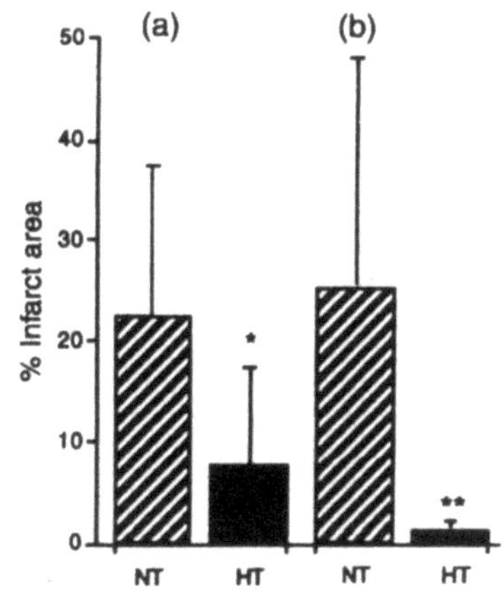

Fig. 1. (Left) Coronal section at the optic chiasm in the normothermic (NT) and hypothermic (HT) group of rat brains, illustrating the distribution of ischemic lesions. Block areas are ischemic core and shaded areas show ischemic penumbra. (from [17], with permission)

Fig. 2. (Right) Percentage infarct area is significantly reduced in the HT group at 24h (**a**, n=10) and 10d (**b**, n=7) after reperfusion compared with that in the NT group (**a**, n=10; **b**, n=8) (from [18], with permission)

Gene, Sanko Junyaku Co.,Ltd., Tokyo, Japan). The pellet obtained was washed with 70% ethanol and dried under vacuum and dissolved in 10mM TE buffer. The DNA content was measured at a wavelength of 260nm. The DNA laddering pattern was analysed by 1.5% and 0.5% agarose gel [21].

The rats treated with 1h ischemia were decapitated after 2 and 24h and the brains were quickly removed (NT, n=6; HT, n=6). The ischemic portion of the brains was carefully isolated on an ice-cold platform. The contralateral side of the brain was used as negative controls. The DNA was extracted using a kit (Sepa Gene, Sanko Junyaku Co.,Ltd., Tokyo, Japan). The pellet obtained was washed with 70% ethanol and dried under vacuum and dissolved in 10mM TE buffer. The DNA content was measured at a wavelength of 260nm. The DNA laddering pattern was analysed by 1.5% and 0.5% agarose gel [21].

Results

Maximum ischemic lesions were detected in the striatum at the level of the optic chiasm. Ischemic infarcts were clearly observed as pale areas with damaged neurons and sponginess of neuropil. In the NT group, the lesion often extended to the lateral cerebral cortex (Fig. 1). In the HT group, the small spongy lesions were

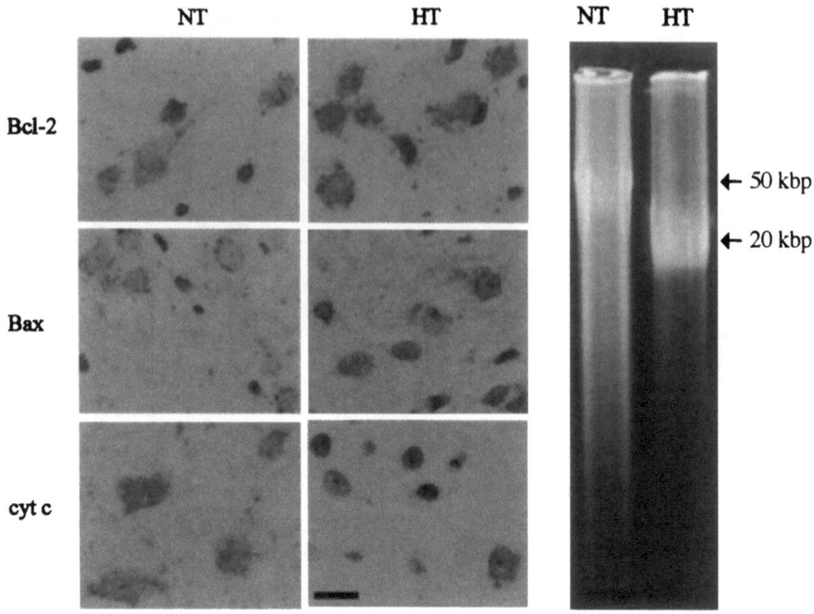

Fig. 3. (Left) Immunohistochemistry to Bcl-2, Bax and cytochrome c proteins in the ischemic penumbra demonstrating different expression patterns in NT and HT groups of rats, 24h after reperfusion. (from [17], with permission)

Fig. 4. (Right) Genomic DNA laddering in the ipsilateral striatum at 2h by 0.5% agarose gel electrophoresis, showing a 50kbp ladder in NT (a) and a 20kbp in HT (b) groups.

recognized, but their severity was less prominent. The lesion was mostly limited to the piriform cortex. The percentage infarct area (PIA) at 24h after reperfusion was 22.4±15.1 (n=10) in NT group, 7.7±9.7 (n=10) in HT group and 10 days after reperfusion was 25.2±22.9 (n=8) in NT, 1.2±1.0 (n=7) in HT group. The PIA was significantly reduced at 24h ($p>0.05$) and 10 days ($p>0.01$) after reperfusion in HT group (Fig. 2).

Histologically, most of the neurons in the ischemic core showed extensive damage in the NT group. Twenty-four hours after reperfusion, these neurons displayed definite lethal changes, including eosinophilic cytoplasm, nuclear condensation and fragmented condensed bodies. The neurons in the lesions of the HT group showed selective damage that included both the lethal and unaffected changes. After 4 days of reperfusion, numerous macrophage and increased blood vessels were evident in the NT group lesion, while the reactive changes were not evident in the HT group. After 10 days of reperfusion, ischemic lesions showed definite atrophy compared with the contralateral side in the NT group. The lethal neurons in the lesions remained, and infiltration of the reactive cells were not recognizable in the HT group.

Immunoreactivity was not present on the side contralateral to the MCAo in both groups or in the section processed without primary antibody. The immunoreactivity of Bcl-2, Bax, cytochrome c and Fas was detectable as early as 5h in the cytoplasm of a few selective neurons. Twenty-four hours after reperfusion, the population of immunoreactive cells was definitely increased. The distribution patterns of positive cells were variable in the ischemic core and the border zone, possibly due to difference in tissue vulnerability and hypothermic effect. Bcl-2 positive cells were localized mainly at the border zone in the NT group and in the HT lesion. In contrast, the expression of Bax, cytochrom c, Fas and caspase-3 was evident at core and penumbra lesions in the NT group, and to a lesser extent in the HT group (Fig. 3).

TUNEL-positive cells were found in greater numbers in the NT group than the HT group.

The DNA extracted from 1h ischemia 24h reperfusion showed DNA fragmentation into low molecular ladders of 180bp integral multiples on 1.5% agarose gel, and a 50kbp ladder in the NT group and a 20kbp ladder in the HT group on 0.5% agarose gel from 1h ischemia 2h reperfusion (Fig. 4).

Discussion

The present study provides evidence for the protective effect of hypothermia induced by MCAo. The severity and size of the infarcts was significantly reduced in the HT group of rats, similar to reports by Morikawa et al [11]. Additionally, we observed both type of neurons, viable and lethal, in lesions of the HT group, 24h, 4d and 10d after reperfusion. In these lesions, the reactive changes such as macrophage infiltration and increased microvessels are minimal or absent, suggesting that the mechanism of lesion repair system is suppressed in the rat with mild hypothermia [14,16].

Recent advances in the knowledge regarding molecular mechanisms in apoptotic cell death have been revealed at least 3 metabolic pathways in affected cells: mitochondrial pathways with or without energy dependency; and Fas-caspase-3 pathway. The mitochondrial pathway with energy dependency involves cytochrome c release and caspase activation, where the cytochrome c release is accelerated by Bax expression and suppressed by Bcl-2 expression [3]. The mitochondrial pathway without energy dependency acts via AIF, which is released into cytoplasm and nucleoplasm, causing nuclear condensation and apoptotic cell death [8,9]. Fas- caspase-3 pathway is believed to activate caspase-10 by binding Fas-liagant at the cell surface, and caspase-10 cleaves procaspase-3 to caspase-3 [4-7].

In the present study, we confirmed mitochondrial release of cytochrome c and caspase pathway as well as Fas- caspase-3 pathway in the NT group. In the HT group, the expression of Bcl-2 is increased, and other factors that accelerate cell death pathway are suppressed by hypothermia. However, AIF was not detected in either group. Accordingly, TUNEL positive cells are prominent in the lesions of the NT group and less prominent in the HT group.

Existence of TUNEL positive cells and DNA laddering with 180bp integral multiples and a 20kbp ladder are regarded as hallmarks of DNA fragmentation during apoptotic cell death. Recently, Yao et al [22] reported that ladders of lower molecular and 20kbp ladders were detectable in tissue with ischemic penumbra, and 50kbp ladder was detectable only in ischemic core. Our results confirm this different laddering pattern. Moreover, the higher molecular ladders from the tissue in the HT group were located at the level of 20kbp, indicating that the neuronal cell death in the HT group is categorized as apoptotic death. In contrast, the lesions in the NT group showed small molecular ladders and 50kbp ladder. This finding suggests that lesions in the NT group includes both necrotic and apoptotic cell death. The possibility of two types of lesions should be considered: ischemic core and penumbra lesions, and necrotic cell death accompanying apoptotic cell death. The immunoreactivity of the Bax, cytochrome c and caspace-3 in the cytoplasm of the cells shows the eosinophilic cytoplasm and nuclear pyknosis (as hallmarks of necrotic cell death) were also discernable in the NT lesion. The TUNEL study demonstrates positivity in those necrotic lethal changes in the NT lesions. These results strongly suggest that the protective effects of hypothermia in ischemic neuronal cell death are mediated by the suppression of cell death pathway of apoptosis.

This work was supported by Special Coordination Funds for Promoting Science and Technology from the Ministry of Education, Culture, Sports, Science and Technology of Japan, and from the Frontier Project of Stroke, Research Institute for Brain and Blood Vessels-Akita.

References

1. Graham SH, Chen J (2001) Programmed cell death in cerebral ischemia. J Cereb Blood Flow Metab 21:99-109
2. Finkel E (2001) The mitochondrion: Is it central to apoptosis? Science 292:624-626
3. Kluck RM, Bossy-Wetzel E, Green DR, et al (1997) The release of cytochrome c from mitochondria: A primary site for Bcl-2 regulation of apoptosis. Science 275:1132-1136
4. Namura S, Zhu J, Fink K, et al (1998) Activation and cleavage of caspase-3 in apoptosis induced by experimental cerebral ischemia. J Neurosci 18:3659-3668
5. Suda T, Takahashi T, Golstein P, et al (1993) Molecular cloning and expression of the Fas ligand, a novel member of the tumor necrosis factor family. Cell 75:1169-1178
6. Kawahara A, Enari M, Talanian RV, et al (1998) Fas-induced DNA fragmentation and proteolysis of nuclear proteins. Genes Cells 3:297-306

7. Huang DCS, Hahne M, Schroeter M, et al (1999) Activation of Fas by FasL induces apoptosis by a mechanism that cannot be blocked by Bcl-2 or Bcl-xL. Proc Natl Acad Sci USA 96:14871-14876
8. Susin SA, Lorenzo HK, Zamzami N, et al (1999) Molecular characterization of mitochondrial apoptosis-inducing factor. Nature 397:441-446
9. Lorenzo HK Susin SA, Penninger J, et al (1999) Apoptosis inducing factor (AIF):A phylogenetically old, caspase-independent effector of cell death. Cell Death Differ 6:516-524
10. Yamashita K, Eguchi Y, Kajiwara K, et al (1991) Mild hypothermia ameliorates ubiquitin synthesis and prevents delayed neuronal death in the Gerbil hippocampus. Stroke 22:1574-1581
11. Morikawa E, Ginsberg MD, Dietrich WD, et al (1992) The significance of brain temperature in focal cerebral ischemia: Histopathological consequences of middle cerebral artery occlusion in rat. J Cereb Blood Flow Metab 12:380-389
12. Widmann R, Miyazawa T, Hossmann KA (1993) Protective effect of hypothermia on hippocampal injury after 30 minutes of forebrain ischemia in rats is mediated by post-ischemic recovery of protein synthesis. J Neurochem 61:200-209
13. Kataoka K, Yanase H (1998) Mild hypothermia - a revived countermeasure against ischemic neuronal damages. Neurosci Res 32:103-117
14. Li PA, He QP, Miyashita H, et al (1999) Hypothermia ameliorates ischemic brain damage and suppresses the release of extracellular amino acids in both normo and hypoglycemic subjects. Exp Neurol 158:242-253
15. Busto R, Mordecai Y-T, Globus MD, et al (1989) Effect of mild hypothermia on ischemia-induced release of neurotransmitters and free fatty acids in rat brain. Stroke 20:904-910
16. Lanier WL (1995) Cerebral metabolic rate and hypothermia: Their relationship with ischemic neurologic injury. J Neurosurg Anesthesiol 7:216-221
17. Prakasa PB, Yoshida Y, Su M, et al (2000) Immunohistochemical expression of Bcl-2, Bax and cytochrome c following focal cerebral ischemia and effect of hypothermia in rat. Neurosci Lett 291:196-200
18. Prakasa PB, Yoshida Y, Santana A, et al (2000) Mild hypothermia mitigates post-ischemic neuronal death following focal cerebral ischemia in rat brain: Immunohistochemical study of Fas, caspase-3 and TUNEL. Neuropathology 20:273-282
19. Zea Longa E, Weinstein PR, Carlson S, et al (1989) Reversible middle cerebral artery occlusion without craniectomy in rat. Stroke 20:84-91
20. Garcia JH, Yoshida Y, Chen H, et al (1993) Progression from ischemic injury to infarct following middle cerebral artery occlusion in the rats. Am J Pathol 142:623-635
21. Gavrieli Y, Sherman Y, Sasson SAB (1992) Identification of programmed cell death *in situ* via specific labeling of nuclear fragmentation. J Cell Biol 119:493-501
22. Yao H, Takasawa R, Fukuda K, et al (2001) DNA fragmentation in ischemic core and penumbra in focal cerebral ischemia in rats. Brain Res Mol Brain Res 91:112-118

Neuroprotection by mild hypothermia for temporary or permanent focal ischemia

Hiroji Yanamoto[1, 2], Izumi Nagata[2], Hideki Sakai[2], Yoichi Niitsu[1], Zhiwen Zhang[1], Jing-Hui Xue[1], and Haruhiko Kikuchi[3]

[1]Laboratory for Cerebrovascular Disorders, Research Institute of the NATIONAL CARDIO-VASCULAR CENTER , Suita, Osaka 565-8565, Japan
[2]Department of Cerebrovascular Surgery, Hospital of the [3]NATIONAL CARDIO-VASCULAR CENTER, Suita, Osaka 565-8565, Japan

Summary: The potential of hypothermic brain protection for ischemic stroke has been demonstrated under laboratory conditions. This article reviews our recent progression understanding the efficacy and specific characteristics of prolonged mild hypothermia for ischemic stroke in rats. Using temporary or permanent focal ischemia models, the rats were treated by mild (33 °C) hypothermia at different schedules. The targeted mild hypothermia was applied only intra- or postischemia, or both periods in the temporary focal ischemia model. In permanent focal ischemia, mild hypothermia was achieved at the onset of ischemia, maintained for 2 h under general anesthesia and further maintained using a cold room for a total of 24 h. The infarcted lesion sizes and neurological function were analyzed for a maximum of 30 days following ischemia and compared to that of the normothermia group. In temporary focal ischemia, the infarcted lesion sizes with intraischemic hypothermia, postischemic hypothermia, or combined prolonged intra- and postischemic hypothermia, analyzed on day 2, were 159 ± 25, 141 ± 19, 76 ± 26 mm^3, respectively. The values in the latter two groups were significantly smaller compared to that obtained under normothermia, 211 ± 19 mm^3 (mean ± SEM, $p< 0.05$). The significant difference in lesion sizes and neurological deficits lasted only in the combined hypothermia group on day 30. In permanent focal ischemia, the infarcted lesion 88 ± 15 mm^3 in the hypothermia group was significantly small compared to that in normothermia, 211 ± 19 mm^3 on day 21 ($p< 0.05$). Mild hypothermia did suppress the development of cerebral infarction and neurological deficit in temporary or permanent focal ischemia. To obtain the maximum neuroprotection from mild hypothermia, acute and prolonged application of hypothermia are key factors.

Key words: Hypothermia, Cerebral infarction, Cerebral blood flow, Focal ischemia, Review

Introduction

Since the 1950's it has been known that deep (<30°C) hypothermia protects the brain under severe ischemic conditions, however, moderate (around 30°C) to deep hypothermia usually resulted in severe side effects, especially in regard to blood and cardiac functions, which have yet to be resolved [1-6]. Recently, mild (>around 33°C) hypothermia therapy was found to carry less but still potent neuroprotective effects for the ischemic brain, and was proposed as a new possible intervention for ischemic stroke based on laboratory results *in vivo* [7-14]. In the paradigm of temporary focal ischemia, in which cerebral blood flow is recovered in the acute phase, the use of either intra- or prolonged postischemic mild hypothermia protected neurons from ischemic injury, and reduced the size of cerebral infarction in laboratory investigations [15-19]. However, because of the technical complexity of establishing a reliable model of focal ischemia able to survive for an extensive period, few studies have been performed to clarify the neuroprotective efficacy with both morphological and neuro-functional assessments of prolonged mild hypothermia. This paper reviews our recent progress that characterizes the efficacies of prolonged mild hypothermia for temporary or permanent focal ischemia in rats [20-23]. These studies clarified the chronic outcome of reduced infarcted lesion analyzed at the acute phase following ischemia, as well as the chronic neuro-functional outcome, both by the use of prolonged mild hypothermia therapy for reversible or irreversible focal ischemia. Prior to these studies, it was considered ineffective to use hypothermia therapy to protect the brain against permanent focal ischemia, in which occlusion of the blood vessels responsible for focal ischemia is not recovered in the acute phase [17].

Materials and methods

Experiment I: temporary focal ischemia

Experimental groups

In male Sprague-Dawley rats, weighing 300-350g, temporary focal ischemia was induced using a micro-clip on the left middle cerebral artery in combination with temporary occlusion of the bilateral common carotid arteries for 2 h [24]. The rats were divided into four groups. In the first group, ischemia and reperfusion was maintained under normothermic (N) conditions (N-N). In the second group, ischemia was induced and maintained under hypothermic (H) conditions (32-

33°C) and reperfusion was performed under normothermic conditions (H-N). In the third group, both ischemia and reperfusion were performed under hypothermic conditions (32-33°C for 2 h during surgery and then the rats were housed in a cold room at 6°C for an additional 22 h after surgery, H-22H). The induction of hypothermia was achieved by the application of alcohol to the body during anesthesia. Housing in a low temperature-environment, significantly prevented recovery of normal body temperature and maintained hypothermia under an 'awake' condition [18]. The temperature of the cold room was set at 12°C from 22 h to 46 h after ischemia to avoid the rebound phenomenon in the prolonged postischemic hypothermia group. In the fourth group, ischemia and the initial reperfusion were performed under hypothermic conditions (32-33°C for 3 h postischemia) and then rats were housed in a normothermic room (25°C) (H-3H). In the fifth group, ischemia was induced and maintained under normothermic conditions and reperfusion was performed under hypothermic conditions for 22 h (N-22H). All rats were sacrificed 48 h after the induction of ischemia. In an additional study, the persistency of the effect of the combined hypothermic therapy was assessed. The same normothermic or hypothermic experiments carried out with groups 1, 3 and 4 were performed in groups 7, 8 and 9 and the rats were sacrificed and the volume of cerebral infarct was analyzed 30 days after the induction of ischemia (n=7 each).

Surgical protocols

The surgical procedures used to induce temporary focal neocortical ischemia are described in detail elsewhere [24]. Briefly, anesthesia was induced with halothane. The right femoral artery was cannulated in each rat to monitor mean arterial blood pressure, assay blood gases (PO_2, PCO_2, pH) and measure the concentration of blood sugar. MABP was kept within 100 to 120 mm Hg by adjusting the halothane concentration. Rectal temperature and temporal muscle temperature were monitored. Both temperatures were controlled within 36.5 to 37.5 °C in the normothermic condition and within 32.0 to 33.0 °C in the hypothermic condition using a heating lamp or alcohol application to the body surface respectively.

Analyses of infarcted volume

The brain was removed under deep anesthesia and from the frontal tip cut into 2 mm-thick slices, which were immersed in 2 % solution of 2,3,5-triphenyltetrazolium chloride (TTC) [25]. The infarcted area and hemispheric areas of each section were measured using an image analysis system. An edema index was calculated by dividing the total volume of the hemisphere ipsilateral to the MCA occlusion by the total volume of the contralateral hemisphere [18]. An infarct index, i.e., the actual infarct volume adjusted for edema, was calculated in each animal as the total infarction volume divided by the edema index. Thirty days after ischemia, the surviving neocortical area was assessed by cresyl-violet stain or TTC. The volume of the right normal neocortex was measured and subtracted from the left neocortical volume to calculate the total infarcted volume, since the infarcted area was completely liquefied and absorbed. Before paraffin embedding of the brain slices, the shrinkage (rate) of the brain by dehydration was measured in the unlesioned right hemisphere to calculate the absolute infarction volume. By using glial fibrillary acidic protein (GFAP) staining in the same brain sections, the area of gliosis developed in the missing area was excluded from the area of intact neocortex.

Analyses of cerebral functions

In an additional experiment, cerebral functions (neurological deficits) following ischemia in normothermic or combined and prolonged mild hypothermic groups were analyzed as described below (n=6 in each). Neurological deficits were examined according to the scoring scale described by Yamamoto et al. [26,27] with a modification, 2 days, 1, 2, 3, or 4 weeks after ischemia in the normothermic (N-N) and intraischemic with prolonged (22 h) postischemic hypothermia groups (H-22H). Hemiplegia and posture by tail-lifting were graded using the following criteria: 0, no deficit (symmetrical movement); 1, mild deficit (asymmetrical incomplete flexion of the right forelimb, or leftward twisting tendency of the body); and 2, severe deficit (asymmetrical complete flexion of the right forelimb, or repeated leftward body twisting). The neurological deficits score was the sum of the hemiplegia and posture-grades (from 0 to 4).

Statistics

Physiological data (i.e., blood pressure, gases, blood sugar concentration, and pH), regional cerebral blood flow (rCBF) at each time point, infarct volumes and infarct indexes were analyzed by ANOVA. If multiple comparisons were indicated, the Student-Newman Keuls test was applied. The neurological deficit score at each time point was analyzed by unpaired *t*-test. The results are presented as the mean ± SEM. A value of $p < 0.05$ was considered significant.

Results of experiment I: temporary focal ischemia

Time courses of rectal temperature

Rectal (core) temperatures for 48 h in all groups are shown in Fig. 1. Spontaneous hyperthermia (around 38°C) was observed in rats housed under normothermic conditions 6 h beyond the induction of temporary focal ischemia. Forty-eight hours after the induction of ischemia, the core temperatures were similar in all four groups.

Analyses of infarcted lesion

Two days after ischemia in the H-N, H-22H, and N-22H groups, one of the seven rats died before the assessment of cerebral infarction, the reason being undefined. The average infarction volumes for each group are shown in Fig. 2. The size of the cerebral infarction was significantly reduced by the combined therapies of intra- and postischemic hypothermia. The infarct index for each group is shown in Table 1. The significant differences observed in the infarct volumes among the groups were also observed among the infarct indexes.

No rat died prior to assessment 30 days after ischemia. Thirty days after ischemia, the lesion of cerebral infarct was observed as a shrunken neocortex or a missing area in the neocortex. In the border of the lesion after necrosis, a very thin layer of glial proliferation was observed surrounding the GFAP-negative tissues (data not shown). The infarct index obtained by cresyl-violet stain (corrected by the shrinkage rate: 1.51 on average) is shown in fig. 3A. The infarct index obtained by the TTC stain (before dehydration) is shown in fig. 3B. The absolute infarction values in each analysis were almost identical. In both analyses of cerebral infarction, there were significant differences between groups N-N and H-22H, but not between groups N-N and H-3H.

Analyses of cerebral function

Severe neurological deficits were observed in the acute phase following temporary focal ischemia in the normothermia (N-N) group with a gradual recovery in the observation period (Fig. 4). In the hypothermic group (H-22H), there were slight neurological deficits from the acute phase following ischemia, which were consistent throughout the observation period. There was a significant difference in the neurological deficit scores in each time point between the groups for 4 weeks following the induction of ischemia.

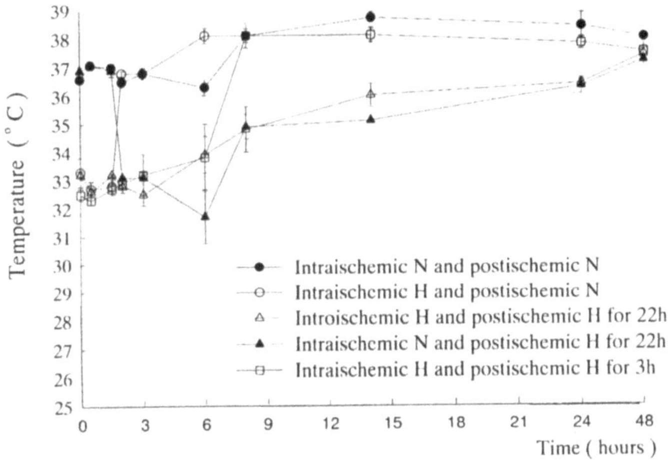

Fig. 1. Time course of the change in rectal temperature in experiment I. There were significant differences in temperature between the two groups over 24 h from the induction of ischemia (from reference [20], with permission).

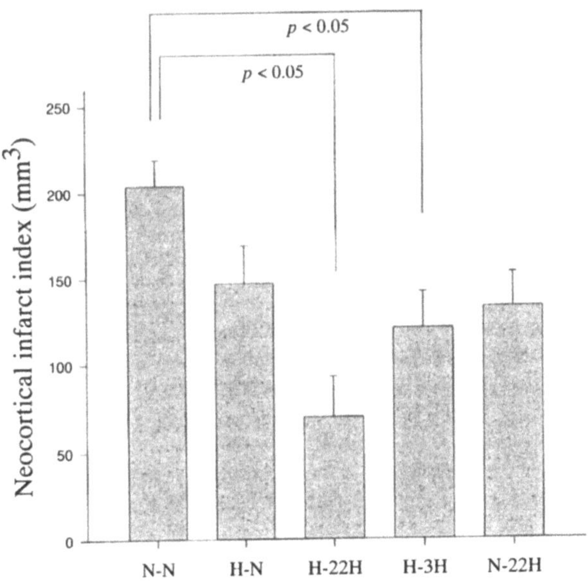

Fig. 2. Total infarct indexes (mm^3) in the experimental groups assessed 2 days after ischemia. Abbreviations: N-N, normothermic ischemia and normothermic reflow; N-H, normothermic ischemia and hypothermic reflow; H-N, hypothermic ischemia and normothermic reflow; H-22H, hypothermic ischemia and prolonged (22 h) hypothermic reflow; H-3H, mild hypothermic ischemia and a short period (3 h) of hypothermic reflow (from reference [20], with permission).

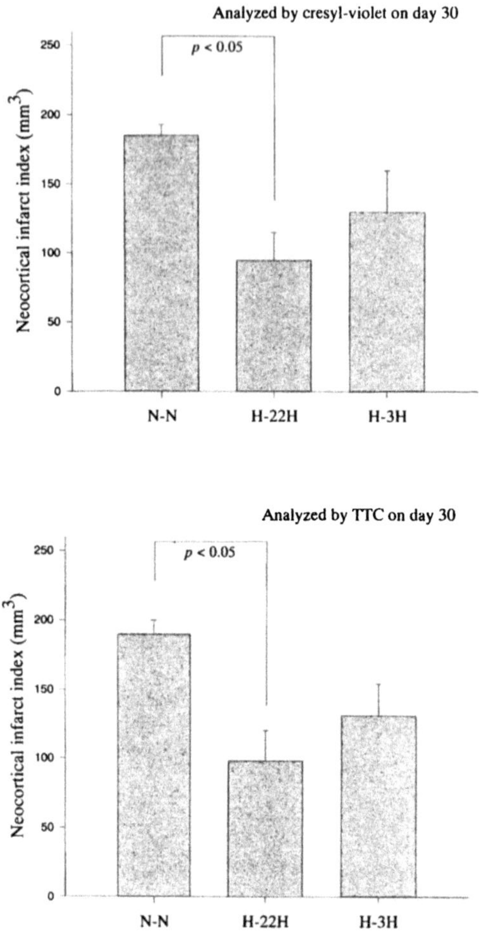

Fig. 3A (upper). Total infarct indexes (mm^3) assessed by cresyl-violet staining. **B (lower).** Total infarct indexes (mm^3) assessed by TTC staining. Significant differences between the group N-N and group H-22H, 30 days after ischemia (from reference [20], with permission).

Table 1. Morphological analyses of infarcted lesion on day 2.

	N-N	H-N	H-22H	H-3H	N-22H
Infarction volume (mm^3)	219 ± 17	159 ± 25	76 ± 26*	127 ± 26*	141 ± 23
Infarct index (mm^3)	204± 15	147 ± 22	70 ± 23*	121 ± 23*	133 ± 20

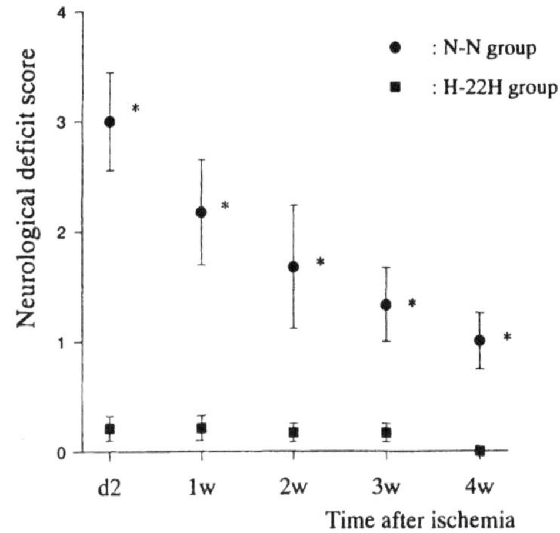

Fig. 4. Time course of neurological deficit scores following temporary focal ischemia in the left middle cerebral arterial territory in N-N and H-22H groups, assessed 2 days, 1, 2, 3, and 4 weeks after ischemia. There were significant differences between the groups during the observation period (from reference [20], with permission).

Experiment II: permanent focal ischemia

Surgical protocols

Male Sprague-Dawley rats, weighing 300 - 350g, anesthetized with halothane, were ventilated mechanically via endotracheal intubation, and the right femoral artery was cannulated to monitor blood pressure, blood sugar, and blood gases (PO_2, PCO_2, pH). The MABP was kept to within 100 to 120 mm Hg by adjusting the halothane concentration (0.5-1.0%). Rectal temperature and temporal muscle temperature were simultaneously monitored. To prolong rat survival following permanent focal ischemia, a newly developed permanent ischemia model was used [21]. In which, 4 vessels of the left middle cerebral artery, the left external and internal carotid arteries, and the right internal carotid artery were occluded permanently. By retaining the blood flow of the right external artery and interrupting the cross-flow between left internal and external carotid arteries after occlusion it was possible to induce a consistent, reliable neocortical infarction and reduce the mortality rate, essentially to the level of zero.

Mild (33 °C) hypothermia was induced on initiation of permanent ischemia and maintained for 2 h. After surgery, hypothermia was maintained using the cold room as described. In the normothermia group, ischemia was induced under normothermia conditions (37 ± 0.5 °C) and the animal was maintained under these normothermic conditions. Rats were sacrificed 2 (n=6 each) or 21 days (n=6 each) after the induction of ischemia, and infarcted volume and the time course of neurological deficits were analyzed as described.

Analyses of infarcted volume

When the assessment of cerebral infarction was carried out at the chronic stage, 21 days after ischemia in experiment 2, the surviving neocortical area was assessed by TTC or double staining with cresyl-violet and glial fibrillary acidic protein (GFAP) as in experiment I. To confirm the consistency in the baseline volume of the non-ischemic right hemisphere following permanent ischemia, age-matched normal rats (n=6) were used to obtain a normal volume of the right hemisphere.

Measurement of regional cerebral blood flow

Regional cerebral blood flow (rCBF) under normothermic or hypothermic conditions were monitored before and during focal ischemia using a laser-Doppler flowmetry system in a separate set of 20 animals pre- and after the induction of permanent ischemia. The region of measurement was the lateral border of the cerebral infarction (penumbra), or 5 mm distal to the point along the MCA artery (ischemic core).

Results of experiment II: permanent focal ischemia

Analyses of infarcted lesion

The physiological parameters except the temporal and rectal temperature were controlled within the physiological range. There were no significant differences in the parameters among the groups (data not shown). No rat died prior to the assessment of cerebral infarction after ischemia.

Core temperatures for 48 h are shown in Fig. 5. In the hypothermia group, the core temperature was significantly lower for the initial 14 h. Average rectal temperature was 2.6 °C-lower in the mild hypothermic group than the normothermia group during the initial 24 h. The average infarction volume for each group is shown in Table 2. Although the size of the cerebral infarction was smaller in the hypothermia group on day 2, there was no significant difference between the two (Table 2). The edema ratio was significantly smaller in the hypothermia than normothermia group on day 2. The infarct index obtained by cresyl-violet staining, corrected by the shrinkage rate as a result of the dehydration procedure in the staining; 1.41 on average, was 186 ± 15 mm^3 in the normothermia group. (This shrinkage of the brain tissue and infarcted lesion should always be corrected to obtain absolute values in the assessment of infarcted lesions when carried out by conventional staining methods after tissue-dehydration [20]). The total infarction volume in the hypothermia group, 96 ± 17 mm^3, was again significantly smaller than that of the normothermia group (p <0.05). In comparison of infarcted lesion size for day 2 and day 21 in the normothermia group, the infarcted lesion size on day 21 was significantly larger than on day 2.

The volume of the non-ischemic hemisphere, used for estimating the volume of normal brain, was 667 ± 25 mm^3, being almost the same as the age-matched normal volume of the right hemisphere, 670 ± 25 mm^3.

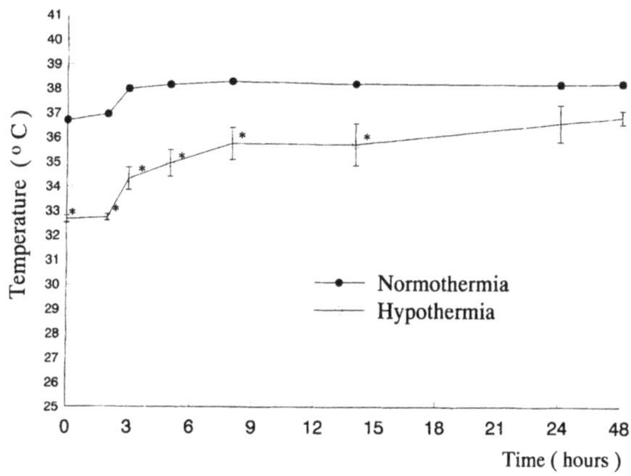

Fig. 5. Time course of the change in rectal temperature in the normothermic and hypothermic groups in experiment II. There were significant differences in temperature between the two groups over 14 h from the induction of ischemia (from reference [21], with permission).

Analyses of cerebral function

Severe neurological deficits were observed in the normothermia group (Fig. 6). In contrast, neurological deficits were mild throughout the observation period in the hypothermia group. There was a significant difference in the scores for each time point between the groups over the 3 weeks. There were similar tendencies of gradual recovery in both groups.

Table 2. The cerebral infarction volume and the infarct index (without edema) values of rats subjected to permanent focal neocortical ischemia. *: A significant difference compared to the value of the normothermic group ($p < 0.05$). ( ): Volume of neocortical infarct.

	Day 2		Day 21	
	Norm	**Hypo**	**Norm**	**Hypo**
Infarction volume (mm^3)	139 ± 21 (139 ± 21)	77 ± 20 (77 ± 20)	-	-
Edema ratio (%)	10 ± 1	5 ± 2*	-	-
Infarct index (mm^3)	127 ± 21	73 ± 19	211 ± 19	88 ± 15*

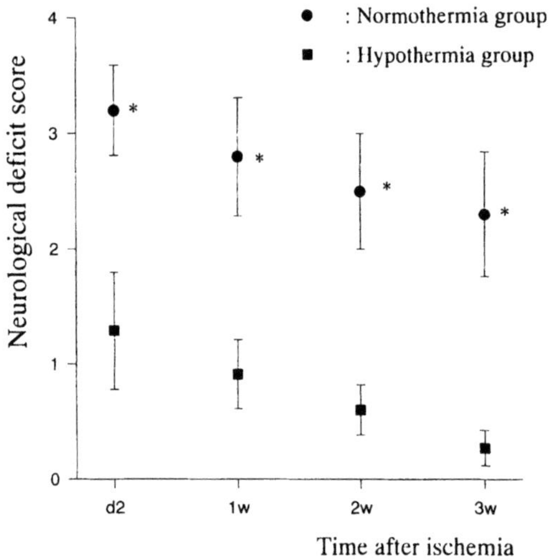

Fig. 6. Time course of neurological deficit scores following permanent focal ischemia in the territory of the left middle cerebral arterial in the normothermia and hypothermia groups, assessed 2 days, and 1, 2, 3 weeks after ischemia. There were significant differences between the groups at each time point (from reference [21], with permission).

Regional CBF measurement

The results of the rCBF measurement in the ischemic core and penumbra are shown in Fig. 7A (normothermia group) and 7B (hypothermia group). In the normothermia group, rCBF increased in both the ischemic core and penumbra 3 h after the induction of ischemia (Fig. 7A). Under hypothermic condition, the initial level of ischemia did not differ from that under normothermic condition, however, the relief of ischemic level was less prominent. In both groups, the reduced rCBF recovered to a level of more than 50% of the preischemic baseline value in the penumbra, and to more than 30% in the core region.

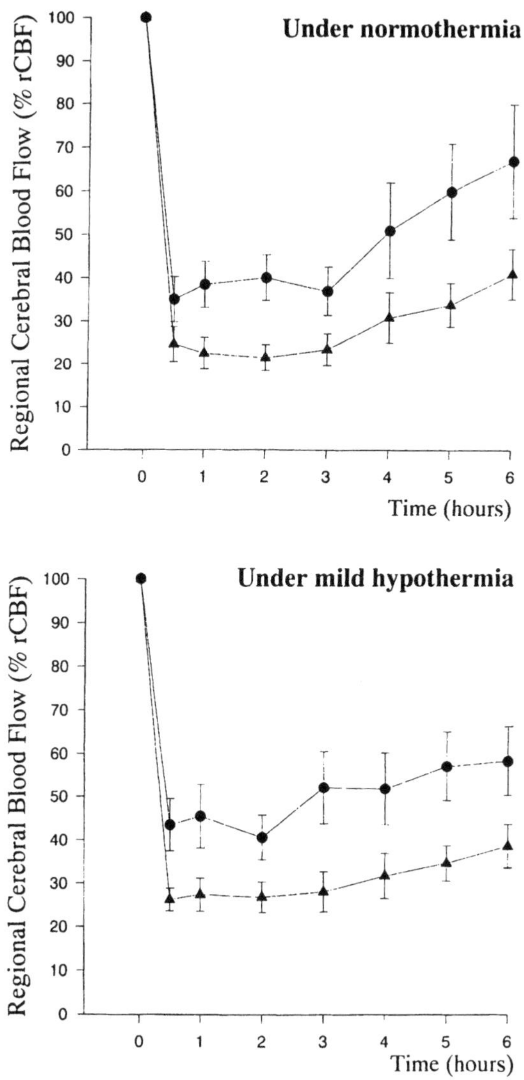

Fig. 7. The rCBF values for the ischemic core and penumbra region after the induction of permanent focal ischemia under normothermic **(A: upper)** or hypothermic **(B: lower)** conditions in experiment II (from reference [21], with permission).

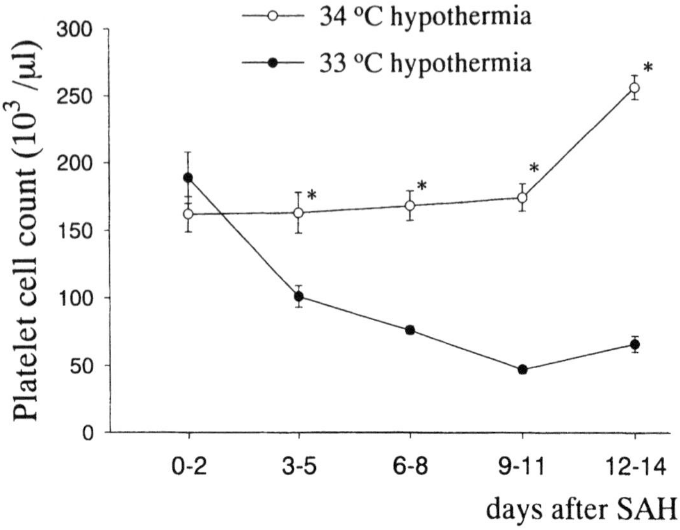

Fig. 8. Time course of the platelet cell counts in the blood from patients with severe subarachnoid hemorrhage during hypothermia therapy in the acute phase in which body temperature was regulated at 33 °C for 7 to 10 days (3 patients) with therapeutic platelets-infusions, or 34 °C for 3 to 5 days (5 patients) without any platelets-infusion, respectively. The reduction of platelet cell counts were significantly prevented in patients at under 34 °C hypothermia compared to that under 33 °C.

Discussion

In temporary focal ischemia, it was reported that postischemic moderate (31 °C) hypothermia for 3 h significantly reduced infarction volume to 39% of the control value, however, the lesion was assessed only 3 h after ischemia because of the high mortality rate under general anesthesia [28]. Since that time, however, several controversial results appeared in the literature, i.e. when postischemic hypothermia was delayed or applied only for a brief period, the neuroprotective effect varied [10,28-31]. Using immediate and moderate (30 °C) post-ischemic hypothermia for 3 h after focal ischemia, the neocortical infarct was significantly reduced when assessed 7 days after ischemia [29]. In contrast, Welsh et al. reported that acute (within 10 min into reperfusion) and deep (23°C) postischemic hypothermia for 2 h failed to protect hippocampal CA1 neurons assessed 7 days after global ischemia in gerbils [32]. Dietrich et al. found that acute (within 3 min into reperfusion) postischemic moderate (30 °C) hypothermia for 3 h failed to protect CA1 neurons assessed 7 days or 2 months after global ischemia in rats [33]. Later, the neuroprotective effects of immediate and prolonged postischemic hypothermia were shown to protect brain in temporary focal ischemia [18,34,35], but still analyzed at the acute phase following the induction of ischemia. In the assessment of neuroprotection, a chronic observation was found to be an essential factor in global ischemia models [14,19,36], and similarly it was also warranted in the assessment of hypothermic interventions for focal ischemia.

To conclude on the efficacy of mild hypothermia for temporary or permanent focal ischemia, the experiments presented here and the study carried out by Corbett et al. clearly demonstrate that only prolonged mild hypothermia for 24 to 48 h persistently protects the brain [20,21,37]. In contrast, brief periods (shorter than 3 h) of mild hypothermia were less effective, and do not have persistent neuroprotection in temporary or permanent ischemia [18,20,21]. In the comparison of intra and postischemic hypothermia therapies, the postischemic mild hypothermia for 22 h had a greater neuroprotective effect compared to that of intraischemic mild hypothermia [20], however, both therapies were less effective than that of combined hypothermia therapy for 5 h (2 h of intraischemic hypothermia plus 3 h of postischemic hypothermia), and the combined therapy (2h+3h) could not achieve significant neuroprotection when assessed at 30 days [20] (Fig. 2, Table 1). Although, the number of animals used were small in each group, only the striking reduction rate of 66%, observed in the combined and prolonged (2h+22h) hypothermia therapy induced at the acute phase, could achieve persistent neuroprotection with a significant reduction rate, 50% at 30 days.

It had been postulated that ischemic cerebral injury is an ongoing process from the induction of global ischemia through the acute reperfusion period [18,31,38]. A delay in the development of cerebral infarction has also been reported after mild focal ischemia [39]. It was noteworthy that the infracted lesion of the permanent focal ischemia increased up to 166% of its initial size assessed at the acute phase, 19 days further on, under normothermic conditions, although the functional impairments in both experiments were not deteriorated, rather they had improved (Fig. 7). Therefore, an improved clinical assessment based on the neurological deficit score supposedly to represent the severity of the ischemic brain lesions, does not always demonstrate that the size of the infracted lesion is stable. The reason for the developing infracted lesion in spite of the acute recovery of ischemia in the rCBF is unknown, however, the progression of intravascular thrombosis as well as the progression of cerebral edema formation in the infracted and peri-infarcted area could be possible mechanisms for the chronic enlargement of the infracted lesion.

It remains under investigation how hypothermic treatment protects neurons from lethal ischemic stress. When intraischemic hypothermia was applied, no significant difference was reported in high-energy phosphate depletion or in levels of lactate accumulation at the end of the ischemic insult [9,40]. Several mechanisms in regard to hypothermic brain protection have been postulated, including the decreased production of free radicals [41,42], and reduced abnormal enhancement of the blood brain barrier (BBB) following ischemia [43-46].

Regarding acute brain injury treated by mild (33°C) hypothermia in humans, 8 h-delayed (in average, for the achievement of the target temperature), continued for 48 h with a subsequent rewarming period for 18 h (in average), failed to improve the outcome of patients with severe traumatic brain injury [47]. Although the pathophysiology between traumatic and ischemic brain injuries differ, a delay of 2 h in rats is the maximum limit to achieve permanent neuroprotection against focal ischemia using mild hypothermia [48], and which could not always achieve permanent neuroprotection [20]. Fundamentally, the standard time for pathological processes in the brain should differ between species. We consider 1.5 h in mice, 2 h in rats, and 6 h in humans being 3 times longer than that of rats, as the time needed for the primary development of cerebral infarction following ischemic induction [24,49-51]. In this context, induction of hypothermia at 6 h from ischemic onset may be too late to obtain any persistent neuroprotective effect from mild hypothermia on the primary ischemic injury in humans. In the same clinical study on severe brain injury, it was found that patients with acute spontaneous hypothermia should be maintained after hospitalization; otherwise acute normalization of body temperature significantly worsened the patients' outcome [47]. Which indirectly indicated the beneficial effects of very early or immediate hypothermia therapy for patients with severe brain injury. Regarding the duration of hypothermia for ischemic injury, 24 h to 48 h was necessary in gerbils and rats [18,20,21,31,37], which can be interpreted as 3 to 6 days for humans. At the end of hypothermia, careful rewarming should be proceeded by confirming that the intracranial pressure (ICP) remains under control. In the study for severe traumatic brain injury, it was shown that temporary control of ICP limited for 48 h failed to maintain normalized ICP beyond the hypothermic period, nor did it improve the outcome of these patients [47]. Recently, we found that 34°C hypothermia better prevented the reduction of platelet cell counts, a critical side effect of mild hypothermia, than that of 33°C when used in patients with severe subarachnoid hemorrhage (Fig. 8). Within this range of hypothermia, it may be possible to prolong the duration more safely from 48 to 72 h, or more.

Although the window for initiating reperfusion therapy following severe focal ischemia is only 3 to 6 h in humans [50,51], the window for induction of mild hypothermia therapy may be larger. A recent small clinical trial demonstrated that mild (33 °C) hypothermia therapy for 2 to 3 days reduced mortality rate from 78 to 44% in patients with severe cerebral infarction due to sudden MCA occlusion, when it was introduced 14 h (in average) after the onset of ischemic symptoms [52]. The existence of delayed; probably the secondary increase of the infarcted lesion after permanent vessel occlusion that is prevented by the prolonged mild hypothermia as shown in experimental study II [21], may be a good target for mild hypothermia therapy in patients with ischemic stroke caused by irreversible blood vessel occlusion.

In summary, acute and prolonged mild hypothermia therapy has the potential to be a powerful intervention therapy for ischemic stroke triggered by sudden reversible or irreversible occlusion of brain blood vessels. The design of an optimal protocol using mild hypothermia for acute ischemic stroke with minimum side effects, as well as a controlled clinical trial are needed.

Acknowledgments: These studies were supported by Special Coordination Funds for the Promotion of Science and Technology, a Grant-in-Aid for Scientific Research, from the Ministry of Education, Culture, Sports, Science and Technology (MEXT) of Japan, and a grant from the Japan Health Sciences Foundation. We acknowledge the valuable assistance of Yasuda T, Okuno A, Kurimoto M, and Nishimori K.

References

1. Schubert A (1995) Side effects of mild hypothermia. J Neurosurg Anesthesiol 7:139-147
2. Hubert L, Rosomoff L (1956) Hypothermia and cerebral vascular lesions I. Experimental interruption of the middle cerebral artery during hypothermia. J Neurosurg 13:244-255
3. Michenfelder JD, Milde JH (1977) Failure of prolonged hypocapnia, hypothermia or hypertension to favorably alter acute stroke in primates. Stroke 8:87-91
4. Steen PA, Milde JH, Michenfelder JD (1980) The detrimental effect of prolonged hypothermia and rewarming in the dog. Anesthesiology 52:224-234
5. Zimmerman JM, Spencer FC (1959) The influence of hypothermia on cerebral injury resulting from circulatory occlusion. Surg Forum 9:216-218
6. Little DM (1959) Hypothermia. Anesthesiology 20:842-877
7. Berntman L, Welch FA, Harp JR (1981) Cerebral protective effect of low-grade hypothermia. Anesthesiology 55:495-498
8. Buchan A, Pulsinelli WA (1990) Hypothermia but not the N-methyl-D-aspartate antagonist, MK-801, attenuates neuronal damage in gerbils subjected to transient global ischemia. J Neurosci 10:311-316
9. Busto R, Dietrich WD, Globus MY, et al (1987) Small differences in intraischemic brain temperature critically determine the extent of ischemic neuronal injury. J Cereb Blood Flow Metab 7:729-738
10. Busto R, Dietrich WD, Globus MY, et al (1989) The importance of brain temperature in cerebral ischemic injury. Stroke 20:1113-1114
11. Busto R, Dietrich WD, Globus MY, et al (1989) Postischemic moderate hypothermia inhibits CA1 hippocampal ischemic neuronal injury. Neurosci Lett 101:299-304
12. Chen H, Chopp M, Zhang ZG, et al (1992) The effect of hypothermia on transient middle cerebral artery occlusion in the rat. J Cereb Blood Flow Metab 12:621-628
13. Chopp M, Chen H, Dereski MO, et al (1991) Mild hypothermic intervention after graded ischemic stress in rats. Stroke 22:37-43

14. Dietrich WD, Busto R, Alonso O, et al (1993) Intraischemic but not postischemic brain hypothermia protects chronically following global forebrain ischemia in rats. J Cereb Blood Flow Metab 13:541-549
15. Goto Y, Kassell NF, Hiramatsu K, et al (1993) Effects of intraischemic hypothermia on cerebral damage in a model of reversible focal ischemia. Neurosurgery 32:980-985
16. Morikawa E, Ginsberg MD, Dietrich WD, et al (1992) The significance of brain temperature in focal cerebral ischemia: Histopathological consequences of middle cerebral artery occlusion in the rat. J Cereb Blood Flow Metab 12:380-389
17. Ridenour TR, Warner DS, Todd MM, et al (1992) Mild hypothermia reduces infarct size resulting from temporary but not permanent focal ischemia in rats. Stroke 23:733-738
18. Yanamoto H, Hong S-C, Soleau S, et al (1996) Mild postischemic hypothermia limits cerebral injury following transient focal ischemia in rat neocortex. Brain Res 718:207-211
19. Colbourne F, Sutherland G, Corbett D (1997) Postischemic hypothermia. A critical appraisal with implications for clinical treatment. Mol Biol 14:171-201
20. Yanamoto H, Nagata I, Nakahara I, et al (1999) Combination of intraischemic and postischemic hypothermia provides potent and persistent neuroprotection against temporary focal ischemia in rats. Stroke 30:2720-2726
21. Yanamoto H, Nagata I, Niitsu Y, et al (2001) Prolonged mild hypothermia therapy protects the brain against permanent focal ischemia. Stroke 32:232-239
22. Yanamoto H, Nagata I, Nakahara I, et al (1999) Prolonged moderate hypothermia suppresses the extension for cerebral infarction for 48 hours following severe permanent focal ischemia. Soc Neurosci Abst 25:235.6
23. Yanamoto H, Nagata I, Niitsu Y, et al (2001) Suppression of cerebral injury due to permanent focal ischemia by prolonged hypothermia therapy in rats. J Cereb Blood Flow Metab 21:S448
24. Yanamoto H, Nagata I, Hashimoto N, et al (1998) Three-vessel occlusion using a micro-clip for the proximal left middle cerebral artery produces a reliable neocortical infarct in rats. Brain Res Protoc 3:209-220
25. Bederson JB, Pitts LH, Germano SM, et al (1986) Evaluation of 2,3,5-triphenyltetrazolium chloride as a stain for detection and quantification of experimental cerebral infarction in rats. Stroke 17:1304-1308
26. Yamamoto M, Tamura A, Kirino T, et al (1989) Effect of a new thyrotropin-releasing hormone analogue administered in rats 1 week after middle cerebral artery occlusion. Stroke 20:1089-1091
27. Yamamoto M, Tamura A, Kirino T, et al (1988) Behavioral changes after focal cerebral ischemia by left middle cerebral artery occlusion in rats. Brain Res 452:323-328
28. Xue D, Huang ZG, Smith KE, et al (1992) Immediate or delayed mild hypothermia prevents focal cerebral infarction. Brain Res 587:66-72
29. Zhang ZG, Chopp M, Chen H (1993) Duration dependent post-ischemic hypothermia alleviates cortical damage after transient middle cerebral artery occlusion in the rat. J Neurol Sci 117:240-244
30. Zhang RL, Chopp M, Chen H, et al (1993) Postischemic (1 hour) hypothermia significantly reduces ischemic cell damage in rats subjected to 2 hours of middle cerebral artery occlusion. Stroke 24:1235-1240

31. Colbourne F, Corbert D (1994) Delayed and prolonged post-ischemic hypothermia is neuroprotective in the gerbil. Brain Res 654:265-272
32. Welsh FA, Harris VA (1991) Postischemic hypothermia fails to reduce ischemic injury in gerbil hippocampus. J Cereb Blood Flow Metab 11:617-620
33. Dietrich WD, Busto R, Alonso O, et al (1993) Intraischemic but not postischemic brain hypothermia protects chronically following global forebrain ischemia in rats. J Cereb Blood Flow Metab 13:541-549
34. Kawai N, Okauchi M, Morisaki K, et al (2000) Effects of delayed intraischemic and postischemic hypothermia on a focal model of transient cerebral ischemia in rats. Stroke 31:1982-1989
35. Huh PW, Belayev L, Zhao W, et al (2000) Comparative neuroprotective efficacy of prolonged moderate intraischemic and postischemic hypothermia in focal cerebral ischemia. J Neurosurg 92:91-99
36. Colbourne F, Corbett D (1995) Delayed postischemic hypothermia: A six month survival study using behavioral and histological assessments of neuroprotection. J Neurosci 15:7250-7260
37. Corbett D, Hamilton M, Colbourne F (2000) Persistent neuroprotection with prolonged postischemic hypothermia in adult rats subjected to transient middle cerebral artery occlusion. Exp Neurol 163:200-206
38. Coimbra C, Drake M, Boris-Moller F, et al (1996) Long-lasting neuroprotective effect of postischemic hypothermia and treatment with an anti-inflammatory/antipyretic drug. Evidence for chronic encephalopathic processes following ischemia. Stroke 27:1578-1585
39. Du C, Hu R, Csernansky CA, et al (1996) Very delayed infarction after mild focal cerebral ischemia: A role for apoptosis? J Cereb Blood Flow Metab 16:195-201
40. Natale JE, D'Alecy LG (1989) Protection from cerebral ischemia by brain cooling without reduced lactate accumulation in dogs. Stroke 20:770-777
41. Globus MYT, Busto R, Lin B, et al (1995) Detection of free radical activity during transient global ischemia and recirculation: effects of intraischemic brain temperature modulation. J Neurochem 65:1250-1256
42. Kil HY, Zhang J, Piantadosi CA (1996) Brain temperature alters hydroxyl radical production during cerebral ischemia/reperfusion in rats. J Cereb Blood Flow Metab 16:100-106
43. Dietrich WD, Busto R, Halley M, et al (1990) The importance of brain temperature in alterations of the blood-brain barrier following cerebral ischemia. J Neuropathol Exp Neurol 49:486-497
44. Karibe H, Zarow GJ, Graham SH, et al (1994) Mild intraischemic hypothermia reduces postischemic hyperperfusion, delayed postischemic hypoperfusion, blood-brain barrier disruption, brain edema, and neuronal damage volume after temporary focal cerebral ischemia in rats. J Cereb Blood Flow Metab 14:620-627
45. Krantis A (1983) Hypothermia-induced reduction in the permeation of radiolabelled tracer substances across the blood-brain barrier. Acta Neuropath (Berl) 60:61-69
46. Yanamoto H, Hashimoto N, Kassell NF, et al (1996) Disruption of blood brain barrier triggered by reperfusion following transient focal ischemia in rats. Soc Neurosci Abst 22:838.3
47. Clifton GL, Miller ER, Choi SC, et al (2001) Lack of effect of induction of hypothermia after acute brain injury. N Engl J Med 344:556-563

48. Maier CM, Sun GH, Kunis D, et al (2001) Delayed induction and long-term effects of mild hypothermia in a focal model of transient cerebral ischemia: neurological outcome and infarct size. J Neurosurg 94:90-96
49. Yanamoto H, Nagata I, Niitsu Y, et al (2001) A new mouse model of neocortical infarct caused by temporary focal ischemia. J Cereb Blood Flow Metab 21:S516
50. The National Institute of Neurological Disorders and Stroke (NINDS) rt-PA Stroke Study Group (1995) Tissue plasminogen activator for acute ischemic stroke. N Eng J Med 333:1581-1587
51. Hacke W, Kaste M, Fieschi C, et al (1995) The efficacy of IV-rtPA in acute ischemic stroke: first results of the ECASS Group: intravenous thrombolysis with recombinant tissue plasminogen activator for acute hemispheric stroke: the European Cooperative Acute Stroke Study (ECASS). JAMA 274:1017-1025
52. Schwab S, Schwarz S, Spranger M, et al (1998) Moderate hypothermia in the treatment of patients with severe middle cerebral artery infarction. Stroke 29:2461-2466

6. Strategies for cerebral aneurysm and vasospasm

The roles of MMPs for cerebral aneurysm formation

Masafumi Morimoto[1], Noriaki Kume[2], Susumu Miyamoto[1], Akira Mizoguchi[3], Kazuhiko Nozaki[1], Nobutake Sadamasa[1], Toru Kita[2], and Nobuo Hashimoto[1]

Department of [1]Neurosurgery, [2]Geriatric Medicine and [3]Anatomy, Graduate School of Medicine, Kyoto University, 54 Kawahara-cho, Shogoin, Sakyo-ku, Kyoto 606-8507, Japan

Summary: Cerebral aneurysm (CA) is histologically characterized by fragmentation of the internal elastic lamina and thinning of the medial smooth muscle cell layer. Its occurrence can be linked to the destruction of the connective tissue by matrix metalloproteinases (MMPs). Among the MMP family, gelatinases (MMP-2 and -9) in particular degrade numerous extracellular matrix components of the vessel wall, such as elastin and type IV collagen. By using animal models of experimentally induced CA, we examined whether MMPs play an important role in CA formation. Our findings showed that the expressions of both MMP-2 and -9 were increased with the progression of CA and that the progression of CA tended to be suppressed in MMP-$2^{-/-}$ or -$9^{-/-}$ mice when compared to wild-type mice. Moreover, we are examining whether the inhibitor of MMPs including MMP-2 and -9, might have a potential for the protection of CA development. Taken together, our data suggest that MMP-2 and -9 might play an important role in CA formation and their blocked-agents might have a new therapeutic potential in preventing the development and rupture of CA.

Key words: Cerebral aneurysm, Extracellular matrix, Matrix metalloproteinase (MMP)

Introduction

Cerebral aneurysm (CA) is the major cause of subarachnoid hemorrhage, which brings about a fatal, catastrophic condition. Although the pathogenesis of CA has been extensively studied for many years [1-4], its molecular mechanisms still remain to be elucidated because human specimens are often too mature or deformed to examine the developmental process of CA.

We have produced experimentally induced CAs in rats and monkeys [5-7], which recapitulate the essential features of human saccular CA. By analyzing these animal models, we have shown the characteristic microscopic findings of the pathological changes in CA formation [5-11]. Recently, we have also developed saccular CAs in mice, which makes it possible to study the pathogenesis of CA in view of the genetic aspect (data submitted).

In the present report, we focus on the degradation of extracellular matrix by matrix metalloproteinases (MMPs), which may prove to be an essential remodeling step in CA formation [12-14]. Using our animal models, we are examining the expressions and functions of MMP-2 and -9, which paticipate in the destruction of the vascular wall which includes collagen and elastin. We provide several new insights into the contributions of these MMPs to this complex disease and show that they might be potentially useful in preventing the growth of CA.

Animal models of saccular cerebral aneurysm

Numerous reports have demonstrated various experimental models of saccular CA, by a vein pouch or a vein patch [15-17], direct injury [18], and toxic agents [19,20], but none of them were spontaneously induced in intracranial arteries. We have developed a method of inducing CAs in rats and monkeys, which have a morphological and pathological similarity to human saccular CAs, by ligating one common carotid artery and rendering the animals hypertensive [5-8]. We have sometimes added beta-aminoproprionitrile, which induces a variety of connective tissue disorders. CAs are often observed in the anterior cerebral artery (ACA)-olfactory artery (OA) bifurcations on the contralateral side of the common carotid artery ligation (Fig.1a,b). In the early stage of CAs, the initial changes were localized almost exclusively at the intimal pad and its neighboring distal portion. The characteristic pathological findings are the thinning of the medial smooth muscle cell layer and the disappearance of internal elastic lamina (Fig.2a). In the advanced stage, the vascular wall protrusion was remarkable and the aneurysmal wall consisted mainly of degenerated connective tissue (Fig.2b). Smooth muscle cells and internal elastic lamina had almost disappeared.

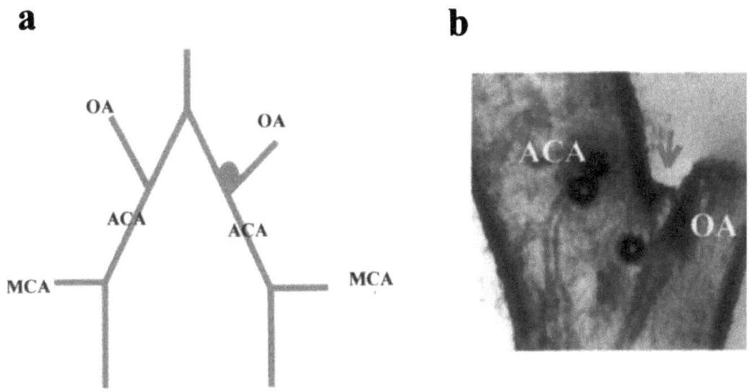

Fig.1a,b. Cerebral aneurysm is spontaneously induced at the anterior cerebral artery (ACA) – olfactory artery (OA) bifurcation in the Willis circle of a SD rat (arrow head). MCA: middle cerebral artery, IC: internal carotid artery.

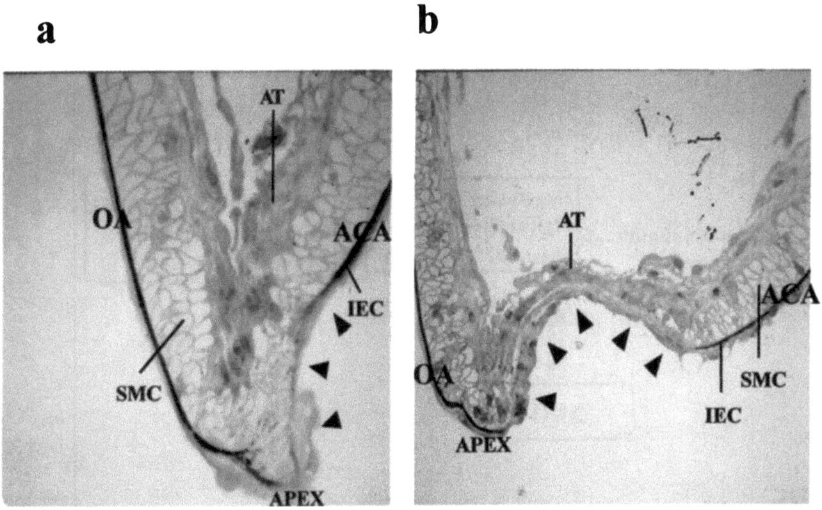

Fig. 2a, b. a In early stages, the wall does not significantly protrude, which shows initial changes as does the fragmentation of internal elastic lamina (IEL) and slight thinning of the medial smooth muscle cells (SMCs) layer. **b** In advanced stages, the wall was remarkably protruded and consisted mainly of degenerated adventitia tissue (AT), accompanied with the absence of internal elastic lamina (IEL) and medial smooth muscle cells (SMCs) layer.

Destruction of extracellular matrix in cerebral aneurysm formarion

With our animal model, we have demonstrated that the three essential pathological changes of CA formation seeme to be as follows: 1.disappearance of the internal elastic lamina, 2.thinning of the smooth muscle cell layer, and 3.degeneration of the adventitial connective tissue [11,21]. All of the changes seem to be mainly caused by the destruction of the connective tissue, including the extracellular matrix. Matrix metalloproteinases (MMPs) are reported as being a family of regulated enzymes that play an important role in the degradation of the extracellular matrix (collagen, elastin, etc,) [22-24]. Many reports have shown that this type of tissue remodeling by MMPs might contribute to the development and rupture of CA [12-14,25] (Fig.3). Within the MMP family, gelatinases (MMP-2 and -9) can especially degrade numerous extracellular matrix components of the vessel wall, such as elastin and type IV collagen [23, 26], and they have often been reported being related to CA formation [4, 12-14, 27]. However, most of the

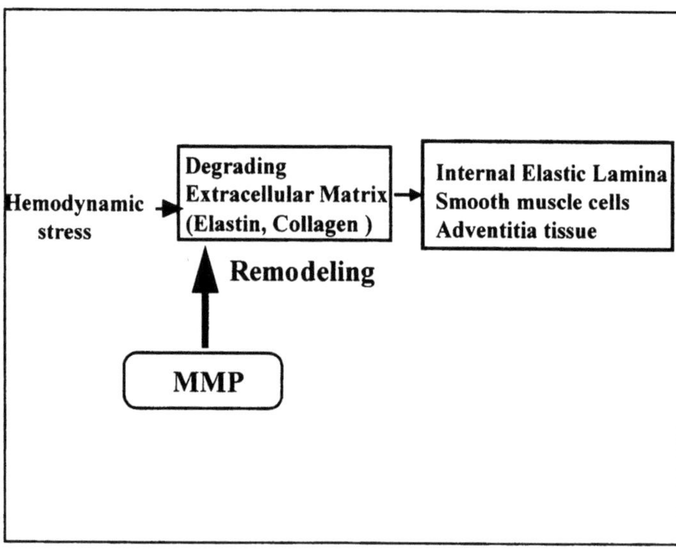

Fig.3 The destruction of arterial wall by hemodynamic stress in the aneurysm development, may be mediated by degrading of extracellular matrix, in which elastin and collagen are major structural components. The dissolution of them requires the activation of specific MMPs.

reports have shown only indirect evidence such that the expressions of MMPs were increased in human CA specimens, most of which are classified as the advanced stage of CA. How their expressions in the aneurymal wall change with the development of CA formation, and whether they are necessary in CA development has never been demonstrated.

Expressions of Gelatinases (MMP-2 and -9) in the wall of cerebral aneurysm

Various stages of CAs can be experimentally produced in our rat models. We observed the expression of MMP-2 and -9 from an early stage in the development process of CA. By immnohistochemistry, MMP-2 was slightly expressed at ACA-OA bifurcations in the control group (Fig.4a), although MMP-9 was not detected (data not shown). This might be because the anti-MMP-2 antibody used also detected pro-MMP-2 in the control sections, even though anti-MMP-9 antibody didin't detect pro-MMP-9. However, to date, we have not yet been able to define it due to the lack of an anti activated-MMP-2 antibody. In the early stage of CA, both MMP-2 and –9 were expressed in each layer of aneurysmal wall, including in the residual endothelial cell layer, the thinning smooth muscle cell layer, and the degenerative adventitia (Fig.4b). MMP-9 was also expressed as the same as MMP-2 (data not shown). On the other hand, in the advanced stage, their expressions were much more active in the aneurysmal wall than in the early stage (Fig.4c). These results provided the new insight that the expressions of MMP-2 and -9 increased with the progress of the CA formation, suggesting that they might play more important role in the progression rather than in the initiation of CA.

a

b

c

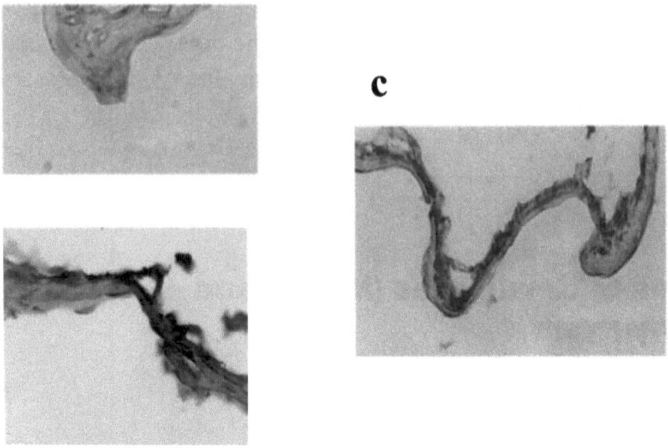

Fig.4 a,b,c The serial changes of MMP-2 expression **a** In the control group, MMP-2 was slightly expressed at ACA-OA bifurcations. **b** In the early stages, MMP-2 was expressed in each layer of wall, residual endothelial cells layer, thinning smooth muscle cells layer, and degenerative adventitia. **c** In the advanced stages, MMP-2 was mainly expressed at the degenerated adventitia and its expression was much more active than in the early stage. X1000

Relationship between MMPs and aneurysm-infiltrating macrophages

Inflammation response within a degenerated wall is a prominent feature of ruptured CA [28], suggesting that inflammatory cells may participate in the connective tissue destruction associated with an aneurysmal formation. Although macrophage infiltration into the aneurysmal wall might play a key role in the rupture of CA [28], the relationship between macrophages and MMPs has not been reported yet. We have already found some MMPs might be co-localized with rupture of CA [28], the relationship between macrophages and MMPs has not been reported yet. We have already found some MMPs might be co-localized with macrophage cells in the CA development (data unsubmitted). The fact would support the hypothesis that MMPs may be strongly related to macrophage cells and play a unique role in CA formation in connection to inflammatory response.

The mechanisms that attract macrophages to the arterial walls of CA are unknown. However, adhesion of blood cells to the damaged endothelium and invasion of the wall by macrophages and leukocytes were commonly observed in the fragile wall of a ruptured aneurysm [28]. These facts suggest that inflammatory cells might produce a variety of biologically active substances including MMPs and play a critical role in CA formation. We need to study other inflammatory responses related to the induction of proteases.

Cerebral aneurysm formation suppressed in MMPs-deficient mice

The functions and obligatory roles of MMP-2 and -9 in CA formation should be clarified by blocking these proteinases or by using genetically altered mice. To study the effects of complex determinants on CA formation in such gene-deficient mice, we have produced a new mouse model of experimentally induced CA, which resembles human saccular CA, as a rat model (data submitted). We are now examining the susceptibility of MMP-deficient mice to CA formation.

In this mouse study, we classified induced-aneurysms into two stages, as mentioned above (Fig.2), according to the pathological findings of a light microscopic study as follows: no change (grade 0); early stages (grade 1), discontinuous internal elastic lamina (IEL) and mild smooth muscle cells (SMCs) damage; advanced stages (grade 2), almost complete disappearance of IEL and SMCs with degenerated adventitia. Our preliminary data showed that the production of advanced-staged CAs tended to be inhibited in both MMP-$2^{-/-}$ and -$9^{-/-}$ mice compared to wild-type mice (wild-type: 50% (6/12), MMP-$2^{-/-}$: 14% (1/7), MMP-$9^{-/-}$: 25% (3/12)). On the other hand, the occurrence of early pathological changes was not significantly different between MMPs$^{-/-}$ and wild-type mice (Table.1). In addition to the immunohistochemical results, these findings support the hypothesis that MMPs might play an essential role in the progression rather than in the initiation of CA, however, we need further studies to show a significant difference between wild-type and MMP-deficient mice.

Table.1 Inhibiting effect on induced aneurysms formation in MMP-deficient mice

	No	No change(0)	Early(1)	Advanced(2)	
Wild-type	12	1(8%)	5(42%)	6(50%)	
$MMP-2^{-/-}$	7	2(29%)	4(57%)	1(14%)	*
$MMP-9^{-/-}$	12	3(25%)	6(50%)	3(25%)	**

* P= 0.097; **P= 0.077 vs Wild-type (Mann-Whitney U test for the grade of Aneurysm)

New therapeutic potential of the inhibitor of MMPs

To examine the effect of MMP inhibitors on the progression of CA, we fed Sprague-Dawley rats with an inhibitor of MMPs including MMP-2 and -9 [29], for 4 months after surgical intervention. We fed the control group a diet with 8% saline, and we fed the treated group a diet with 8% saline and the inhibitor of MMPs.

We are now examining whether this inhibitor can effectively protect the production of advanced-stage CAs compared to the control group. These findings may suggest that MMP-blocked agents might have the potential as a new medical therapy for CA in place of clipping or other disruptive surgeries. However, this MMPs inhibitor used cannot only inhibit the activation of MMP-2 and –9 but also inhibited the functions of other MMPs at the same time. We have to further examine the effects of each specific MMP inhibitor, which might be targeted as a key factor in CA formation.

Summary and perspective

In the present study, we have demonstrated that the expressions of both MMP-2 and -9 are increased with the progress of CA. In addition, in a gene-targeted study with MMP-2and -9 deficient mice, we have provided direct genetic evidence that they might have crucial roles in the progression rather than the initiation of CA formation, and our data using an MMP inhibitor may support the hypothesis that they might be suitable targets for a new therapeutic strategy for preventing the rupture of CA.

Vascular remodeling in the process of CA formation should be caused by two major mechanisms, the degradation of the connective tissue including the extracellular matrix, and a decrease in medial SMCs. In this report, we have provided new insights to the mechanisms of extracellular matrix destruction.

decrease of SMCs, such as apoptosis or the production of nitric oxide (NO) through inducible NO synthase (iNOS) [30,31].

Many reports have shown that increased hemodynamic stress might be a requisite for CA formation [32-34]. We also showed, using rat models [35], in the previous paper that the wall shear stress was the highest at the distal end of the aneurysmal wall. In addition, we found that wall remodeling was especially active at the distal end of the aneurysmal wall in the mouse model. These findings provide evidence that the major changes in CA might be initially caused by an increase of hemodynamic stress, which may activate complex pathways and multiple mediators, following the production of matrix degradation proteinases, such as MMPs. Further studies are needed to clarify whether other factors including cytokines, growth factors, and chemokines, might participate in the recruitment and migration of inflammatory cells.

References

1. Sekher LN, Heros RC (1981) Origin, growth, and rupture of saccular aneurysm: A review. Neurosurgery 8 : 248-60
2. Ostergaard JR (1989) Risk factors in intracranial saccular aneurysms. Aspects on the formation and rupture of aneurysms, and development of cerebral vasospasms. Acta Neurol Scand 80 : 81-98
3. Stehbens WE (1989) Etiology of intracranial berry aneurysms. J Nuerosurg 70 : 823-31
4. Inci S, Spetzler FR (2000) Intracranial aneurysms and arterial hypertension: A review and hypothesis. Surg Neurol 53 : 530-42
5. Hashimoto N, Handa H, Hazama F (1978) Experimentally induced cerebral aneurysm in rats. Surg Neurol 10: 3-8
6. Hashimoto N, Kim C, Kikuchi H, et al (1987) Experimental induction of cerebral aneurysms in monkeys. J Neurosurg 67: 903-905
7. Nagata I, Handa H, Hashimoto N, et al (1980) Experimentally induced cerebral aneurysms in rats: Part IV. Hypertension. Surg Neurol 14: 477-79
8. Kim C, Kikuchi H, Hashimoto N, et al (1989) Histopathological study of induced cerebral aneurysms in primates. Surg Neurol 32: 45-50
9. Hazama F, Kataoka H, Yamada E, et al (1986) Early changes of experimentally induced cerebral aneurysms in rats. Light-microscopic study. Am J Pathol. 124: 399-404
10. Kojima M, Handa H, Hashimoto N, et al (1986) Early changes of experimentally induced cerebral aneurysms in rats: scanning electron microscopic study. Stroke 17: 835-41
11. Kim C, Kikuchi H, Hashimoto N, et al (1988) Involvement of induced cerebral aneurysms in rats. Stroke 19: 507-11
12. Kim SC, Singh M, Huang J, et al (1997) Matrix metalloproteinase-9 in cerebral aneurysms. Neurosurgery 41: 642-46

13. Chyatte D, Lewis I (1997) Gelatinase activity in the occurrence of cerebral aneurysms. Stroke 28: 799-804
14. Bruno G, Todor R, Lewis I, et al (1998) Vascular extracellular matrix remodeling in cerebral aneurysms. J Neurosurg 89: 431-40
15. German WJ, Black SPW (1954) Experimental production of carotid aneurysms. New Engl J Med 250: 104-6
16. Stehbens WE (1973) Experimentally production of aneurysms by microvascular surgery in rabbits. Vasc Surg 7: 165-75
17. Nishikawa M, Smith RD, Yonekawa Y (1977) Experimentally intracranial aneurysms. Surg Neurol 7: 241-44
18. van Alphen HA, Go YE, Kamphorst W (1990) An acute experimental model of saccular aneurysms in the rat. Neurol Res 12: 256-9
19. Handa H (1961) The neurosurgical treatment of intracranial vascular malformations. Particularly with the use of plastics and polarographic measurements. Clin Neurosurg 9: 223-244
20. White JC, Sayer GP, Whisnant IP (1961) Experimental destruction of the media for the production of intracranial arterial aneurysms. J Neurosurg 18: 741-5
21. Kim C, Cervos-Navarro J, Kikuchi H, et al(1992) Alternations in cerebral vessels in experimental animals and their possible relationship to the development of aneurysms. Surg Neurol 38: 331-7
22. Murphy G (1995) Matrix metalloproteinases and their inhibitors. Acta Orthop Scand 66: 55-60
23. Dollery CM, McEwan JR, Henney AM (1996) Matrix metalloproteinases and cardiovascular disease. Circ Res 77: 863-68
24. Mignatti P, Rifkin DB (1996) Plasminogen activators and matrix metalloproteinases in angiogenesis. Enzyme protein 49: 117-137
25. van den Berg JSP, Pals G, Arwert F, et al (1999) Type III Collagen Deficiency in saccular intracranial aneurysms. Stroke 30: 1628-31
26. Sakalihasan N, Delvenne P, Nusgens BV, et al (1996) Activated forms of MMP2 and MMP9 in abdominal aortic aneurysms. J Vasc Surg 24: 127-33
27. Peters GP, Kassam A, Jean PLS (1999) Functional Polymorphism in the matrix metalloproteinase-9 promoter as a potential risk factor for intracranial aneurysm. Stroke 30: 2612-16
28. Kataoka K, Taneda M, Asai T, et al (1999) Structural fragility and inflammatory response of ruptured cerebral aneurysms. Stroke 30: 1396-1401
29. kenji Sugita (1999) Recent advances in inhibitors of matrix metalloproteinases for cancer theraphy. I Drug 4: 327-339
30. Kondo S, Hashimoto N, Kikuchi H,et al (1998) Apoptosis of medical smooth muscle cells in the development of saccular cerebral aneurysms in rats. Stroke 29: 181-89
31. Fukuda S, Hashimoto N, Kikuchi H, et al (2000) Prevention of rat cerebral aneurysm formation by inhibition of nitric oxide synthase. Circulation 101: 2532-38
32. Dyste GN, Beck DW (1989) De novo aneurysm formation following carotid ligation: case report and review of the literature. Neurosurgery 24: 88-92
33. Tognetti F, Limoni P, Testa C (1983) Aneurysm growth and hemodynamic stress. Surg Neurol 20:74-78
34. Strother CM, Graves VB, Rappe A (1992) Aneurysm hemodynamics: An experimental study. AJNR Am J Neuroradiol 13: 1089-95

35. Nakatani H, Hashimoto N, Kang Y, et al (1991) Cerebral blood flow patterns at major vessel bifurcations and aneurysms in rats. J Neurosurg 74: 258-62

Systemically administered thrombin inhibitors can prevent neointimal formation and cerebral vasospasm: The possible role of thrombin and PDGF-BB in vascular pathogeneses

Izumi Nagata[1], Zhiwen Zhang[2], Motoshi Sawada[2], Nobuo Hashimoto[4], Haruhiko Kikuchi[3], and Hiroji Yanamoto[1, 2]

[1]Department of Cerebrovascular Surgery, Hospital of the NATIONAL CARDIO-VASCULAR CENTER, Suita, Osaka 565-8565, Japan
[2]Laboratory for Cerebrovascular Disorders, Research Institute of the [3]NATIONAL CARDIO-VASCULAR CENTER
[4]Department of Neurosurgery, Kyoto University Graduate School of Medicine, Kyoto 606-8507, Japan

Summary: Thrombin and the complement system are activated in vascular lesions during the process of atherosclerosis or pathologic proliferation of smooth muscle cells, and in the subarachnoid space during the development of cerebral vasospasm following subarachnoid hemorrhage (SAH). This article reviews the effects of a potent inhibitor of the complement system and/or thrombin on vascular neointimal formation in the carotid artery of rats, and the development of cerebral vasospasm following subarachnoid hemorrhage (SAH) in rabbits. Carotid balloon dilation injury induced in rats was treated with FUT-175 for 7 days. In rabbits, SAH was treated with FUT-175, or argatroban for 48 h. In addition, recombinant PDGF-BB was injected into the cisterna magna of normal rabbits to observe the calibers of the basilar arteries for 48 h. Neointimal formation after balloon injury was significantly reduced by the treatment with FUT-175. Development of cerebral vasospasm was prevented by FUT-175 or argatroban. In the histological examination, effective doses of FUT-175 or argatroban suppressed the expression of PDGF-BB in the neointimal lesions. Exogenous PDGF-BB resulted in delayed and prolonged vasoconstriction in normal basilar arteries. The complement system and/or thrombin activation following balloon dilation injury or SAH was demonstrated to play a critical role in the development of vascular lesion formation. In the cascade downstream of the protease activation, the production of PDGF-BB was indicated.

Key words: Neointimal formation, Cerebral vasospasm, Thrombin, Serine protease, Platelet-derived growth factor, Review

Introduction

The pathological thickening of arterial walls in the development of atherosclerosis or following vascular injury, or pathologic arterial narrowing (cerebral vasospasm) following subarachnoid hemorrhage (SAH) generate serious vascular stenosis that ultimately causes ischemic disorders [1,2]. In terms of the thickening of the vascular wall, evidences of the activation of thrombin and proteases in the complement system have been accumulating [3-12]. Thrombin, a serine protease cleaved from prothrombin in plasma, is not only a potent stimulator of platelet aggregation, but also acts as a growth factor for vascular smooth muscle cells (VSMC) via specific thrombin receptor *in vitro* [3,13]. An increased expression of thrombin receptors was observed in lesions of atherosclerosis and in VSMC after balloon injury [4,14]. The complement system is a self-defense mechanism that destroys non-self or injured cells, and which is also known to be activated in the process of atherosclerosis [5-7,10-12]. On the other hand, the coagulation and the complement systems are both activated in the subarachnoid space prior to the development of cerebral vasospasm following SAH [15-20]. However, it was unknown whether the activation of thrombin and the complement system is an essential factor in neointimal formation or for the development of cerebral vasospasm following SAH, or purely an inflammatory epiphenomenon during the processes toward vascular lesion formation. This paper reviews our previous studies following the hypothesis that the activation of the complement system and/or thrombin in the coagulation system is necessary for stenotic vascular lesion formation in neointimal or cerebral vasospasm.

To study the role of activated proteases in the two different vascular lesion formations in vivo, we used a specific broad spectrum, non-selective serine protease inhibitor: FUT-175 (nafamostat mesilate), or a selective serine protease inhibitor targeting thrombin: argatroban in a rat balloon injury-neointimal model and a rabbit SAH-vasospasm model [21,22]. In addition, the role of platelet-derived growth factor-BB (PDGF-BB): a growth factor induced by thrombin-activation *in vivo* was studied on the arterial wall following mechanical vascular injury or SAH [23,24].

I. Inhibition of neointimal formation

Materials and methods

Carotid balloon-injury model

Balloon injury to the carotid artery was induced in male Sprague-Dawley rats, weighing 350 to 400 g, based on the method described by Clowes et al. [25,26]. The left common (CCA), internal (ICA) and external carotid (ECA) arteries were exposed under a surgical microscope. A 2 French balloon catheter was introduced from the ECA into the aortic arch through the CCA. An inflated balloon in the aortic arch was slowly pulled back from the aortic arch toward the ECA, 3 times [21].

Inhibitory drug treatment protocol

A synthetic serine protease inhibitor FUT-175 (nafamostat mesilate; 6-amidino-2-naphthyl p-guanidinobenzonate; molecular weight, 539.58) was used to inhibit the activations of thrombin and the compliment system *in vivo* (Futhan®, Torii Pharmaceutical Co., Tokyo, Japan) [27]. FUT-175 competitively, and specifically blocks the active sites of multiple serine proteases including, the complement components, Clr, Cls, B factor, D factor; a component of the coagulation system, thrombin, and a component of the fibrinolytic system; plasmin [27,28]. The protocol design of FUT-175 administration was based on the reported pharmacological properties and kinetics (specific inhibition of serine proteases) studied *in vitro* and *in vivo* [27-30]. The safety of this drug was confirmed in a clinical phase 1-study for the treatment of DIC or acute pancreatitis in humans [31].

FUT-175 (0.5 mg, 1 mg, 2 mg) or vehicle (1 ml of saline) was injected intraperitoneally each day for 7 days, starting immediately after the balloon injury (n=8 each), since it is known that VSMC proliferation to form neointima reaches maximum 4 days after injury in this model [32]. In a sham control group (n=5), the left CCA was exposed but not balloon-dilated.

Morphometric study

Five cross-sections (4 mm length) from the left CCA were stained with hematoxylin and eosin (HE) or Masson trichrome (MTC). Cross-sectional areas of the medial smooth muscle cell layer and neointimal layer were calculated as described elsewhere [21]. The data are expressed as the means ± standard errors of the mean. Statistical analysis was performed by one-way analysis of variance (ANOVA). If multiple comparisons were indicated, the Student-Newman Keuls test was applied. The results are presented in the text as mean ± SEM. A value of $p < 0.05$ was considered significant.

Immunohistochemical study of the rat carotid artery

At the end of the treatment, i.e. 7 days after the balloon injury or the sham-operation treated with or without 2 mg/day of FUT-175 for 7 days, the CCAs were cut into 4 mm-thick segments. The murine monoclonal antibody PGF-007 (a gift from Mochida Pharmaceutical Co., Tokyo) was used for PDGF-BB immunostaining as described elsewhere [33-35].

Results (I)

Morphometric study

In the vehicle-treated group (Fig. 1A, B), neointimal thickening with proliferated-migrated smooth muscle cells in a malarranged inner layer was prominent, accompanied by a normal-appearing medial smooth muscle layer and adventitia (smooth muscle cells, red; collagen fibers, blue), whereas in all rats treated with FUT-175 (Fig. 1C-H), the formation of the neointimal layer was suppressed.

The ratios of the neointima/medial area are shown in Fig. 2. The ratios after treatment with FUT-175 were all significantly smaller than those in the vehicle group. Regarding dose dependency, there were significant differences between each pair of FUT-175-treated groups.

Immunohistochemical analysis of the rat carotid artery

Strong immunoreactivity for PDGF-BB was observed in the neointimal and medial layer 7 days after balloon injury (Fig. 3A, B). After treatment with 2 mg/day of FUT-175, the immunoreactivity was reduced (Fig. 3C, D). In the sham-operated group (Fig. 3E, F), there was neither neointimal formation nor immunoreactivity for PDGF-BB in the medial smooth muscle cell layer.

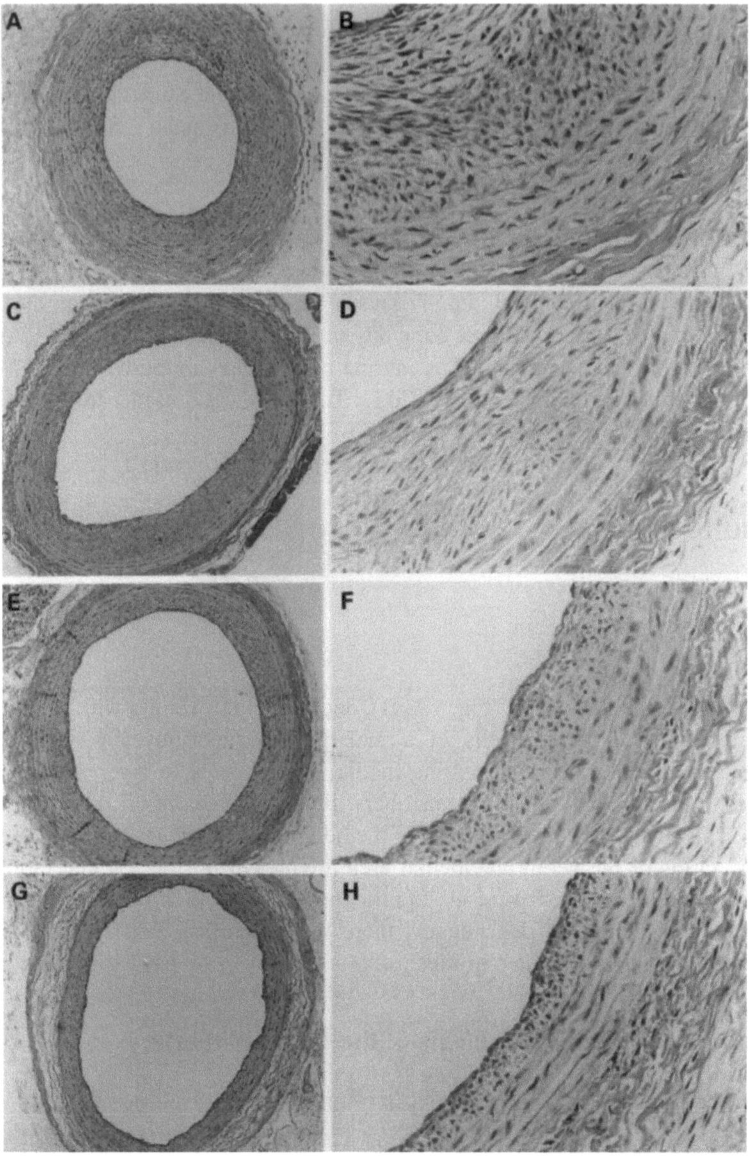

Fig. 1. Cross-sections of rat carotid artery 14 days after balloon-injury and treated with vehicle (A, B), or low dose (C, D), medium dose (E, F) or high dose (G, H) of FUT-175. Thick neointimal formation composed of proliferated smooth muscle cells were seen in the inner layer in all sections. The thickness of the neointimal layer was suppressed in the FUT-175-treated groups (B-H) compared to the vehicle-treated group (A, B) (magnification: × 40, × 100, original; Masson trichrome) (from reference [21], with permission).

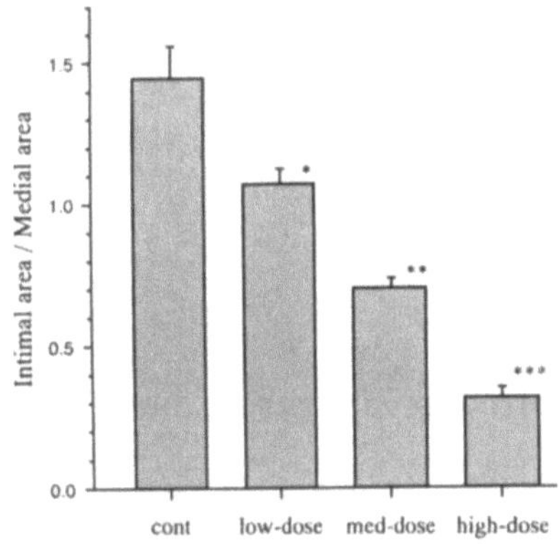

Fig. 2. The ratio of neointima/medial area. The systemic administration of FUT-175 inhibited neointimal formation (*: $p < 0.05$) (from reference [21], with permission).

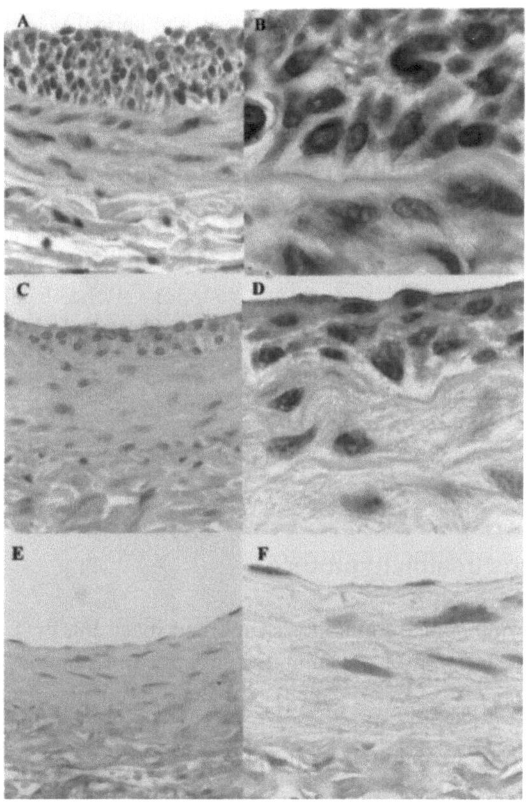

Fig. 3. Immunostaining for PDGF-BB on balloon-injured rat carotid artery. A, B: vehicle-treated group. C, D: treated with FUT-175 (2 mg/day for 7 days). E, F: sham-operated group (magnification: × 200, × 600) (from reference [21], with permission).

II. Inhibition of cerebral vasospasm

Materials and methods

Subarachnoid hemorrhage-vasospasm model

SAH was simulated by transcutaneous single injection of autologous non-heparinized arterial blood in male Japanese white rabbits weighing 3.0 to 3.5 kg (n=92 total) [22]. One ml of fresh arterial blood aspirated via a catheter inserted from the right femoral artery was injected into the cisterna magna after an aspiration of 1.0 ml of normal cerebrospinal fluid, in a precise head-down prone position under anesthesia. After the injection, the animal was maintained in the same position for 40 minutes to allow the injected blood, following a mixture with CSF, to completely coagulate around the targeted basilar artery.

Angiographic examination on cerebral vasospasm

A 4 F-angiographic catheter was inserted from the right femoral artery into the left vertebral artery by fluoroscopy under general anesthesia. The contrast material was injected manually to obtain a fronto-posterior vertebro-basilar angiogram in constant exposure condition and at constant magnification [36,37]. Angiography was performed before SAH (day 0) to determine the baseline caliber of the basilar artery and then repeated 48 h after SAH (day 2). The caliber of the basilar artery was measured at the three corresponding cross sections in a blind manner using a computer-assisted image analysis system, and the mean value in each group was expressed on day 0 and 2.

Inhibitory drugs treatment protocol

The synthetic serine protease inhibitor with broad spectrum, FUT-175 (nafamostat mesilate) and the serine protease inhibitor, argatroban (Slonnon® or Novastan®, Mitsubishi Pharma Co. Osaka, Japan), competitively and selectively block the active site of thrombin [38-41]. Fifty-four rabbits were randomly divided into nine groups (n=6, each) and used for the following experiments.

Experiment A:

FUT-175 (2.5, 5.0, 10, 20 mg / day) or the same volume (480 μl) of saline (vehicle) was infused intravenously via an osmotic mini-pump for 48 h, which was designed to infuse at a speed of 10 μl per hour. The mini-pump was implanted under the femoral skin with the tip of the infusion catheter set in the proximal right femoral vein under a surgical microscope starting 40 min after the induction of SAH. Non-obstruction of the infusion system was confirmed in each rabbit at the time of sacrifice on day 2.

Experiment B:

Argatroban (1.25, 2.5, 5.0 mg / day) or the same volume (480 μl) of saline (vehicle) was infused using the same intravenous infusion system described above. Argatroban or vehicle was infused continuously for 48 h, and the absence of catheter obstruction was confirmed as described above.

In each animal in experiment A and B, the formation of thick SAH around the basilar artery was confirmed at the time of sacrifice. The protocol for argatroban was designed to inhibit thrombin in consideration of the pharmacological properties and kinetics reported in experimental and human clinical studies [38,41].

Physiological parameters during angiographic examinations

Blood pressure, heart rate, blood pH, blood gases (O_2, CO_2), and blood glucose levels were monitored in a separate set of animals during angiographic examinations before and at 48 h after SAH in groups treated with the highest volumes of FUT-175 (20 mg / day), argatroban (5.0 mg / day), and in a group without drug treatment (n=4 each).

Immunohistochemical analysis of the rabbit basilar artery

All SAH rabbits used for angiographic examination on day 2 and another 6 normal rabbits were used for immunohistochemical analysis. Cross sections of brain stem with surrounding arteries were processed for immunohistochemistry by indirect immunoperoxidase method using the murine monoclonal antibody, PGF-007.

Effects of PDGF-BB on the diameter of normal basilar arteries

In a separate set of rabbits, the effects of PDGF-BB on the vascular tone of the normal basilar artery were studied. Five μg of recombinant rat PDGF-BB (R&D Systems, Inc) or vehicle (1 ml of saline), both in 0.2% rat albumin as a carrier protein for PDGF-BB, was injected into the cisterna magna (n=10 each). The caliber of each basilar artery was assessed on repeated angiographic images using a computer-assisted image analysis system. During the angiographic examinations, blood pressure, blood pH, and blood gases were monitored.

Results (II)

Angiographic analysis on cerebral vasospasm

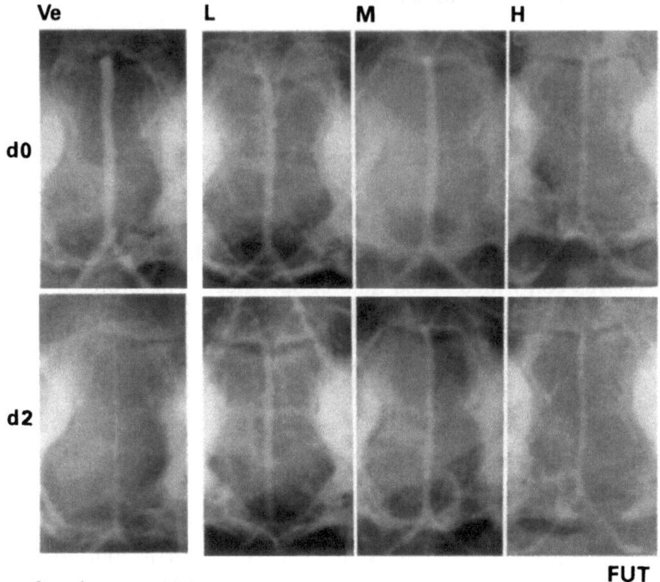

Fig. 4. Sets of angiograms (d 0 and d 2) of rabbit basilar arteries. Severe vasospasm is seen on day 2 in the vehicle-treated group (Ve). The vasoconstriction was reduced in the FUT-175-treated groups (from reference [22], with permission).

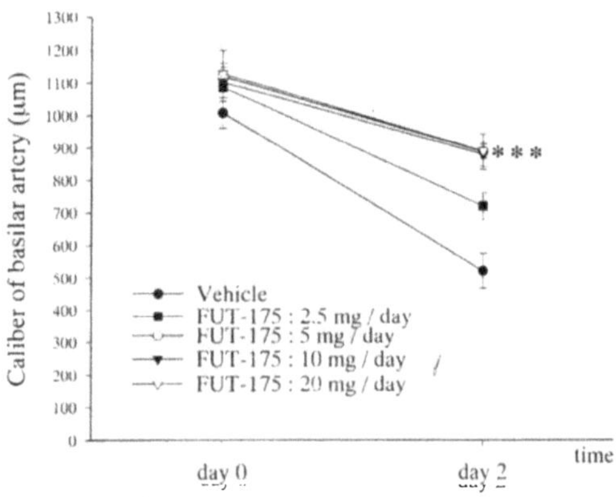

Fig. 5. Angiographic evaluation of cerebral vasospasm in rabbit basilar arteries. There were significant reductions in the development of vasospasm in the three larger volumes of FUT-175-treated groups, but not in the lowest volume (2.5 mg / day) compared to that in the vehicle-treated group (from reference [22], with permission).

Experiment A:

The mean caliber of the basilar artery decreased to 52 ± 5.0 % of the baseline value on day 2 in the vehicle-treated group (Fig. 4, left paired panels and Fig. 5). In those groups treated with the three larger doses of FUT-175 (5.0, 10, or 20 mg / day), there were significant differences in the calibers of basilar arteries compared to those of the vehicle-treated groups on day 2 ($p < 0.05$) (Fig. 4, right three paired panels and Fig. 5). There were no significant differences between the vehicle-treated and the group treated with the lowest dose of FUT-175 (2.5 mg / day) (Fig. 5).

Experiment B:

The mean caliber of the basilar artery decreased to 52 ± 6.4 % of the control value in the vehicle-treated group on day 2 (Fig. 6, 7). In argatroban-treated groups on day 2, there were significant differences in the calibers of basilar arteries in the medium to high dose (2.5 – 5 mg / day) groups, but not in the low dose (1.25 mg / day) group ($p < 0.05$).

Physiologic parameters during angiographic examinations

There were no significant differences in any of the physiological parameters between the groups on day 2, and between before and 2 days after SAH (data not shown).

Immunohistochemical analysis of the rabbit basilar arteries

Two days after SAH, strong immunoreactivity for PDGF-BB was observed in all layers; the endothelial cell, smooth muscle cell and adventitial cell layer in the vehicle-treated SAH group (Fig. 8 upper). In contrast, there was faint, or no immunoreactivity for PDGF-BB detected in the normal basilar artery (Fig. 8 lower). The enhanced immunoreactivity was observed mainly in the nuclei of endothelial and smooth muscle cells.

In groups treated with FUT-175 (Fig. 9), the immunoreactivity in the endothelial and smooth muscle cells were weakly positive compared to that of vehicle-treated vessels (Fig. 8 upper, Fig. 9). Furthermore, the level of immunoreactivity in the smooth muscle cells correlated well to the degree of vascular constriction indicated by corrugation of the internal elastic lamina (Fig. 9).

In groups treated with argatroban (Fig. 10), the level of immunoreactivity for PDGF-BB was highest in the low dose group (1.25 mg / day), and lowest in the high dose group (5 mg / day). The level of immunoreactivity in the smooth muscle cells correlated well to the degree of vascular constriction indicated by corrugation of the internal elastic lamina (Fig. 10).

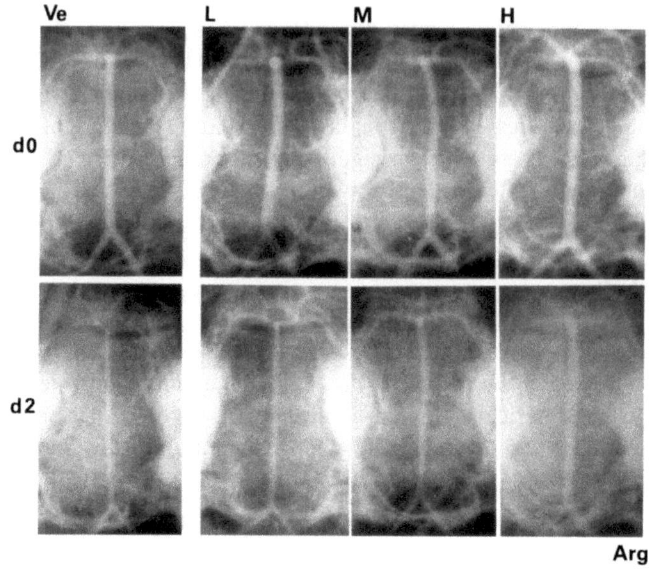

Fig. 6. Sets of angiograms (d 0 and d 2) of rabbit basilar arteries. Severe vasospasm seen on day 2 in the vehicle-treated (Ve) group was reduced in the medium (M: 2.5 mg / day), and high dose (H: 5 mg / day) argatroban-treated groups, but was not apparent in the low dose group (L: 1.25 mg / day) on day 2 (from reference [22], with permission).

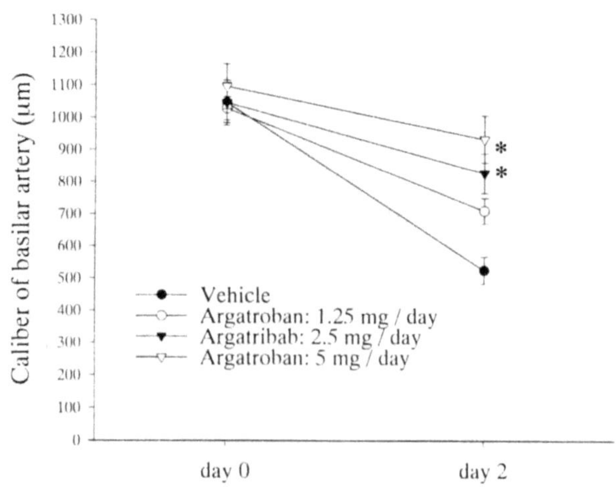

Fig. 7. Angiographic evaluation of cerebral vasospasm in rabbit-basilar artery. There were significant reductions in the development of vasospasm in the medial and high dose (2.5 to 5 mg / day) Argatroban-treated groups, but not in the low dose (1.25 mg / day) group compared to the caliber in the vehicle-treated group (from reference [22], with permission).

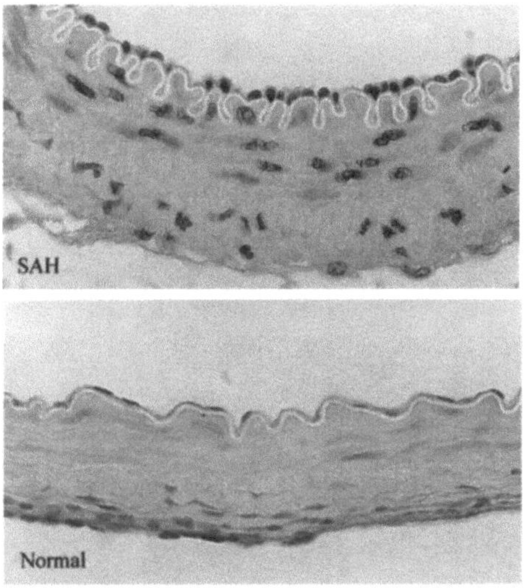

Fig. 8. Immunostaining for PDGF-BB of rabbit basilar artery following SAH (upper panel) or without SAH (lower panel) (×600, originally) (from reference [22], with permission).

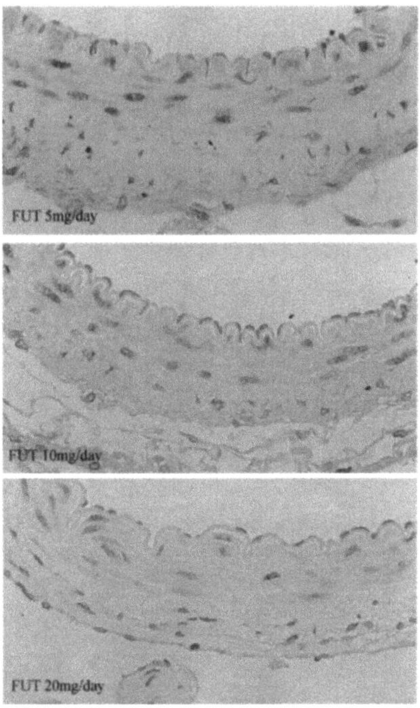

Fig. 9. Immunostaining for PDGF-BB of rabbit basilar artery treated with FUT-175, 5 mg / day (upper), 10 mg / day (middle), or 20 mg / day (lower panel). When the vasoconstriction was moderate (upper panel), the endothelial cell expressed immunoreactivity. (×600, originally) (from reference [22], with permission).

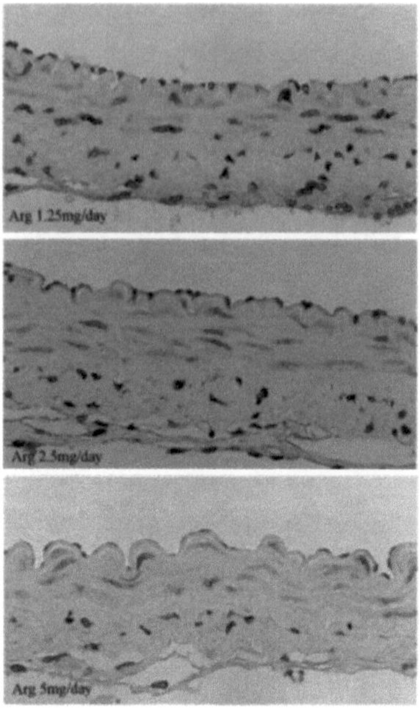

Fig. 10. Immunostaining for PDGF-BB on cross-sections of rabbit basilar artery treated with argatroban, 1.25 mg / day (upper), 2.5 mg / day (middle), or 5 mg / day (lower panel) on day 2. When vasoconstriction was moderate (upper panel, with winding internal elastic lamina and thickened vascular wall), the endothelial cell expressed the immunoreactivity. (×600, originally) (from reference [22], with permission).

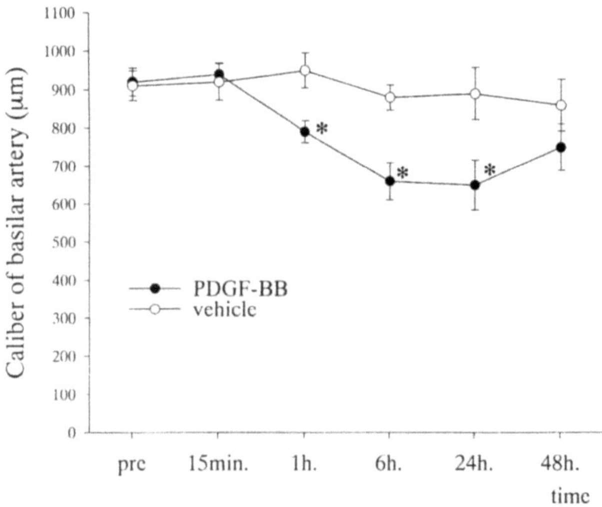

Fig. 11. Time course of the angiographic caliber of the basilar arteries after a cisternal injection of recombinant PDGF-BB or vehicle. (from reference [22], with permission).

Effects of PDGF-BB on the calibers of normal basilar arteries

The basilar arteries slowly constricted following the injection of recombinant PDGF-BB (Fig. 11). The peak of the chronic and long-lasting constriction was at 24 h after the injection. Regarding the physiological parameters, there were no significant differences between PDGF-BB or vehicle injection (data not shown).

Discussion

From the experimental results on the inhibition of rat neointimal formation, it was indicated that the activation of the complement system and/or thrombin is an essential factor in VSMC-proliferation resulting in stenotic lesion after mechanical vascular injury. Injury or loss of integrity of endothelial cells elicits the activation of the complement system, which generates trans-membrane pores on the cell surface and leads to cell dysfunction or ultimately target cell death [5]. The complement components C3 and C5b-9 antigens have been observed in human atherosclerosis lesions [6,7,10-12]. Recently, we confirmed the complement activation (C5b-9 antigen) in the cervical atherosclerosis lesion collected during surgery of human carotid endarterectomy (Fig. 12). The activated complement factor was prominent in the inner layer that was supposed to be a growth cone of atherosclerosis lesion. Platelets possess complement receptors to interact with the complement system [42,43], and the C5b-9 stimulation in the complement system increases platelet prothrombinase activity [44,45]. Therefore, activation of the complement system is considered an enhancer of thrombin activation.

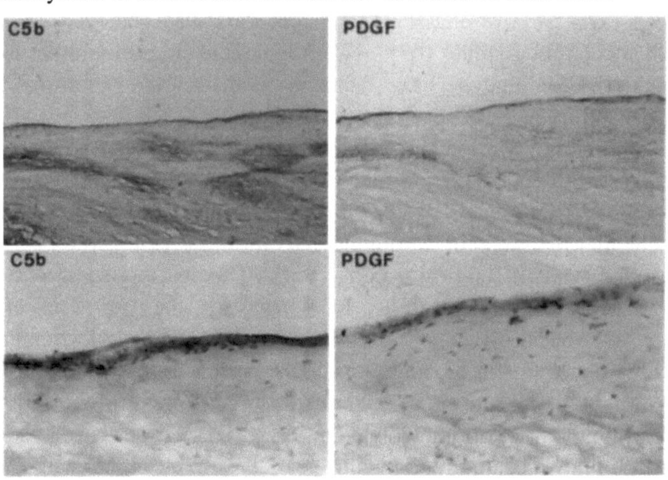

Fig. 12. Immunostaining for C5b: the terminal complement complex, and PDGF-BB on cross-sections of a human carotid lesion of arteriosclerosis. The lesion demonstrates strong immunoreactivity for the terminal complement component (C5b-9) and PDGF-BB in the luminal layer (upper × 50, lower × 200, original).

Thrombin, a multifunctional serine protease generated at the site of vascular injury, is known as a most potent stimulator of platelet aggregation while also exhibiting a host of activating effects on VSMC, vascular endothelial cells, and macrophages [46-50]. Thrombin is chemotactic for monocytes [51] and acts as a mitogen for mesenchymal cells including VSMC *in vitro* [3,3,13]. In a study of human atherosclerotic plaques, the thrombin receptor was widely expressed within the lesions including VSMC and macrophages [4,9]. The multiple cell-activating functions of thrombin can be viewed as a normal remodeling response to vascular injury, by potentiating inflammatory and proliferative cascades in the healing processes [52,53].

In the search for factors downstream of thrombin activation caused by vascular mechanical (balloon) injury, elevated immunoreactivity for PDGF-BB was demonstrated in the endothelial and smooth muscle cells, or following SAH as reviewed above. Studies of PDGF biology revealed that many cell types, including VSMC [14,54,55], macrophages [56,57], and endothelial cells [58] produce PDGF *in vitro*. PDGF is expressed at low or undetectable concentrations in normal adult tissues, but its expression is increased after tissue injury. After vascular injury, VSMC, macrophages, endothelial cells, and fibroblasts in atherosclerosis lesions produce PDGF [23,35,55,59]. PDGF-β receptor mRNA was elevated between 2 and 14 days after carotid injury in rat [60]. Inhibition of the PDGF receptor tyrosine kinase inhibited VSMC migration and proliferation *in vitro* [61]. In a trial for the treatment of neointimal formation in rats, an antibody to PDGF inhibited the neointimal formation after balloon injury [32]. As for the development of atherosclerosis, PDGF B-chain mRNA was detected in the endothelial and neointimal cells in advanced human atherosclerotic plaques [62]. Pronounced expression of PDGF B-type receptors was observed on VSMC in human atherosclerotic plaques [63]. Taken together, the proliferative function of PDGF-BB for VSMC may be a key factor in the disordered neointimal formation after vascular injury and atherosclerosis, although further *in vivo* investigations on thrombin inhibition in relation to the development of atherosclerosis are required.

Regarding thrombin activation and PDGF-BB production following SAH, it has been reported that levels of thrombin-anti-thrombin III complex (TAT) and F1+2, molecular markers of thrombin activation in CSF, were elevated and correlated well with the clinical severity of SAH at the onset and occurrence of cerebral vasospasm [17,18,64,65]. In a trial for the treatment of cerebral vasospasm, intrathecal placement of collagen pellets releasing thrombin inhibitor prevented the development of canine cerebral vasospasm [66]. Although vascular endothelial and smooth muscle cells are capable of expressing thrombin receptor [4], and thrombin causes an immediate contraction of smooth muscle cells via the activated thrombin receptor [67,68], the peak TAT concentration in the CSF of SAH patients was apparently earlier, i.e. on day 2-5, than the development of cerebral vasospasm, indicating that thrombin activation was not a direct cause of arterial narrowing [64,68]. As for a candidate of spasmogens for cerebral vasospasm, it has been reported that levels of PDGF-BB concentration in the cerebrospinal fluid (CSF) in the acute phase of SAH patients were significantly higher in patients with, rather than without, symptomatic vasospasm [69], although the values of PDGF-BB, that is basically insoluble, detected in the CSF do not directly express the PDGF-BB contents in the arterial walls following SAH. Recombinant PDGF-BB has been found to cause a potent concentration-dependent vasoconstriction [70,71]. However, this remained controversial following the finding that PDGF-BB did not constrict rat intracerebral arterioles (perforating arteries) in an *ex-vivo* study [72]. Our latest finding that exogenous PDGF-BB causes delayed and prolonged vasoconstriction in cerebral arteries *in vivo* goes some way to settling the controversies, namely it explains the pathogenesis of cerebral vasospasm based on the slow vasoconstrictive function of PDGF-BB on cerebral arteries.

The pathophysiology of the proliferative or constricting abnormalities, following balloon-injury or bleeding-derived inflammation were considered as different, however, both these vascular responses may have a common cascade through PDGF-BB expression linked to thrombin activation and the subsequent healing process. In conclusion, neointimal formation after vascular injury and cerebral vasospasm following SAH may be caused by a disorder of the normal healing process through thrombin activation and the production of PDGF-BB, or by excessive healing responses, since the thickened arterial walls may be more resistant to second mechanical injury, and the spastic artery may be functioning at least temporarily to prevent re-ruptures of the ruptured cerebral aneurysms by reducing regional cerebral blood flow.

Acknowledgments: These studies were supported by Special Coordination Funds for the Promotion of Science and Technology from the Ministry of Education, Culture, Sports, Science and Technology (MEXT) of Japan. We acknowledge the valuable assistance of Yasuda T, Okuno A, Kurimoto M, and Nishimori K.

References

1. Ross R (1993) The pathogenesis of atherosclerosis: a perspective for the 1990s. Nature 362:801-809
2. Zabramski JM (1997) In: AANS Publications Committee; Bederson JB (editor) Vasospasm after subarachnoid hemorrhage. Subarachnoid hemorrhage: pathophysiology and management. The American Association of Neurological Surgeons pp 127-156
3. McNamara CA, Sarembock IJ, Gimple LW, et al (1993) Thrombin stimulates proliferation of cultured rat aortic smooth muscle cells by a proteolytically activated receptor. J Clin Invest 91:94-98
4. Nelken NA, Soifer SJ, O'keefe J, et al (1992) Thrombin receptor expression in normal and atherosclerotic human arteries. J Clin Invest 90:1614-1621
5. Seifert PS, Kazatchkine MD (1988) The complement system in atherosclerosis. Atherosclerosis 73:91-104

6. Niculescu F, Hugo F, Rus HG, et al (1987) Quantitative evaluation of the terminal C5b-9 complement complex by ELISA in human atherosclerotic arteries. Clin Exp Immunol 69:477-483
7. Vlaicu R, Niculescu F, Rus HG, et al (1985) Immunohistochemical localization of the terminal C5b-9 complement complex in human aortic fibrous plaque. Atherosclerosis 57:163-177
8. Sarembock IJ, Gertz SD, Gimple LW, et al (1991) Effectiveness of recombinant desulphatohirudin in reducing restenosis after balloon angioplasty of atherosclerotic femoral arteries in rabbits. Circulation 84:232-243
9. Dechend R, Mo X, Schulz W, et al (1996) Thrombin receptor and urokinase-type plasminogen activator are colocalized in vascular smooth muscle cells derived from human carotid atherosclerotic plaques. Fibrinolysis 10:41-45
10. Vlaicu R, Rus HG, Niculescu F, et al (1985) Immunoglobulins and complement components in human aortic atherosclerotic intima. Atherosclerosis 55:35-50
11. Hansson GK, Holm J, Kral JG (1984) Accumulation of IgG and complement factor C_3 in human arterial endothelium and atherosclerotic lesions. Acta Pathol Microbiol Immunol Scand Sect A 92:429-435
12. Hollander W, Colombo MA, Kirkpatrick B, et al (1979) Soluble proteins in the human atherosclerotic plaque: with spectral reference to immunoglobulines, C_3-complement component, α_1-antitrypsin and α_2-macroglobulin. Atherosclerosis 34:391-405
13. Chen LB, Buchanan JM (1975) Mitogenic activity of blood components.1. Thrombin and prothrombin. Proc Natl Acad Sci USA 72:131-135
14. Okazaki H, Majesky MW, Harker LA, et al (1992) Regulation of platelet-derived growth factor ligand and receptor gene expression by α-thrombin in vascular smooth muscle cells. Circ Res 71:1285-1293
15. Kasuya H, Shimizu T (1989) Activated complement components C3a and C4a in cerebrospinal fluid and plasma following subarachnoid hemorrhage. J Neurosurg 71:741-746
16. Kasuya H, Shimizu T, Okada T, et al (1988) Activation of the coagulation system in the subarachnoid space after subarachnoid hemorrhage: Serial measurement of fibrinopeptide A and bradykinin of cerebrospinal fluid and plasma in patients with subarachnoid hemorrhage. Acta Neurochir (Wien) 91:120-125
17. Suzuki M, Ogawa A, Sakurai Y, et al (1992) Thrombin activity in cerebrospinal fluid after subarachnoid hemorrhage. Stroke 23:1181-1182
18. Peltonen S, Juvela S, Kaste M, et al (1997) Hemostasis and fibrinolysis activation after subarachnoid hemorrhage. J Neurosurg 87:207-214
19. Ikeda K, Asakura H, Futani K, et al (1997) Coagulative and fibrinolytic activation in cerebrospinal fluid after subarachnoid hemorrhage. Neurosurgery 41:344-349
20. Suzuki M, Kudo A, Otawara Y, et al (1999) Extrinsic pathway of blood coagulation and thrombin in the cerebrospinal fluid after subarachnoid hemorrhage. Neurosurgery 44:483-493
21. Sawada M, Yanamoto H, Nagata I, et al (1999) Prevention of neointimal formation by a serine protease inhibitor, FUT-175, after carotid balloon injury in rats. Stroke 30:644-650
22. Zhang Z, Nagata I, Kikuchi H, et al (2001) Broad-spectrum and selective serine protease inhibitors prevent expression of platelet-derived growth factor-BB and cerebral vasospasm after subarachnoid hemorrhage: vasospasm caused by cisternal injection of recombinant platelet-derived growth factor-BB. Stroke 32:1665-1672

23. Ross R, Raines EW, Bowen-Pope DF (1986) The biology of platelet-derived growth factor. Cell 46:155-169
24. Shultz PJ, Knauss TC, Mené P, et al (1989) Mitogenic signals for thrombin in mesangial cells: regulation of phospholipase C and PDGF genes. Am J Physiol 257:F366-F374
25. Clowes AW, Reidy MA, Clowes MM (1983) Mechanisms of stenosis after arterial injury. Lab Invest 49:208-215
26. Morishita R, Gibbons GH, Kaneda Y, et al (1993) Novel and effective gene transfer technique for study of vascular renin angiotensin system. J Clin Invest 91:2580-2585
27. Ikari N, Sakai Y, Hitomi Y, et al (1983) New synthetic inhibitor to the alternative complement pathway. Immunology 49:685-691
28. Hitomi Y, Fujii S (1982) Inhibition of various immunological reactions in vivo by a new synthetic complement inhibitor. Int Archs Allergy Appl Immunol 69:262-267
29. Koshiyama Y, Ozeki K, Motoyashi A, et al (1984) Pharmacological studies of FUT-175, nafamostat mesilate. Nippon Yakurigaku Zasshi 84:417-428
30. Aoyama T, Ino Y, Ozeki M, et al (1984) Pharmacological studies of FUT-175, nafamostat mesilate. 1.inhibition of protease activity in vitro and in vivo experiments. Jpn J Pharmacol 35:203-227
31. Abe T, Kinoshita T, Matsuda S, et al (1984) Phase 1 study of FUT-175. Single and multiple dose study. Jpn Pharmacol Ther 12:4941-4964
32. Ferns GA, Raines EW, Sprugel KH, et al (1991) Inhibition of neointimal smooth muscle accumulation after angioplasty by an antibody to PDGF. Science 253:1129-1132
33. Johnson RJ, Raines EW, Floege J, et al (1992) Inhibition of mesangial cell proliferation and matrix expansion in glomerulonephritis in the rat by antibody to platelet-derived growth factor. J Exp Med 175:1413-1416
34. Floege J, Burns MW, Alpers CE, et al (1992) Glomerular cell proliferation and PDGF expression precede glomerulosclerosis in the remnant kidney model. Kidney Int 41:297-309
35. Ross R, Masuda J, Raines EW, et al (1990) Localization of PDGF-B protein in macrophages in all phases of atherogenesis. Science 248:1009-1012
36. Yanamoto H, Kikuchi H, Okamoto S, et al (1992) Preventive effect of synthetic serine protease inhibitor, FUT-175, on cerebral vasospasm in rabbits. Neurosurgery 30:351-357
37. Yanamoto H, Kikuchi H, Okamoto S, et al (1994) Cerebral vasospasm caused by cisternal injection of polystyrene latex beads in rabbits is inhibited by a serine protease inhibitor. Surg Neurol 42:374-381
38. Hantgan RR, Jerome WG, Hursting MJ (1998) No effect of clot age or thrombolysis on argatroban's inhibition of thrombin. Blood 92:2064-2074
39. Kikumoto R, Tamao Y, Tezuka T, et al (1984) Selective inhibition of thrombin by (2R, 4R)-4-methyl-1-[N^2-[(3-methyl-1,2,3,4-tetrahydro-8-quinolinyl)sulfonyl]-L-arginyl]-2-piperidinecarbosylic acid. Biochemistry 23:85-90
40. Kikumoto R, Hara H, Ninomiya K, et al (1990) Syntheses and platelet aggregation inhibitory and antithrombotic properties of [2-[(omega-aminoalkoxy) phenyl] ethyl]benzenes. J Med Chem 33:1818-1823
41. Okamoto S, Hijikata A, Kikumoto R, et al (1981) Potent inhibition of thrombin by the newly synthesized arginine derivative No.805. The importance of stereo-structure of its hydrophobic carboxamide portion. Biochem Biophys Res Comm 101:440-446

42. Peerschke EI, Ghebrehiwet B (1987) Human blood platelets possess specific binding sites for C1q. J Immunol 138:1537-1541
43. Vik DP, Fearon DT (1987) Cellular distribution of complement receptor type 4 (CR4): expression on human platelets. J Immunol 138:254-258
44. Wiedmer T, Esmon CT, Sims PJ (1986) Complement proteins C5b-9 stimulate procoagulant activity through platelet prothrombinase. Blood 68:875-880
45. Wiedmer T, Esman CT, Sims PJ (1986) On the mechanism by which complement proteins C5b-9 increase platelet prothrombinase activity. J Biol Chem 261:14587-14592
46. Clowes AW, Reidy MA, Clowes MM (1983) Kinetics of cellular proliferation after arterial injury: I. smooth muscle growth in the absence of endothelium. Lab Invest 49:327-333
47. Harker LA, Hanson SR, Runge MS (1995) Thrombin hypothesis of thrombus generation and vascular lesion formation. Am J Cardiol 75:12B-17B
48. Coughlin SR (1994) Thrombin receptor function and cardiovascular disease. Trends Cardiovasc Med 4:77-83
49. Coughlin SR, Vu T-KH, Hung DT, et al (1992) Characterization of a functional thrombin receptor. J Clin Invest 89:351-355
50. Fenton II JW (1981) Thrombin specificity. Ann NY Acad Sci 370:468-495
51. Shuman MA (1986) Thrombin-cellular Interactions. Ann NY Acad Sci 485:228-239
52. Gibbons GH, Dzau VJ (1994) The emerging concept of vascular remodeling. New Eng J Med 330:1431-1438
53. McNamara CA, Sarembock IJ, Bachhuber BG, et al (1996) Thrombin and vascular smooth muscle cell proliferation: implications for atherosclerosis and restenosis. Semin Thromb Hemost 22:139-144
54. Seifert RA, Schwartz SM, Bowen-Pope DF (1984) Developmentally regulated production of platelet-derived growth factor-like molecules. Nature 311:669-671
55. Walker LN, Bowen-Pope DF, Ross R, et al (1986) Production of platelet-derived growth factor-like molecules by cultured arterial smooth muscle cells accompanies proliferation after arterial injury. Proc Natl Acad Sci USA 83:7311-7315
56. Shimokado K, Raines EW, Madtes DK, et al (1985) A significant part of macrophage-derived growth factor consists of at least two forms of PDGF. Cell 43:277-286
57. Martinet Y, Bitterman PB, Mornex J, et al (1986) Activated human monocytes express the c-sis proto-oncogene and release a mediator showing PDGF-like activity. Nature 319:158-160
58. DiCorleto PE (1984) Cultured endothelial cells produce multiple growth factors for connective tissue cells. Exp Cell Res 153:167-172
59. Antoniades HN, Galanopoulos T, Neville-Golden J, et al (1991) Injury induces in vivo expression of platelet-derived growth factor (PDGF) and PDGF receptor mRNAs in skin epithelial cells and PDGF mRNA in connective tissue fibroblasts. Proc Natl Acad Sci USA 88:565-569
60. Majesky MW, Reidy MA, Bowen-Pope DF, et al (1990) PDGF ligand and receptor gene expression during repair of arterial injury. J Cell Biol 111:2149-2158
61. Myllärniemi M, Calderon L, Lemström K, et al (1997) Inhibition of platelet-derived growth factor receptor tyrosine kinase inhibits vascular smooth muscle cell migration and proliferation. FASEB J 11:1119-1126

62. Wilcox JN, Smith KM, Williams LT, et al (1988) Platelet-derived growth factor mRNA detection in human atherosclerotic plaques by in situ hybridization. J Clin Invest 82:1134-1143
63. Rubin K, Tingström A, Hansson GK, et al (1988) Induction of B-type receptors for platelet-derived growth factor in vascular inflammation: possible implications for development of vascular proliferative lesions. Lancet 1:1353-1356
64. Hirashima Y, Nakamura S, Suzuki M, et al (1997) Cerebrospinal fluid tissue factor and thrombin-antithrombin III complex as indicators of tissue injury after subarachnoid hemorrhage. Stroke 28:1666-1670
65. Kasuya H, Shimizu T, Takakura K (1998) Thrombin activity in CSF after SAH is correlated with the degree of SAH the persistence of subarachnoid clot and the development of vasospasm. Acta Neurochir (Wien) 140:579-584
66. Kudo A, Suzuki M, Kubo Y, et al (2000) Intrathecal administration of thrombin inhibitor ameliorates cerebral vasospasm: use of a drug delivery system releasing hirudin. Cerebrovasc Dis 10:424-430
67. Yanagisawa M, Kurihara H, Kimura S, et al (1988) A novel potent vasoconstrictor peptide produced by vascular endothelial cells. Nature 332:411-415
68. Jerius H, Beall A, Woodrum D, et al (1998) Thrombin-induced vasospasm: cellular signaling mechanisms. Surgery 123:46-50
69. Gaetani P, Tancioni F, Grignani G, et al (1997) Platelet derived growth factor and subarachnoid haemorrhage: a study on cisternal cerebrospinal fluid. Acta Neurochir (Wien) 139:319-324
70. Berk BC, Alexander RW, Brock TA, et al (1986) Vasoconstriction: a new activity for platelet-derived growth factor. Science 232:87-89
71. Sachinidis A, Locher R, Hoppe J, et al (1990) The platelet-derived growth factor isomers, PDGF-AA, PDGF-AB and PDGF-BB, induce contraction of vascular smooth muscle cells by different intracellular mechanisms. FEBS Lett 275:95-98
72. Bassett JE, Bowen-Pope DF, Takayasu M, et al (1988) Platelet-derived growth factor does not constrict rat intracerebral arterioles *in vitro*. Microvasc Res 35:368-373

Cerebral vasospasm induced by the interaction between macrophage and oxidized membrane of erythrocyte

Taro Komuro[1,2], Soichi Miwa[3], Yoshifumi Kawanabe[1,2], Xiao-Feng Zhang[1], Tatsuya Sawamura[1], Manabu Fukumoto[4], Haruhiko Kikuchi[2], Tomoh Masaki[1]

Departments of [1]Pharmacology and [2]Neurosurgery, Kyoto University Graduate School of Medicine, Kyoto 606-8501, Japan
[3]Department of Pharmacology, Hokkaido University Graduate School of Medicine, Sapporo 060-8638, Japan
[4]Department of Pathology, Institute of Development, Aging and Cancer, Tohoku University, Sendai 980-8575, Japan

Summary: Cerebral vasospasm after subarachnoid hemorrhage appears when infiltration of macrophages is prominent, however, a causal relationship between the vasospasm and infiltration of macrophages has not been elucidated. A potent vasoconstrictor endothelin is reported to be involved in the cerebral vasospasm, while the origin of the endothelin is unknown. We found and characterized the macrophage-induced constriction of cerebral artery via endothelin in a subarachnoid hemorrhage model. An injection of oxidized but not non-oxidized erythrocyte membranes induced an infiltration of macrophage and a cerebral vasospasm on the day 3. A simultaneous injection of macrophages along with the oxidized membranes induced a cerebral vasospasm immediately and the vasospasm was abolished by co-injection of endothelin-receptor antagonists (FR-139317 for ET_AR or BQ-788 for ET_BR). The direct vasoconstricting action of macrophage along with the oxidized membranes was confirmed with an isometric tension study. Macrophages preferentially recognized and interacted with the oxidized membranes. These data suggest that the infiltrated macrophage induces a cerebral vasospasm via endothelin after it's activation by the interaction with oxidized erythrocyte menbranes.

Key words: Macrophage, Cerebral vasospasm, Erythrocyte, Endothelin

Introduction

Cerebral vasospasm after subarachnoid hemorrhage (SAH) is a pathological vasoconstriction of major cerebral arteries and becomes apparent from 3 to 7 days after SAH and subsides within 2 or 3 weeks. It often causes cerebral infarction and/or ischemia, which often determin the prognosis of SAH patient. A number of substances from subarachnoid clot have so far been suspected as endogenous spasmogens but only a few of them have been established as etiologic factors for the cerebral vasospasm after SAH. Even these factors, i.e., oxyhemoglobin and endothelin, also have some problems as the definitive etiologic factors[1].

Infiltration of macrophages (Mϕs) into the subarachnoid clot and phagocytosis of erythrocytes by Mϕs are prominent histological features of the brain after SAH[2, 3, 4]. The time course of the phagocytotic activity seems to coincide with that of the cerebral vasospasm. It is also known that Mϕs are activated by phagocytosis and gain the potency to secrete vasoconstricting substances[5]. From these data, we hypothesized that Mϕs which have infiltrated into the subarachnoid clot and interacted with erythrocyte (RBC) play a critical role in the cerebral vasospasm after SAH. We found and characterized the macrophage-induced cerebral vasospasm with a subarachnoid hemorrhage model of rabbit.

Materials and methods

Preparations of ox- or non-ox-erythrocyte ghost

RBCs were obtained from Japanese White Rabbits of either sex weighing 3.0 - 3.5 kg and washed twice with PBS containing 0.1% glucose. For preparation of oxidated RBCs (ox-RBCs), RBCs were incubated in PBS containing 0.2 mmol/L $CuSO_4$ and 5 mmol/L ascorbate at 37 °C for 90 minutes[6]. After washing once with PBS containing 0.1% glucose, the ox- or non-oxidated RBCs (non-ox-RBCs) were lysed in 5 volumes of hemolysis buffer (1 mmol/L K^+-EDTA, 10 mmol/L Tris-Cl, 1 mmol/L $MgCl_2$, pH 7.4) and centrifuged at 18,000 x g for 10 minutes. After the supernatant was discarded, floating white pellet was collected and washed four times with 5 volumes of hemolysis buffer and twice with 5 volumes of PBS containing 15 mmol/L $MgCl_2$; this concentration of $MgCl_2$ keeps the ghosts outside-out[7]. For tension study, the ghosts were resuspended in PBS at a density of $0.24 \times 10^8/\mu L$ and added to the suspension of Mϕs on the plastic plate. For intracisternal injection and labeling with Fast DiO (Molecular Probes), the RBC ghosts were resuspended at a density of $4.8 \times 10^9/mL$ and $10^{10}/mL$ in PBS, respectively.

Preparation of macrophage

Thioglycolate medium (4%, 60 mL, Nissui) was injected into peritoneal cavity of the same rabbit from which RBCs were collected and exudated peritoneal cells were collected by lavage of the peritoneal cavity 3 days later. The cells were devided into four parts, and seeded in 100-mm culture dishes containing Roswell Park Memorial Institute 1640 medium (RPMI 1640 medium, Nissui) and kept for 20 minutes in a CO_2 incubator containing 5 %CO_2 in air. After the incubation, the dishes were washed vigorously with phosphate-buffered saline (PBS) 3-5 times to remove non-adherent cells (non-Mϕ cells). The adherent cells were cultured for 4 hours in RPMI 1640 medium supplemented with 10% autoserum which had been heat-inactivated by incubating it at 56 °C for 30 minutes. The dishes were washed vigorously 3 times with PBS, the cells were harvested and resuspended in PBS. This usually yielded 1-2.5 x 10^6 peritoneal exudated cells, and we confirmed that over 90% of the cells were Mϕs. When more than 6 x 10^6 peritoneal Mϕs were obtained, the Mϕs were discarded. For the experiments to investigate the interaction of Mϕs with RBC ghosts, the Mϕs attached to the dishes were used after washing with PBS. For tension study, the cells were harvested with 5 mmol/L EGTA, spun down and resuspended in PBS containing 0.1% glucose at a density of 2 x 10^6 cells/10 μL. For application of Mϕs to aortic ring specimens, a layer of Mϕs was prepared by placing 10 μL of the Mϕs suspension on a plastic plate (4 x 3 mm) for 15 minutes. The plate was put directly on the adventitia of the ring specimens with the Mϕs being in contact with the adventitia.

Isometric tension study

Isometric tension recording was performed with rabbit aorta as described previously[8].

Preparation of labeled erythrocyte ghost

The non-ox- or ox-RBC ghosts were incubated with a fluorescent dye Fast DiO (1 nmol/L) in PBS for 5 minutes and washed 4 times with PBS. The Mϕs were incubated for 20 minutes with the labeled non-ox- or ox-RBC ghosts and washed 4 times before microscopic examinations.

Intracisternal injection of erythrocyte ghost and cerebral angiography in rabbits

The cisterna magna of rabbits were punctured with 25-gauge needle. After 1-mL of cerebrospinal fluid had been removed, 1-mL aliquot of the ghost and/or Mϕ suspension (2×10^6 cells/mL) were injected. For assessment of cerebral vasospasm, cerebral angiography was performed before and after the injection of RBC ghosts, and the caliber of basilar artery was measured on ten-times magnified X-ray film.

Histological study

Three days after the intracisternal injection of RBC ghosts, rabbits euthanized by pentobarbital were perfused through the left ventricle of heart with PBS followed by 4% paraformaldehyde/PBS. The brainstem with basilar artery and arachnoid membrane was removed, dehydrated, fixed in 4% paraformaldehyde and stained with hematoxylin and eosin.

Statistical analysis

Data are presented as means ± standard deviation. Pairs of means were compared by Student's or Welch's *t* test for unpaired values. A provability level of $P<0.01$ was considered to be statistically significant. Numbers of experiments were five unless otherwise mentioned.

Prevention of cruelty to animal

All experiments with rabbits were performed according to the guideline for animal experiments in Kyoto University. General anesthesia with pentobarbital (30 mg/kg, IV) in all experiments and local anesthesia with small amount of 0.25% lidocaine in some steps were used.

Results

Since it is known that Mφs phagocytose senescent or oxidatively damaged erythrocyte *in vitro* by recognizing the changes in molecules on the cell membrane[6], we attempted to experimentally induce infiltration of Mφs by injecting ox-RBC ghosts instead of intact RBCs into cisterna magna of rabbits (Fig. 1) and examined whether the infiltration was accompanied by a cerebral vasospasm (Fig. 2-A, 2-B).

Histological findings of the brain section on the 3rd day after the injection of ox-RBC ghosts showed that the dominant cells infiltrating into clusters of the ox-RBC ghosts were Mφs, while infiltration of polymorphonuclear leukocytes or lymphocytes was almost negligible. Notably many Mφs phagocytosed the ghosts. On the other hand, infiltration of Mφs was less in clusters of the ox-RBC ghosts at

2.5 hours, 8 hours and the 7th day (data not shown), and also in clusters of non-ox-RBC ghosts throughout the postinjection period.

At 2.5 or 8 hours following the injection of ox-RBC ghosts, the caliber of the basilar artery assessed by cerebral angiography was not significantly changed, but on the 3rd day it was reduced to 70 ± 9.7% of the control value before injection (also different from the vehicle group). On the 7th day, it recovered (89 ± 9.5% of controls; also not significantly different from vehicle group). Injection of non-ox-RBC ghosts was without effect up to the 7th day. The time course and severity of the vasoconstrictions after the injection of ox-RBC ghosts were essentially similar to those of experimental vasospasm in rabbits induced by injection of whole blood[9].

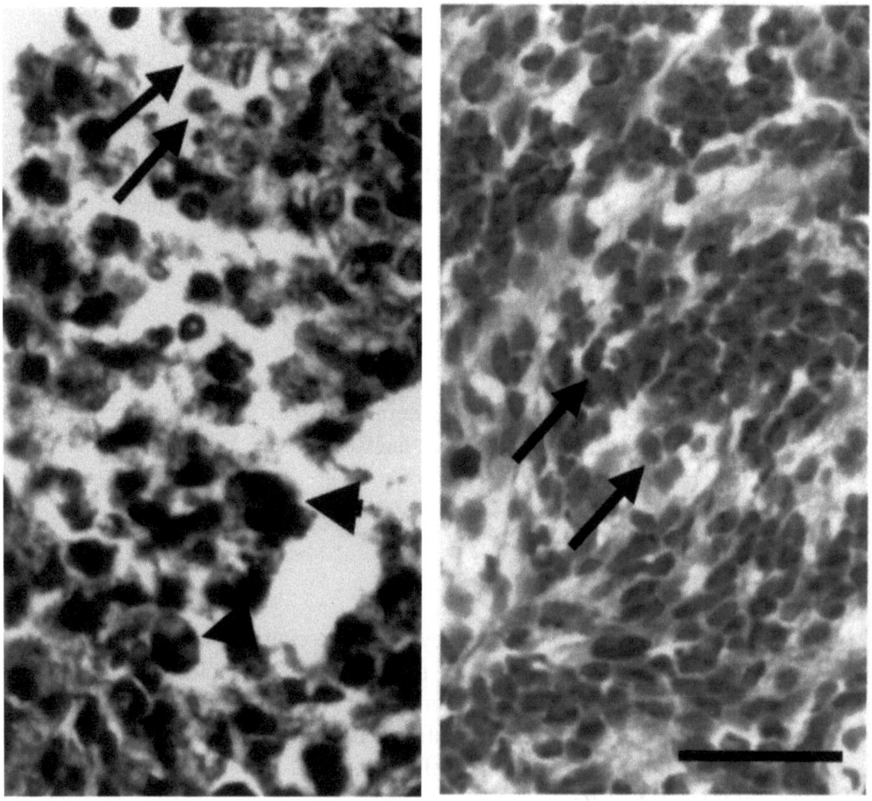

Fig. 1. Histological study of subarachnoid clots on the 3rd day. Small arrows; clusters of RBC ghosts, Large arrowheads; Mϕs, Scale bar; 25 μm, ox-RBC ghosts (left), non-ox-RBC ghosts (right) H.E. staining.

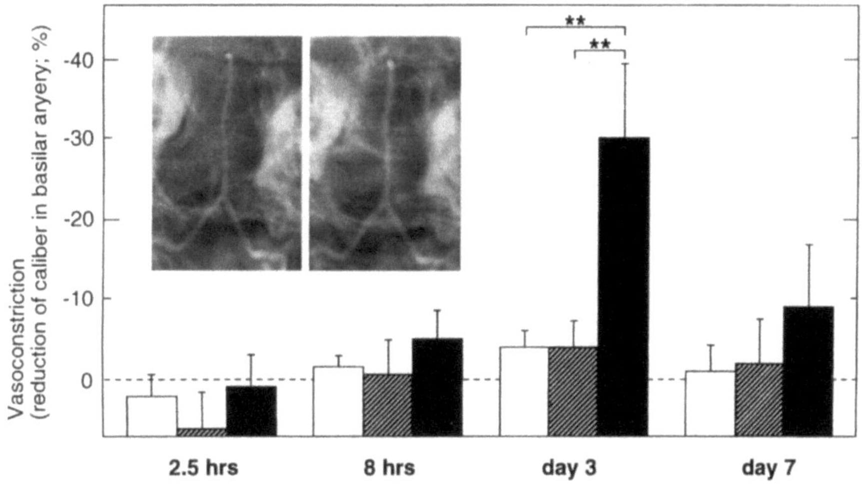

Fig. 2. Vasoconstricting effects of intracisternal injection of RBC ghosts. Vehicle alone (PBS, open circles), non-ox-RBC ghosts (hatched squares), ox-RBC ghosts (closed squares) were injected and cerebral angiograms were performed before and at some time points (2.5 hrs, 8 hrs, day 3 and day 7) after the injections. The values mean the percentages of calibers after the injection to those before the injection. (Negative value means "vasoconstriction" .) Each point represents the mean ± SD of 5 experiments. $^{**}P < 0.01$: significantly different from control (vehicle alone). **Inlets**. Representative cerebral angiograms after the cisternal injection of ox-RBC ghosts (left) and non-ox-RBC ghosts (right).

To clarify the roles of Mφs and their interaction with RBC ghosts in the vasospasm, we examined the immediate effect of simultaneous administration of the ox- or non-ox-RBC ghosts along with exudated peritoneal Mφs (Fig. 3). The intracisternal injection of ox-RBC ghosts along with Mφs induced cerebral vasospasm far earlier than that induced by the injection of ox-RBC ghosts alone: the time to reach the maximal vasoconstriction (82 ± 4.5% of control values, significantly different from vehicle group) was markedly shortened to around 2.5 hours. The injection of non-ox-RBC ghosts plus Mφs was without effect on the caliber of basilar artery, as was the injection of ox-RBC ghosts, non-ox-RBC ghosts or Mφs alone (data not shown).

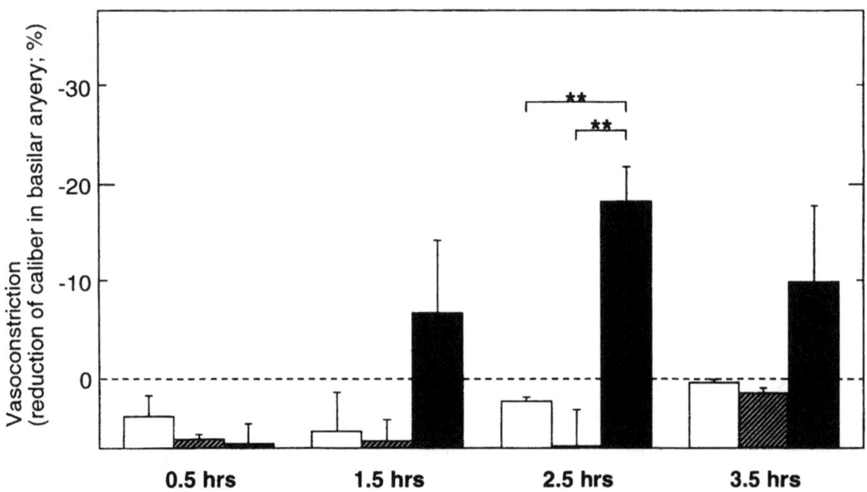

Fig. 3. Vasoconstricting actions by "Mφs along with RBC ghosts" on cerebral artery *in vivo*. Time courses of changes in caliber of rabbit basilar artery after "PBS", "non-ox-RBC ghosts + Mφs" or "ox-RBC ghosts + Mφs" were injected. Symbols are same as Fig.2. The values mean the percentages of calibers at each time points after the injection to those before the injection. Each point or bar represents the mean ± SD of 5 experiments. $^{**}P < 0.01$: significantly different from control.

Mφs are reported to synthesize and release a potent vasoconstricting peptide endothelin[5], the concentration of which is elevated in the cerebrospinal fluid from SAH patients[10]. In addition, several researchers reported that blockers of endothelin type A receptor (ET_AR) and/or ET_BR inhibited experimental cerebral vasospasms[11, 12, 13], although the origin of endothelin has not been elucidated. Therefore, we tested the effect of a blocker for ET_AR (FR-139317, 1 μmol/L) or for ET_BR (BQ-788, 10 μmol/L) on our models induced by coinjection of Mϕs and ox-RBC ghosts. Notably, either FR-139317 or BQ-788 reversed the vasospasm (120 ± 5.3 or 105 ± 7.6% of the caliber before the injection, respectively; significantly different from Mϕ + ox-RBC group: 82 ± 4.5%), whereas these blockers by themselves produced no effect on control arteries. These results suggest that endothelins released from Mϕs in subarachnoid space induce the cerebral vasospasm via ET_AR and ET_BR.

To verify that the vasoconstriction is induced by direct interaction of Mϕs with arteries, we attempted to reproduce the Mϕs-induced vasoconstriction with isolated rabbit thoracic aortic rings *in vitro* (Fig. 4). As in the experiments *in vivo*, application of Mϕs in combination with ox-RBC ghosts directly induced a significant vasoconstriction (6.6 ± 2.7% of 10 μmol/L-noradrenaline-induced vasoconstriction), whereas that of either non-ox-RBC ghosts, ox-RBC ghosts, Mϕs or Mϕs plus non-ox-RBC ghosts had little effect on the tension (not detected, not detected, 0.5 ± 0.3 or 0.7 ± 0.4% of 10 μmol/L-noradrenaline-induced vasoconstriction, respectively; significantly different from Mϕ + ox-RBC group). The magnitude of this vasoconstriction is relatively small, however, it was reproducible and significant.

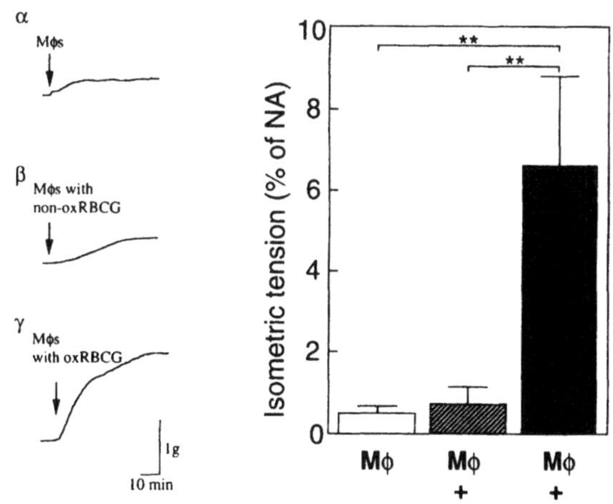

Fig. 4. Direct vasoconstricting action of "Mϕs with or without ox- or non-oxRBC ghosts" on isometric tension of rabbit aorta. Representative tracings of vasoconstriction by Mϕs with or without ox- or non-oxRBC ghosts (left α, β, γ). The values mean the percentages to the induced tension with 1 μmol/L noradrenaline. Each bar represents the mean ± SD of 5 experiments. $**P < 0.01$: significantly different from control.

To investigate the interaction between Mϕs and RBC ghosts, peritoneal Mϕs were incubated with fluorescent-dye-labeled ox- or non-ox-RBC ghosts. After the incubation with ox-RBC ghosts, many Mϕs showed the fluorescence derived from the ghosts which were either bound or phagocytosed (Fig. 5 α and β). In contrast, in the case of the non-ox-RBC ghosts, few of Mϕs showed significant fluorescence (Fig. 5 γ and δ). These data show that the ox-RBC ghosts were preferentially recognized by Mϕs.

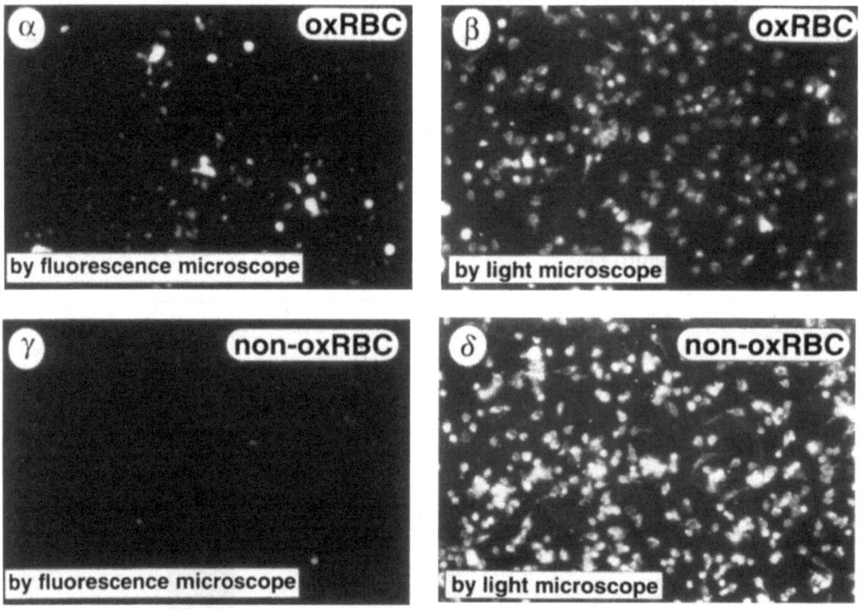

Fig. 5. Interaction between Mϕs and RBC ghosts. α, β; Recognitions of Fast DiO-labeled ox-RBC ghosts to Mϕs. γ, δ.; Recognitions of Fast DiO-labeled non-ox-RBC ghosts to Mϕs. Mϕs were incubated with the RBC ghosts prelabeled with Fast DiO at 37 °C for 20 min and photographed with fluorescent (α, γ) or light (β, δ) microscopy in a magnifying power (x40).

Discussion

Reactive infiltration of Mϕ into the blood clot in the subarachnoid space and phagocytosis of RBCs by Mϕ are one of the prominent histological features of the brain after SAH[2, 3, 4]. Some investigators pointed that the time course of the phagocytotic activity of Mϕ seems to coincide with that of vasospasm[14, 15], however, the causal relationship between Mϕ and cerebral vasospasm has never been clarified. In the present study, we showed that infiltrated Mϕs into subarachnoid space induced a delayed cerebral vasospasm. The vasoactivity was promoted by the interaction with ox-RBC ghosts. We confirmed the direct vasoconstricting activity of Mϕ by isometric tension study with rabbit aorta in the present study because rabbit basilar artery is not suitable for the measurement of isometric tension or perfusion pressure with Mϕ and RBC ghosts because of technical problems. It was too small to attach to the pellet of Mϕ and RBC ghosts stably.

Monocyte in blood is known to infiltrate into inflammatory focus, mature to Mϕ and is activated after inflammatory stimulations, so that there is an interval before a significant monocyte-mediating inflammation. It is known that expression of monocyte chemoattractant peptide and beginning of infiltration of Mϕ take 6 hours after trauma in central nervous system[18]. When foreign body is injected into subarachnoid space, Mϕ is recognized to be infiltrated there on the day 2 and the infiltration becomes remarkable on the day 4[19]. In this study, the significant infiltration of Mϕ were recognized on the day 3 but not at 8 hours after an intracisternal injection of ox-RBC ghosts. Our results are consistent with those past results about the time course for infiltration of Mϕ. On the other hand, a simultaneous injection of exudated Mϕ with ox-RBC ghosts showed a significant vasoconstriction much earlier than the vasoconstriction by injection of ox-RBC ghosts alone. But it did not appear instantly, actually took about 2.5 hours to induce a maximal vasoconstriction. The Mϕs seems to take around 2.5 hours for the maximal activation by the interaction with ox-RBC. According to these all findings, Mϕ needs certain periods for infiltration and activation after SAH. If we can regard the Mϕ-induced vasospasm as one of the etiologic factors for the cerebral vasospasm after SAH, these periods may explain the delay of the onset of cerebral vasospasm after SAH, like the period for hemolysis which produces vasoconstricter oxyhemoglobin explains the delayed onset of the vasospasm.

Endothelin has been suspected as one of the most important spasmogens and numerous groups reported that experimental cerebral vasospasms after SAH were significantly inhibited by endothelin receptor inhibitors[11, 12, 13]. Our results are consistent with these experiments. Although it was reported that thrombin or oxyhemoglobin increased endothelin secretion from cultured endothelial cell[20, 21], endothelial cell may not be the most important origin of endothelin as an ethiologic factor of cerebral vasospasm after SAH because extra-arterial application of endothelin seems to be much more effective to constrict artery than intraarterial application of it[22]. So it may be reasonable to consider infiltrated Mϕ in subarachnoid space as the main origin of endothelin in the cerebral vasospasm after SAH.

Further understanding of the Mϕ-induced vasoconstriction may be important not only for the study of cerebral vasospasm after SAH but for the studies of other vascular diseases.

References

1. Weir B, Macdonald L, Stoodley M (1999) Ethiology of cerebral vasospasm. Acta Neurochir 72: 27-46
2. Hammes Jr EM (1944) Reaction of the meninges to blood. Arch Neurol Psychiat 52: 505-514
3. Jackson IJ (1949) Aseptic hemogenic meningitis. Arch Neurol Psychiat 62:572-589
4. Hughes JT, Schianchi PM (1978) Cerebral artery spasm. J Neurosurg 48:515-525
5. Martin-Nizard F, Houssaini HS, Lestavel-Delattre S, et al (1991) Modified low density lipoproteins activate human macrophages to secrete immunoreactive endothelin. FEBS Lett 293:127-130
6. Sambrano GR, Parthasarathy S, Steinberg D (1994) Recognition of oxidatively damaged erythrocytes by a macrophage receptor with specificity for oxidized low density lipoprotein. Proc Natl Acad Sci USA 91:3265-3269
7. McEvoy L, Williamson P, Schlegel RA (1986) Membrane phospholipid asymmetry as a determinant of erythrocyte recognition by macrophages. Proc Natl Acad Sci USA 83:3311-3315
8. Komuro T, Miwa S, Minowa T, et al (1997) The involvement of a novel mechanism distinct from the thrombin receptor in the vasocontraction induced by trypsin. Br J Pharmacol 120:851-856
9. Yanamoto H, Kikuchi H, Okamoto S (1992) Preventive effect of synthetic serine protease inhibitor, FUT-175, on cerebral vasospasm in rabbits. Neurosurgery 30:351-357
10. Suzuki H, Sato S, Suzuki Y, et al (1990) Increased endothelin concentration in CSF from patients with subarachnoid hemorrhage. Acta Neurol Scand 81:553-554
11. Zimmermann M, Seifert V (1998) Endothelin and subarachnoid hemorrhage: an overview. Neurosurgery 43:863-876
12. Nirei H, Hamada K, Shoubo M, et al (1993) An endothelin ETA receptor antagonist, FR139317, ameliorates cerebral vasospasm in dogs. Life Sci 52:1869-1874
13. Zuccarello M, Boccaletti R, Romano A, et al (1998) Endothelin B receptor antagonists attenuate subarachnoid hemorrhage-induced cerebral vasospasm. Stroke 29:1924-1929
14. Jackowski J, Crockard A, Burnstock R, et al (1990) The time course of intracranial changes following experimental subarachnoid hemorrhage in rat. J Cereb Blood Flow Metab 10:835-849
15. Kubota T, Handa Y, Tsuchida A, et al (1993) The kinetics of lymphocyte subsets and macrophages in subarachnoid hemorrhage in rats. Stroke 24:1993-2001
16. Zubukov Y, Rollins S, Parent D, et al (2000) Mechanism of endothelin-1-induced contraction in rabbit basilar artery. Stroke 31: 526-533

17. Komuro T, Miwa S, Zhang X-F, et al (1997) A physiological role of Ca2+-permeable nonselective cation channel in endothelin-1-induced contraction of rabbit aorta. J Cardiovasc Pharmacol 30:504-509
18. Berman JW, Guida MP, Warren J, et al (1996) Localization of monocyte chemoattractant peptide-1 expression in the central nervous system in experimental autoimmune encephalomyelitis and trauma in the rat. J Immunol 156:3017-3023
19. Yanamoto H, Kikuchi H, Okamoto S, et al (1994) Cerebral vasospasm caused by cisternal injection of polystyrene latex beads in rabbits is inhibited by a serine protease inhibitor. Surg Neurol 42:374-381
20. Yanagisawa M, Kurihara H, Kimura S, et al (1988) T A novel potent vasoconstrictor peptide produced by vascular endothelial cells. Nature 332:411-415
21. Cocks TM, Malta E, King SJ, et al (1991) Oxyhemoglobin increases the production of endothelin-1 by endothelial cells in culture Eur J Pharmacol. 196:177-182
22. Shigeno T, Mima T, Takakura K, et al (1989) Endothelin-1 acts in cerebral arteries from the adventitial but not from the luminal side. J Cardiovasc Pharmacol 13:S174-S176

7. Developments in brain-imaging technology

Evaluation and analysis of brain attack using MR functional imaging

Chuzo Tanaka, Toshihiko Ebisu, Masahiro Umeda , Ichio Aoki , Masaki Fukunaga, Yasuharu Watanabe, Yoshiaki Someya , Yuki Mori, and Shoji Naruse

Medical MR Center, Meiji University of Oriental Medicine, Hiyoshi-cho, Funai-gun, Kyoto 629-0392, Japan

Summary: Recent advances in magnetic resonance (MR) have made possible not only anatomical but functional mapping of the brain. The advantages of functional mapping with MRI are that the procedure is non-invasive, gives high temporal and spatial resolution, and makes use of equipment widely in the clinic. We introduce several new methods of detecting stroke lesions and evaluating the pathophysiology of cerebral ischemic disorders using a clinical 1.5T and an experimental 4.7T MR apparatus, including 1) a MR diffusion technique to detect acute stroke, 2) a MR perfusion technique to evaluate stroke areas using both spin labeling and Gd-dynamic susceptibility methods, 3) the basic and clinical application of fMRI, 4) activity-induced manganese (AIM) MRI for functional mapping and detecting acute ischemic lesions in experimental animals, and 5) multi-slice MR spectroscopic imaging to observe brain metabolites of cerebral ischemia and brain tumors. We emphasize that MR functional mapping of the brain has excellent potential for detecting acute stroke lesions and evaluating cerebral perfusion, cerebral function, and cerebral metabolism in clinical fields. Moreover, these methods should be useful for analyzing the pathophysiolgy of ischemic brain, especially when determining the therapeutic time window in acute cerebral ischemia.

Key words: Brain attack, Cerebral perfusion, Diffusion weighted image, fMRI, MRS

Diffusion-weighted imaging of acute stroke

With the report by Moseley, et al. [1, 2] that diffusion-weighted magnetic resonance imaging (DWI) sensitively detected super acute ischemic stroke within minutes after vascular occlusion in animals [1-3], DWI was predicted to become a useful tool for detecting very early ischemic injury in patients [4, 5]. The ultra fast capabilities of echo planar imaging (EPI) without motion artifacts have made this form of DWI a routine clinical examination for brain attack [6]. In patients with super acute infarction within 6 hours after the onset of symptoms, changes that have not been depicted on T2-weighted images are detectable with DWI [6, 7]. It was also reported that the DWI technique helped discriminate areas of acute infarction (decreased apparent diffusion coefficient [ADC]) from chronic infarction (increased ADC) [7, 8] (Fig. 1). Diffusion-weighted imaging (DWI) is now a promising technique for the early detection of cerebral infarction in routine clinical practice.

From the point of view of acute stroke, discriminating acute infarction from acute cerebral hemorrhage is important because these diseases require quite different therapies. Since conventional magnetic resonance imaging (MRI) modalities have difficulty in diagnosing hemorrhage in the first 24 hours, conventional computed tomography (CT) is currently used [9].

In this study, we determine if diffusion-weighted EPI (DWEPI) and T2-weighted EPI (T2WEPI) can detect acute hemorrhagic stroke, including acute intracerebral hemorrhage and hemorrhagic infarction, as well as acute nonhemorrhagic infarction, and distinguish between them. Our additional aim was to compare hemorrhagic stroke with nonhemorrhagic stroke in the temporal evolution of ADC and signal intensity of T2WEPI.

Materials and methods

Patient Selection: Overall, 118 MRI examinations were performed. Eighty-nine examinations were performed on 27 nonhemorrhagic infarctions in 19 patients at various intervals after the onset. Twenty-nine examinations were also performed on 7 hemorrhagic strokes in 6 patients. This group included 11 examinations on 4 intracerebral hemorrhages and 18 examinations on 3 hemorrhagic infarctions. The patient population consisted of 12 males and 7 females, aged 36-88 (mean, 68.6) years for nonhemorrhagic stroke; and 4 males and 2 females, aged 51 - 80 years (mean, 69.0 years) for hemorrhagic stroke. Four stages of evolving hemorrhagic and nonhemorrhagic stroke were defined: acute (first 3 days), subacute (4 - 10 days), early chronic (11 - 30 days), and late chronic (older than 31 days). To obtain information as to whether hemorrhage truly occurred, some of the following imaging modalities were performed in all patients: T1-weighted spin echo (T1WSE) at 3 - 13 days, T2-weighted fast spin echo (T2WFSE) later than 14 days, and CT scan within 3 days.

MR Imaging: All MRI studies were performed using a 1.5-T whole-body imager (Signa Horizon; GE Medical Systems, Milwaukee, WI) capable of EPI. Single shot DWEPI (b = 1736 s/mm2) and T2WEPI (b = 0 s/mm2) images were obtained in all 118 examinations. Imaging parameters for spin echo DW- and T2WEPI were repetition time (TR) = 6500 ms, echo time (TE) =120 ms, field of view (FOV) = 40 cm, matrix = 128x128 pixels, slice thickness = 7 mm, and 15 to 20 axial multislices with no gap. The five b values used were 0, 108, 434, 976, and 1736 s/mm^2. These gradients were applied in the anterior-to-posterior (phase-encoding) direction. The ADC map was calculated from the 5 different b values. The region of interest (ROI) was taken from the central core of the lesion and a comparably contralateral area. The relative ADC (rADC) and relative T2WEPI (rT2W), the ratio of lesion-to-control regions, were calculated for evaluation of ADC and T2WEPI signal intensities to compensate the global differences in each MR parameter that are independent of pathological changes. In the core with heterogeneous intensity, average values were used for these evaluations. Both T1WSE (TR/TE = 400 ms/9 ms, FOV = 24 cm, matrix = 256 x 256 pixels) and T2WFSE (TR/TE = 3000 ms/126 ms, echo-train length [ETL] = 12, FOV = 24 cm, matrix = 256 x 256 pixels) images were also obtained from the same slices used for DWEPI and T2WEPI.

Results

Acute and Subacute Stages: All acute nonhemorrhagic stroke lesions (n = 20) displayed hyperintensity on DWEPI and a decreased ADC relative to normal brain tissue within 2.5 hours of the onset (Fig. 1, 2). However, isointensity relative to the contralateral control was detected in 6 of 20 measurements (30%) on T2WEPI, and in 4 of 19 (21 %) on T2WFSE. In the first 15 hours, isointensity was evident in 4 of 5 measurements (80%) on T2WEPI and in 3 of 4 (75%) on T2WFSE .

Similarly, hemorrhagic stroke including intracerebral hemorrhage and hemorrhagic infarction at acute and subacute stages, also demonstrated hyperintensity or heterogeneous hyperintensity on DWEPI within 4 hours. The ADC was also decreased in the core of the lesions, similar to nonhemorrhagic stroke at the same stages (Fig. 3). However, in contrast to nonhemorrhagic stroke showing isointensity or hyperintensity on T2WEPI, hypointensity mixed with hyperintensity was demonstrated in hemorrhagic stroke on T2WEPI (Fig. 3).

Early and Late Chronic Stages: The nonhemorrhagic stroke showed DWEPI hyperintensity in only 14 of 25 lesions (56%) during the early chronic stage and none of 30 lesions (0 %) during the late chronic stage, although hyperintensity was shown in 22 of 25 lesions (88%) on T2WEPI and all 24 lesions (100%) on T2WFSE during the early chronic stage and in all 30 lesions (100%) on both T2WEPI and T2WFSE during the late chronic stage. In contrast, all 9 hemorrhagic lesions including both intracerebral hemorrhage and hemorrhagic infarction showed hyperintensity or heterogeneous hyperintensity on DWEPI and mixed hypointensity with hyperintensity on T2WEPI during the early chronic stage. During the late chronic stage (>31 days), hemorrhagic lesions still showed hyperintensity or hyperintensity with hypointensity on DWEPI in 9 of 13 examinations (69%).

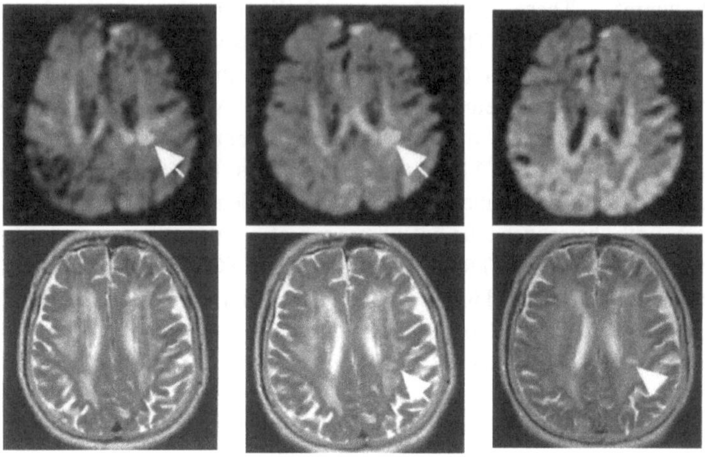

a 13 hours **b 7 days** **c 90 days**

Fig. 1a, b, c Time course of cerebral infarction in images of DWI (upper) and T2w (lower). In the super acute (**a** 13h after onset) and subacute (**b** 7 days after onset) stages, the infarcted area exibits high signal intensity in the DW images (arrow), however in the chronic (**c** 90 days after onset) stage, the area shows isointensity. On the other hand, T2w images did not show this area in the super acute stage but showed the high intensity area in the subacute and chronic stages (arrow).

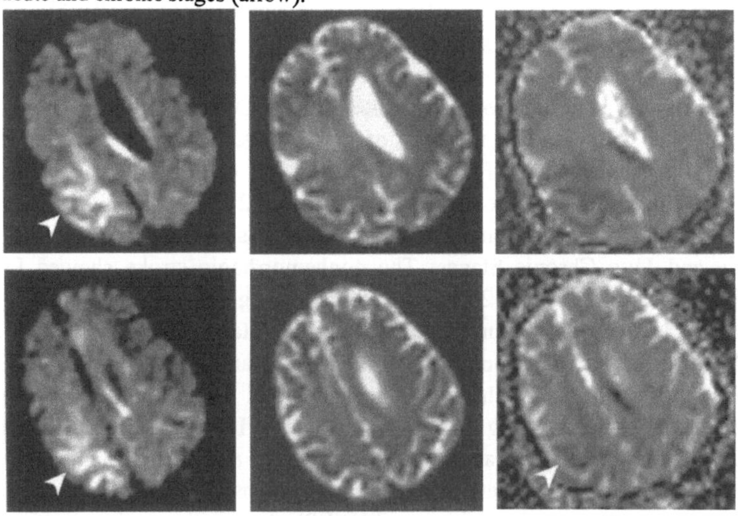

a DWI **b T2w image** **c ADC images**

Fig. 2a, b, c Images of acute infarction were obtained in a 76-year-old female patient at 2.5 hours after the onset of a sudden loss of consciousness, right-ward conjugate deviation, and left hemiplegia. **a** Diffusion-weighted EPI (b = 1736) demonstrated gyral hyperintensity in the right frontoparietal area (arrows). Hyperintensity due to anisotropy was also evident on the other side of the deep white matter and corpus callosum. **b** In contrast to diffusion-weighted EPI, T2-weighted EPI showed signal of normal intensity in this lesion. **c** The calculated ADC map showed decreased ADC in this lesion.

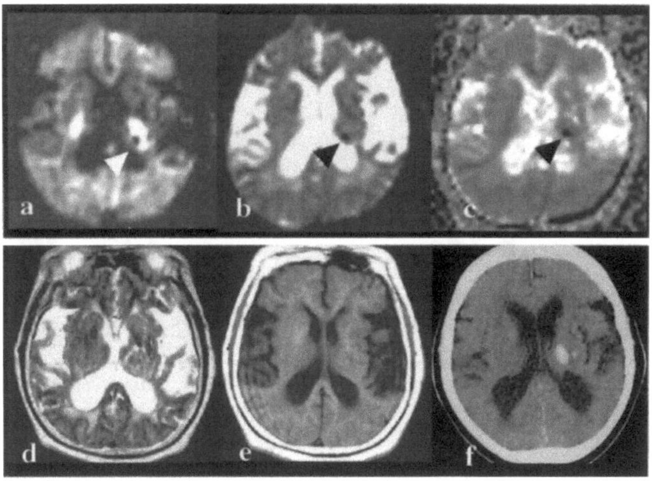

Fig. 3a, b, c, d, e, and f Images of left thalamic hemorrhage were obtained in an 80-year-old female patient at 4 hours after the onset of sudden right hemiplegia and gait disturbance without loss of consciousness. **a** Diffusion-weighted EPI (b=1736) indicated hyperintensity, together with some hypointensity (arrow) in the upper part of the left thalamus and deep white matter, although the outer zone of this area may include hyperintensity due to white matter anisotropy. This finding was also observed on the other side of the deep white matter. Markedly atrophic hemispheres were also evident. **b** T2-weighted EPI showed heterogeneous signal intensities including hypointensity (aroow), probably due to deoxyhemoglobin-induced magnetic susceptibility in acute hemorrhage. **c** ADC image: The area with a decreased ADC and diffusion-weighted hyperintensity included both hypointensity and (arrow) hyperintensity areas on T2-weighted EPI. **d** T2-weighted FSE showed heterogeneous hyperintensity, not specific for the hemorrhagic condition, in this lesion. **e** No abnormal intensity was evident on T1-weighted SE. **f** A CT scan, just after the MR examination, showed high density spots in this lesion. A similar distribution was observed between areas of high density on CT and decreased ADC.

Evolution of Signal Intensities and ADC: The time course of rADC and rT2W in the core of the nonhemorrhagic infarction, intracerebral hemorrhage, and hemorrhagic infarction is shown in Figure 3 a) and b). Within 10 days of the onset, both nonhemorrhagic and hemorrhagic stroke similarly revealed a decreased rADC. In contrast, large differences in signal intensities on T2WEPI were observed between nonhemorrhagic infarction and hemorrhagic lesions. The rT2W in hemorrhagic stroke was decreased, whereas it was normal to increased in nonhemorrhagic stroke. Subsequently, although rADC gradually increased in nonhemorrhagic infarction, it tended to remain decreased in hemorrhagic lesions even 100 days after the onset. There was also a tendency for rT2W to be consistently lower in hemorrhagic lesions than nonhemorrhagic infarction.

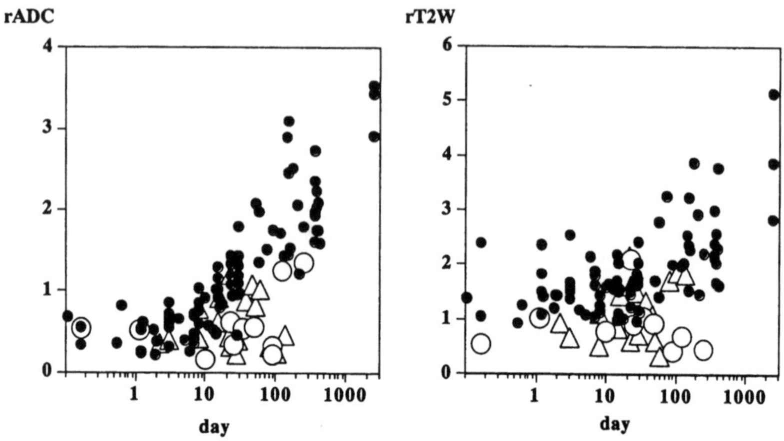

a b

Fig. 4a, b Scatter plots of the time course after the onset versus rADC **(a)** and rT2W **(b)** in patients with nonhemorrhagic infarction (●), intracerebral hemorrhage (○), and hemorrhagic infarction (△). Within 10 days of the onset, all strokes similarly showed decreased rADC. In contrast, the rT2W was decreased in hemorrhagic stroke but increased in nonhemorrhagic stroke. Subsequently, although rADC gradually increased in nonhemorrhagic infarction, it tended to remain decreased in hemorrhagic lesions even 100 days after the onset. The rT2W was consistently lower in hemorrhagic lesions than that nonhemorrhagic infarction.

Discussion

The three major findings of this study were: 1) ADC was decreased in the lesions of acute hemorrhagic stroke, as well as in the lesions of acute nonhemorrhagic stroke. 2) The acute hemorrhagic stroke included a hypointensity area on T2WEPI, in contrast to the normal to increased signal intensity of acute nonhemorrhagic stroke. 3) The decrease in ADC tended to persist longer in hemorrhagic stroke than nonhemorrhagic stroke.

Using conventional MRI, diagnosing acute hemorrhagic lesions, especially within 24 hours of onset, has been reported to be difficult, because hemorrhage in this period predominantly affects intracellular oxyhemoglobin without any paramagnetic effect, resulting in neither T1 nor T2 shortening [9 - 12]. The only finding would be T2-weighted hyperintensity, which is not specific for hemorrhage [9, 12]. In this period, conventional MRI is less sensitive than CT for the detection of hemorrhage [9]. However, in our results, hyperintensity on DWEPI and decreased ADC were demonstrated in the core of acute hemorrhagic stroke, initially at 4 hours, similar to those in nonhemorrhagic stroke. One possible explanation for the decreased ADC in the core of acute hemorrhage is the heavily impeded mobility of water caused by high viscosity [13] in acute hematoma, similar to that in gel. In fresh hematoma, thrombosis progresses, plasma is resorbed, and red blood cells with an intact membrane conglomerate, leading to a high concentration of red blood cells [9, 10 , 12, 14]. These concentrated intact blood cells and the formation of fibrin clots [13] may cause the decrease in ADC. A second axplanation for the decreased ADC in acute hemorrhagic stroke might simply be cytotoxic edema as in nonhemorrhagic stroke; the brain tissue might well become ischemic because blood is leaking out of the capillary bed and perfusion pressure may be locally reduced.

In Fig. 3, the area of decreased ADC was wider than the area of hypointensity on T2WEPI. The former which could indicate fresh gel-like hematoma, may include areas of both oxyhemoglobin-induced heterogeneous hyperintensity on T2WEPI and hypointensity on T2WEPI caused by deoxyhemoglobin, a minor component of hematoma in the first 4 hours [9]. Thus, the ADC map may provide unique information regarding the characteristics, fluid or solid, of hematoma other than hemoglobin evolution.

Acute hemorrhagic and nonhemorrhagic stroke could be discriminated based on T2WEPI signal intensity. Signal intensity was significantly lower in the core of acute hemorrhagic stroke than nonhemorrhagic stroke. Because the EPI sequence is very sensitive to magnetic susceptibility interference[15], this reduction in signal may be caused by a shortening of T2 due to intracellular deoxyhemoglobin [9, 10]. Thus, the combination of DWEPI and T2WEPI may be an excellent tool for the diagnosis of acute cerebrovascular diseases including both hemorrhagic and nonhemorrhagic stroke.

In our experiment on nonhemorrhagic stroke, data on the evolution of DWEPI signal intensity and ADC were consistent with those in previous reports [7]. The decrease in rADC in nonhemorrhagic stroke lasted about 10 days. In contrast, rADC in the core of hemorrhagic stroke was significantly decreased even at early and late chronic stages. A possible explanation for the persistent reduction of ADC in chronic hemorrhagic stroke is the high cellularity of infiltrative inflammatory cells and macrophages with or without hemosiderin and ferritin as well as concentrated hematoma clots with high viscosity [9, 10, 16]. In our recent reports, the pus fluid in the core of a brain abscess also showed markedly decreased ADC [17]. Thus, it is speculated that persistent reduction of ADC in the chronic hemorrhage could be caused by the high cellularity of infiltrative inflammatory cells and high viscosity, similar to pus fluid. In Fig. 3, the area with decreased ADC was wider than the area of hyperintensity with a rim of hypointensity on T2WEPI and T2WFSE. Furthermore, a decrease in ADC was observed in areas of both hyperintensity and hypointensity in these sequences. Therefore, the decrease in ADC in the chronic stage may not be caused by intracellular methemoglobin, extracellular methemoglobin or hemosiderin.

Because of the limited sample size for hemorrhagic cases especially at the acute stage, further study based on a large population may be needed. Despite this limitation, our findings are consistent with the hypothesis that a combination of DWEPI and T2WEPI may be an excellent diagnostic tool for acute cerebrovascular diseases including both nonhemorrhagic and hemorrhagic stroke

[18]. Furthermore, a knowledge of DWEPI hyperintensity in acute hemorrhagic stroke may be important in avoiding mis-diagnoses of acute DWI hyperintensity.

Cerebral perfusion imaging of cerebral disorders

Cerebral perfusion imaging with FAIR: Acetazolamide effects and clinical applications

Recently, cerebral perfusion MRI without contrast medium has been performed using an ultra fast imaging technique, echo planar imaging (EPI) [19, 20]. Cerebral perfusion-weighted images with FAIR (flow-sensitive alternation inversion recovery) employs a very simple pulse sequence to detect perfused blood in the brain. Thus, with the FAIR technique, two images are acquired consecutively, each after a fixed delay period subsequent to the inversion pulse; in one, the inversion pulse is slab selective and in the other it is non-selective. The difference image generated from this pair is a flow-sensitive image. Fig. 5 shows a normal human cerebral perfusion-weighted image (PWI). In this image, cerebral cortex, basal ganglia, and thalamus were clearly demonstrated, though white matter showed no or very low signal intensity due to the poor S/N ratio of perfused blood. However, only a few reports have examined the basic clinical usefulness of this type of perfusion imaging. The purpose of this study is to determine if MR perfusion imaging can demonstrate the effect of acetazolamide on human cerebral blood flow, and to examine its clinical usefulness in various cerebral disorders.

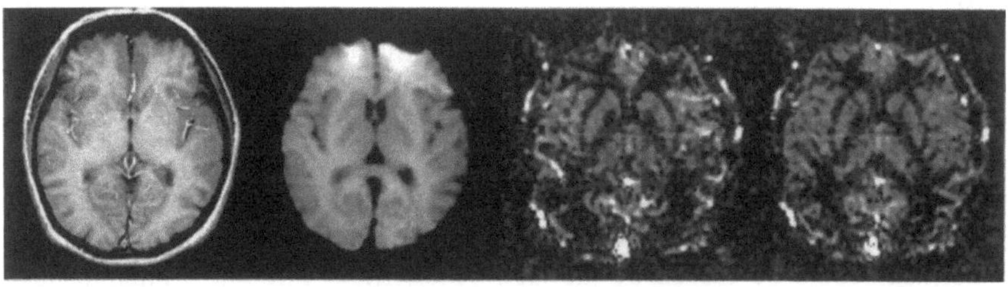

SPGR **IR-EPI** **TI=900ms** **TI=1200ms**

Fig .5. FAIR images of normal brain. SPGR: Gradient echo image, IR-EPI: Original Image, TI (inversion time)=900 ms and 1200 ms: FAIR images at different TIs. The original image was T1w using the inversion recovery method and though it showed white matter with high signal intensity, FAIR images showed no signal in white matter due to low perfusion. With a long TI, cortical signal was strengthed by peripheral labeling spins.

Materials and methods

Cerebral perfusion images with FAIR were obtained using a standard head coil on a 1.5 T clinical MRI scanner (Signa Horizon, GE). Six healthy volunteers were studied before and after intravenous administration of 500 mg of acetazolamide

(Lederle, Inc.). Measurements were performed 3 or 4 times before and 10 times after the administration of acetazolamide every 6 min. Forty-one clinical patients, including 22 with cerebral infarction (15 acute and 7 chronic), 2 with hematomas (1 acute and 1 old), 3 with TIA or RIND, 3 with IC occlusion, 6 with brain tumors, and 5with miscellaneous , were also studied by the FAIR technique.

Parameters for the FAIR sequence were Tr/Te/TI: 2 s/21 ms/1.2 s, slice thickness/slice thickness of a selective inversion:10/16.5 mm, matrix: 96x96 and FOV (field of view): 24 cm. Selected inversion was conducted using an adiabatic pulse. The number of acquisitions was 25 and 50 images for acetazolamide and clinical experiments. Statistical analyses of the results of the acetazolamide experiment were performed by repeated ANOVA using Stat-View software (Abacus Concepts, Inc.) on a Macintosh computer (Apple Computer, Inc.).

Results

1) Acetazolamide experiment: the signal intensity in the perfusion-weighted images increased after the administration of acetazolamide in bilateral occipital cortices, thalamus and putamen (Fig. 6). The ROIs in these regions showed p values of <0.001, <0.5 and <0.1, respectively. This result was consistent with the well-known effect of acetazolamide to increase cerebral blood flow in brain tissue.

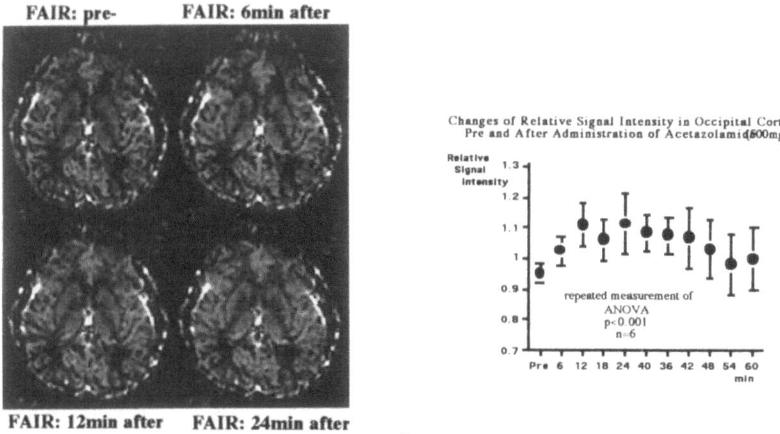

a b

Fig. 6a, b Effect of acetazolamide (500mg, iv) detected using FAIR. **a** FAIR images of pre- and post- (6, 12, 24 min) administration. Signal intensity increased after acetazolamide administration. **b** The signal intensity of the occipital cortex was significantly increased by the administration, resulting in increased cerebral blood flow.

2) Clinical application of perfusion-weighted images: the acute cerebral infarction of lacuna type, was detected as an area of low perfusion in three cases within 5 days of a stroke (Fig. 7a). An acute embolic stroke lesion was detected as an area of high perfusion in three cases within 7 days and in one case within 1 month of a stroke (Fig. 7b). Lesions of an old cortical infarction or old

intracerebral hemorrhage were detected as areas of low perfusion. However, one old lacuna infarction could not be detected. A bifrontal arachnoid cyst showed no perfusion. A cerebellar cystic metastatic tumor showed low perfusion and a parasagittal small meningioma showed hyper perfusion. A large metastatic tumor, a glioblastoma and a convexity meningioma showed a heterogeneous intensity due to heterogeneously perfused areas.

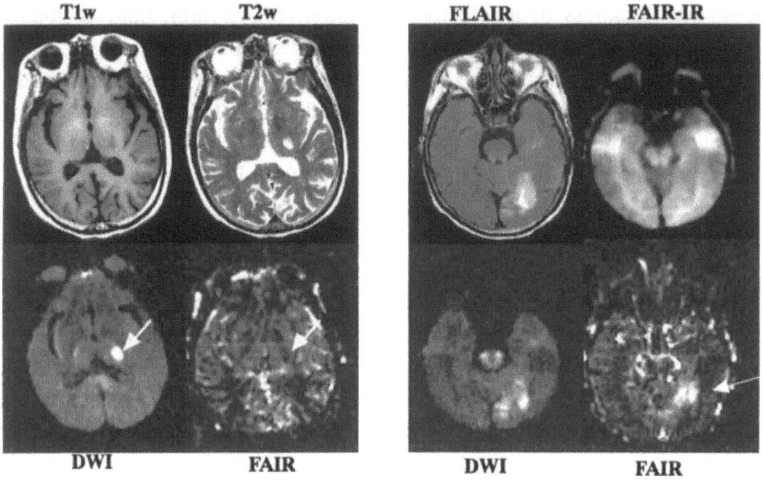

a b

Fig. 7a, b FAIR images of cerebral thrombosis and cerebral embolism . **a** A small right thalamic infarction (arrow), 4 days after onset, is well demonstrated by a loss of signal in this FAIR image. **b** Left occipital embolic infarction, 3 days after onset, showed hyperperfusion, which was detected as an area of high signal intensity, using FAIR.

Discussion

Using FAIR technique, we obtained perfusion-weighted images in all cases with a clinical MR apparatus. The images showed high signal intensity in the thalamus, basal ganglia and cerebral cortex and low signal intensity in white matter. These results correlated well with obtained by other methods like PET and SPECT. The great advantage of MR perfusion imaging is it provides images without a contrast medium. Moreover, with perfusion imaging it is easy to observe the time course of ischemia after a stroke. In a few cases, the images failed to show cerebral blood flow because of motion artifacts in restless patients. The FAIR technique has a relatively low S/N ratio compared with Gd-dynamic contrast imaging, so more technical improvements are necessary before if can be put to general use.

After the acetazolamide administration, perfusion images showed no remarkable signal changes in white matter. Moreover, in the case of lacuna infarction, perfusion-weighted images did not reveal the ischemic regions in white matter, which showed low intensity in T1W and high intensity in T2W images. These findings mean that it was difficult to detect low perfusion lesions in low perfusion areas like white matter using perfusion-weighted imaging.

In conclusion, perfusion imaging has excellent potential for the diagnosis of various diseases, examinations of pathophysiology and evaluatation of treatment.

Clinical applications of cerebral perfusion imaging using Gd-dynamic susceptibility method

Recently, a method of cerebral perfusion imaging with or without contrast medium has been established using MRI [19 - 23]. However, only a few basic studies on the clinical usefulness of perfusion imaging have been reported.

The purpose of this study is to compare the results of various types of MR perfusion-weighted imaging (PWI), namely FAIR or Peak images, CBV (cerebral blood volume) images, relative CBF (cerebral blood flow) images, MTT (mean transient time) images, and TTP (time to peak) images, using Gd-dynamic contrast in clinical practice.

Materials and methods

Cerebral perfusion imaging with a Gd-susceptibility contrast method was performed using a standard head coil on a 1.5 T clinical MRI scanner (Signa Horizon, GE). Twenty eight clinical patients, including 12 with cerebral infarction (9 acute and 3 chronic), 1 with acute hematoma , 3 with TIA or RIND, 3 with IC occlusion, 6 with brain tumors, and 3 with miscellaneous, were studied by MR perfusion imaging using a FAIR and Gd-dynamic contrast method.

The parameters of FAIR were as above. The parameters for the Gd-susceptibility contrast method were Tr/Te: 2 s/21 ms, slice thickness/slices:5 mm/6, matrix:128x128 and FOV:24 cm. After the recording of 10 consecutive images, 0.2 mmol/Kg of Gd-DTPA (Magnevist; Shering) was injected manually within 4-8 seconds and a total of 60 images per slice were taken in 2 minutes. Image processing for the Gd-dynamic study was performed by both gamma fitting and poly fitting using MRVision software (MRVision Inc.) on a Sun ultra30 computer (Sun Microsystems, Inc.) and each perfusion image, including a Peak image, CBV image, relative CBF image, MTT image, and TTP image, was calculated.

Results

Both FAIR and Gd-perfusion imaging could detect areas of low perfusion in acute cortical infarction 3 hours after onset (Fig. 8). In two cases of internal carotid artery occlusion, an abnormal perfused area was evident in the territory of the middle cerebral artery (MCA) in the Gd-perfusion but not the FAIR image. In one case an abnormal perfused region was detected only in the TTP image and this region was almost the same as that in the CBF image obtained by PET (Fig. 9). All acute cortical infarctions showed a abnormal perfused region in every image. A small cerebral infarction of lacuna type was not detected using either the Gd-perfusion or FAIR image. Brain tumors showed heterogeneous perfused regions in all the perfusion images.

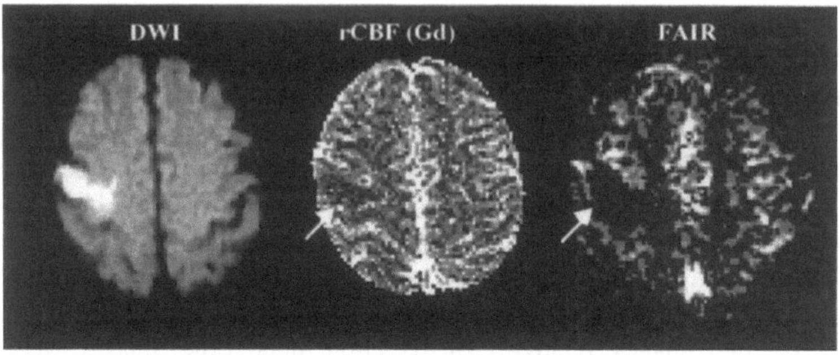

Fig. 8. Right frontal cortical infarction 3 hours after onset. The DW image shows an area of markedly high intensity in the frontal cortex whereas both the Gd-PW (middle) and FAIR images (right) show low intensity, as low perfusion, in the area (arrow).

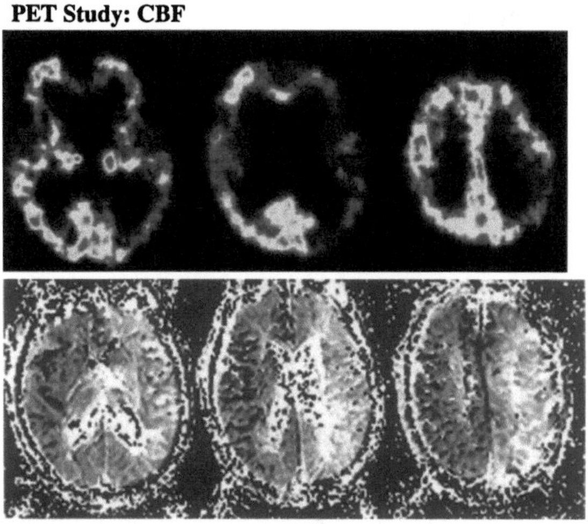

Fig. 9. PET and Perfusion-weighted images for a left MCA occlusion. Both images show low cerebral blood flow in the left MCA territory. The patient had symptoms of dementia.

Discussion

In this study, we obtained perfusion-weighted images using both the Gd-dynamic and FAIR methods. In particular, Gd-susceptibility contrast imaging provided very interesting findings in case of acute stroke including low perfusion of IC occlusion, no changes in TIA, and a focal hyperemic response to subacute cortical infarction. Both perfusion-weighted images had limitations for detecting a low perfused area in the case of lacuna infarction in white matter. Though the quantitative analysis of cerebral blood flow was difficult using Gd-susceptibility methods [24], these techniques are easy to use clinically and take only a few minutes.

In conclusion, perfusion imaging has good potential for the diagnosis of disease, for examining pathophysiology and for evaluating treatment.

Functional MRI and its clinical applications

Functional magnetic resonance imaging (fMRI) is a useful tool for the functional mapping and analysis of activated brain [25, 26]. FMRI is based on BOLD (blood oxygen level dependent) contrast, first described by Ogawa, et al [27] in rat brain studies and subsequently used to generate functional images in human brain. BOLD contrast originates from the intravoxel magnetic field inhomogeneity induced by paramagnetic deoxyhemoglobin in red blood cells. Magnetic susceptibility differences between deoxyhemoglobin-containing compartments (blood vessels) and the surrounding area generate magnetic field gradients across and near the boundaries of these compartments. Therefore, signal intensities in MR images sensitized to BOLD contrast are altered if the regional deoxyhemoglobin content is perturbed. This occurs in the brain because of spatially specific metabolic and hemodynamic responses to enhanced neuronal activity; it has been suggested that regional blood flow (CBF) increases but the oxygen consumption rate ($CMRO_2$) is not elevated in the same way [28, 29], and as a result there is a lower deoxyhemoglobin content per unit volume of brain tissue. Consequently, the signal intensity in BOLD sensitive images increases in regions of the brain activated by a "task" compared to areas in a resting, basal state.

In clinical examinations for neurosurgery, the presurgical evaluation of the location of the eloquent cortex and tumor or AVM is important [30]. Recently, Mueller et al. used fMRI in patients in which more than 2 cm separated the border of the tumor from the activated motor area and no decline in motor function occurred after surgical resection [31]. Other clinical studies using fMRI examined the central sulcus and lateralization of the dominant hemisphere [32, 33]. However, motion artifacts can affect the clinical application of fMRI. As it is difficult for patients with neurological deficits to keep their head still during motor tasks, sensory stimulation is useful for determination of the sensoriomotor cortex using fMRI. In this study, we investigated the usefulness of sensory stimulation in clinical fMRI.

Materials and methods

Eleven normal volunteers and 25 patients with neurological disorders were examined in an activation study using clinical a 1.5 T MRI (Signa Horizon; GE-YMS). Using gradient echo echo planar imaging (GE-EPI), fMRI provided 120 images per slice with the following parameters; Tr/Te/FA/slices: 2000ms/50ms/90o/5-7, FOV: 24c, and Matrix: 96 x 96. The slice thickness was 5mm and 20 slices covered the brain. Brain activation was achieved using sensory stimulation, including somatosensory stimulation, visual stimulation with a checkerboard pattern using a projector, and auditory stimulation with earphones. Patients with lesions near the motor cortex were examined using two kinds of activation tasks, finger opposition and somatosensory stimulation. For somatosensory stimulation, the patient's hand or foot was rubbed with a sponge every 20 seconds. Anatomical images were also obtained using a conventional 2D and 3D imaging sequence. The parameters of the spin echo T1w image were Tr/Te/FOV = 500ms/9ms/24cm and of the 3D gradient echo image were Tr/Te/FA//thickness = 11.4ms/2.1ms/15o/1mm. Statistical analysis was performed by a cross correlation method using MRVision software (MRVision company) and motion artifacts were analyzed using SPM (Statistical Parametric Mapping: free software; Neurological Institute, London) or MEDx software (Sensory Systems Inc.).

Results

In the control, the central sulcus was detected using the anatomical method in all cases with three dimensional images. fMRI was also performed in all cases using both motor task and somatosensory stimulation. Figure 10 shows the sensoriomotor area activated by finger tapping, which was overlayed on the three dimensional anatomical image with the central sulcus obtained by the anatomical method [34]. The activated area was divided into motor and sensory areas by the central sulcus. This finding showed that the anatomical map of the primary motor and sensory cortex was consistent with the functional map.

In all patients, using somatosensory stimulation of the palm and foot, activated areas in the sensoriomotor cortex were certainly detected using fMRI. Areas activated by the motor task could not be detected in 2 cases. Moreover, to obtain activated areas, subject had to repeat the motor task 2 or 3 times in several cases. In many cases, the area activated by sensory stimulation was of almost the same intensity as that for the motor task. In a 19 year old female with right frontoparietal arteriovenous malformation (AVM), activated areas in both the right and left motor cortices were detected with the left finger opposition task. However, the activated area was only detected in the left sensoriomotor cortex with the right finger opposition task. In this case, the area activated by left finger opposition was also located in the AVM (Fig. 11) [35]. In a case of left temporal malignant glioma, the right-handed patient did not complain of speech disturbance. Using a word listening task, neither Wernicke's area nor the dominant hemisphere could be detected using fMR images and the bilateral temporal lobes were activated (Fig. 12). Furthermore, the functional map superimposed on a 3 D image was very useful for evaluating the relationship between the activated area of the sensoriomotor cortex and the central sulcus.

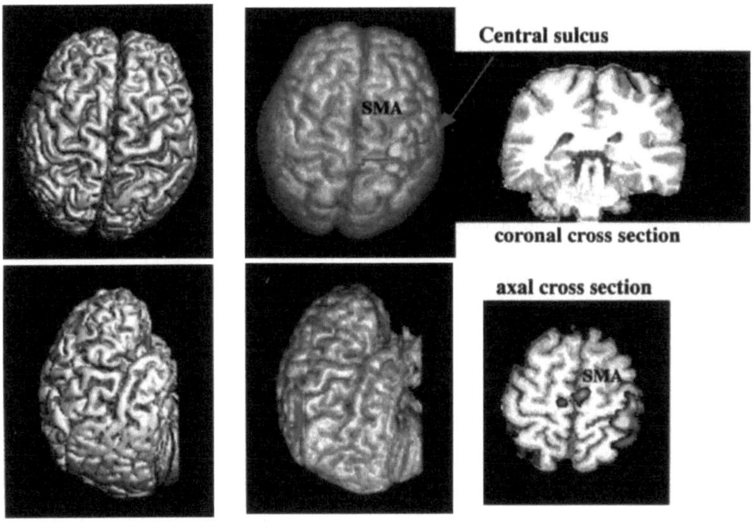

Fig. 10. Functional MRI showing areas activated by the right finger opposition task (orange to yellow) and central sulcus (SC) obtained by an anatomical method (blue line). The left sensoriomotor cortex, supplementary motor area (SMA), and SC were superimposed on 3D surface images and cross-sectional images. The sensoriomotor cortex was divided by the SC same as in the anatomical map.

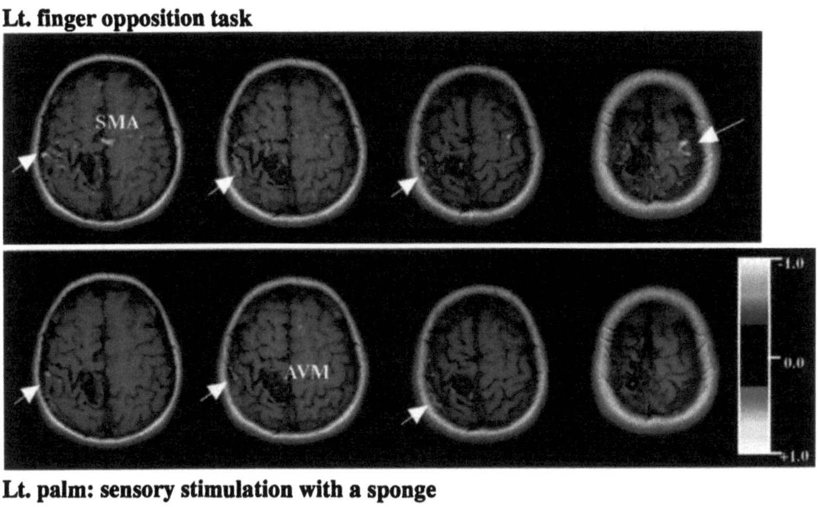

Fig. 11. Functional MRI of the right fronto-parietal AVM (right handedness) using left finger opposition (upper) and left sensory stimulation of palm (lower). Though sensory stimulation activated only the right sensoriomotor cortex, the motor task activated both cortices (arrow). Moreover, the activated area included the AVM itself.

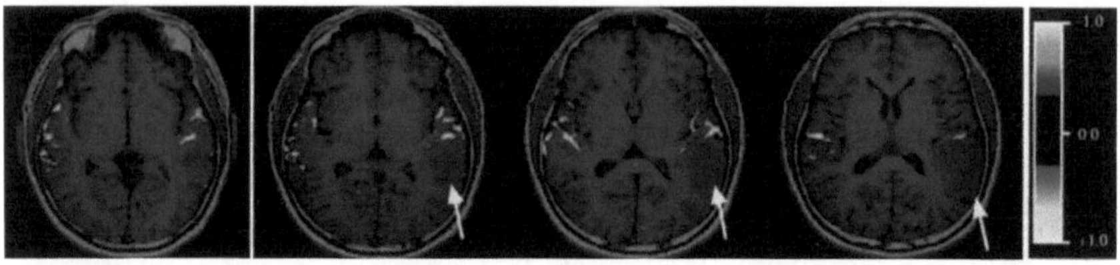

Fig. 12. Functional MRI of left temporal glioblastoma (right handedness) using listening word. The low intensity area (arrow) is a glioblastoma and perifocal edema. Bilateral auditory areas were activated by word listening and no laterality appeares in these images. This patient exhibited no disturbance of speech or hearing function.

Discussion

Functional mapping using sensory stimulation on 3 D images was very useful to determine the relationship between the sensoriomotor cortex and brain tumor or vascular lesions. Three dimensional anatomical images were also useful to confirm the central sulcus using anatomical method. These images were helpful for presurgical evaluation of brain tumors and AVM. However, in previous reports using clinical fMRI, the main activation task was the motor task. Motion artifacts with motor tasks may seriously affect the clinical application of fMRI. Therefore, a standard clinical fMRI study should be performed with a 1.5 MR apparatus. Our recommended activation tasks were sensory, somatosensory, visual, and auditory stimulations to diminish motion artifacts[36].

Detection of acute cerebral ischemic core using AIM MRI

Recently, a new method of functional MRI, named Activity-Induced Manganese dependent (AIM) MRI, has been introduced which is independent of hemodynamic changes [37]. This method uses manganese as an MRI detectable contrast agent. Manganese ion (Mn^{2+}) acts in a manner similar to calcium ion (Ca^{2+}) in many biological systems [38, 39] and is known to enter cells through ligand-gated or voltage-gated Ca^{2+} channels during nerve action potentials [40, 41] In addition, the properties of Mn^{2+} as an MR contrast agent are that it shortens both the T1 and T2 relaxation times of water proton. AIM MRI is expected to map brain activation at high signal-to-noise (SNR), contrast-to-noise (CNR), and spatial/temporal resolution.

In this study, functional mapping to detect the ischemic core of a super acute rat MCAO (middle cerebral artery occlusion) model was performed using AIM MRI.

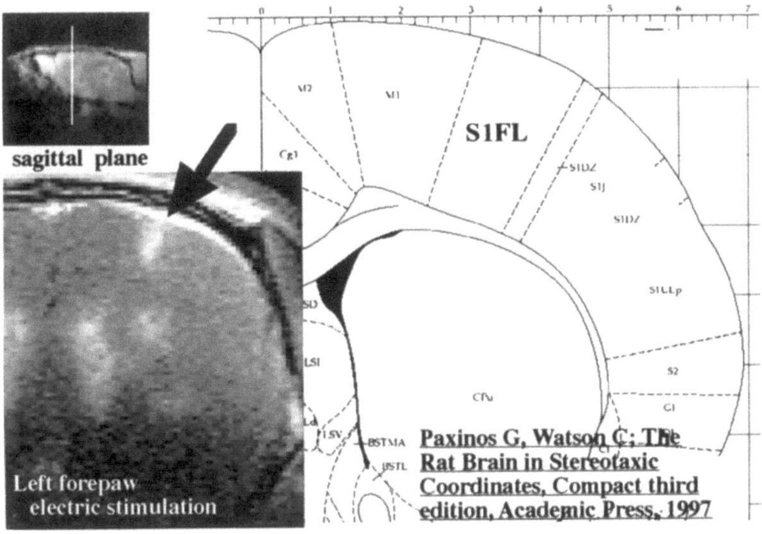

Fig. 13. AIM MRI of left forepaw electric stimulation in rat. S1FL (primary sensory cortex of foreleg) and caudate nucleus were enhanced by Mn administration on opening of the blood brain barrier using electric stimulation.

Materials and methods

Animal preparation: Male Wistar rats (307 ± 14g, Shimizu Experimental Animals, Japan) were divided into 2 groups: a sham operated control (n = 5) and the MCAO model (n = 5). Rats were initially anesthetized with diethyl ether (Nacalai Tesque, Inc., Japan), orally intubated, and then ventilated with a 1.2-1.5 % halothane and 1:1 oxygen / nitrous oxide-oxygen gas mixture using a rodent ventilator (Model 683, Harvard Instruments, MA). Polyethylene catheters (PE-50, Becton Dickinson, MD) were placed in the femoral artery and vein for drug administration and blood pressure monitoring, and in the right external carotid artery for drug administration into the right common carotid artery. In addition, the MCAO suture method was performed via the right common carotid artery. Blood pressure, blood gas, and body temperature were maintained in physiological ranges.

After the operation, pentobarbital (50 mg/kg, Dainippon Pharmaceutical Co. Ltd, Japan) was injected intraperitoneally to suppress neural activation not related to anoxic depolarization by MCAO. A D-mannitol solution (25 %, 5 ml/kg, Sigma, MO) was infused at a speed of 50.0 ml/h from the right external carotid artery into the common carotid artery while maintaning the temperature. At 15 minutes after pentobarbital injection, a manganese chloride solution (10mM, Sigma, MO) was infused at a speed of 60 μmol/h (4.5 ml/h) from the right external carotid artery into the common carotid artery.

MRI Measurements: Data acquisition was performed on a 4.7-T horizontal MRI (CSI-II-Omega, Bruker, Germany) with a shielded gradient coil 65 mm in diameter. A homemade 25 mm surface coil that fitted the head was used. Body temperature was maintained at approximately 37 °C by passing warm air in the magnet-bore during scanning. MRI measurements were started 20 minutes after the occlusion. Two sets of T1-weighted coronal images for which the slice offset was changed (0 or 1 mm), were obtained using a spin-echo sequence with the following parameters: TR/TE= 400/12 ms, matrix size = 256 x 256, FOV = 28 mm, slice thickness = 1 mm, number of acquisitions = 8, number of slices = 8, slice gap = 1 mm, and acquisition time for one set = 13.7 minutes. T2-weighted images and DWI (b value = 1922 mm2/s) were also obtained using the spin-echo sequence at a slice orientation the same as the T1W.

Results

T1-weighted Imaging: Typically, a marked enhancement of signal intensity was observed on the lateral side of the caudate-putamen, and lateral cortex including piriform cortex in the T1W images after manganese administration in the MCAO group (Fig. 14). In contrast, there was no or less signal enhancement in the vertex area of the cortex including the primary and secondary motor cortex, medial side of the caudate putamen, thalamus, hypothalamus and ventricles. There was no peak in the sham group.

Diffusion-weighted Imaging and ADC: While the high intensity area of T1W was restricted to the lateral side of the caudate-putamen and lateral cortex, the hyper intensity area of DWI or the low value area of ADC extended throughout the hemisphere. However it is. difficult to compare them because the scanning time-point was not the same, the high intensity area of T1W was smaller than the and high intensity area of DWI and the low value area of ADC. In the T2W images, signal enhancement that corresponded with the area of high DWI or low ADC was not observed.

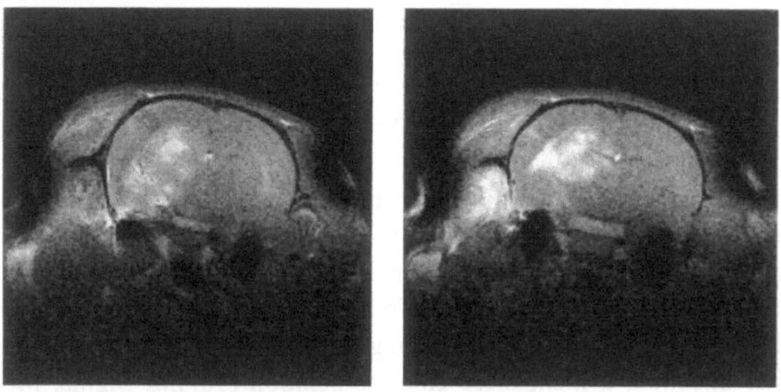

Fig. 14. AIM MRI of right MVAO in rat. In the brain, acute ischemic core was enhanced by Mn administration. It as considered that the enhancement of these regions was caused by anoxic depolarization.

Discussion

The signal enhancement in the MCAO model was detected using manganese enhanced T1W MRI in the rat brain. DWI MRI can detect an acute brain ischemia. However, the whole region that indicates high signal intensity on DWI (or a low value in the ADC map) did not directly correspond with the irreversibility of neurons. In a recent study, ischemic penumbra was considered a region of both mildly increased intensity for DWI and moderately decreased cerebral blood flow. Therefore, the ischemic core and ischemic penumbra could not be detected by the single imaging method. In this study, we identified the ischemic core using manganese-enhanced T1w MRI. This method is clearly a new approach using anoxic depolarization for in vivo experimental cerebral ischemia. In this experiment, deep anesthesia was used to suppress normal depolarization. In addition, no stimulation was used except for occlusion. Therefore, it is quite likely that the influx and accumulation of Mn caused by anoxic depolarization gave the T1W contrast on the MCAO group. Furthermore, it is possible that this enhanced region contains the irreversible area in which necrosis is unavoidable even after reperfusion, or the region that is known as the necrotic infarct core.

Mapping of brain metabolites on brain disorders using multi-slice proton magnetic resonance spectroscopic imaging

Proton magnetic resonance spectroscopy (^{1}H-MRS) using a clinical 1.5T apparatus is a method used to detect cerebral metabolites such as aminoacids, creatine (Cr), choline (Cho), and lactate. In clinical use, ^{1}H-MRS can reveal early ischemic regions with increased lactate signal and decreased N-acetyl aspartate (NAA). Though ^{1}H-MRS has the advantage of detecting cerebral metabolites, it is not yet a common clinical tool due to the single voxel measurement method, which shows brain metabolites in only one small volume within a limited examination time.

Since 1990, MR Spectroscopic Imaging (MRSI) or chemical shit imaging (CSI), a method of making multi voxel measurements by MRS, has been put to clinical use [42, 43]. But this method can measure only one slice [44]. In clinical use, the detection of brain metabolites from whole brain is needed. Therefore, we have performed multi-slice MRSI using a 1.5T clinical MR apparatus (Signa Advantage, GE, Milwaukee).

Materials and methods

Normal volunteers and patients with several kinds of cerebral disorders were examined using the following parameters; Tr/Te=2.3s/280ms, slice thickness/gap/slices=15/3.5mm/4, phase encoding=32 and FOV=24cm. Four slice images of NAA , Cr , Cho and lipid (Lip)/Lac were obtained in about 34 minutes. Water suppression was performed using a CHESS pulse. Outer volume suppression for lipid signals of the scalp was applied with an exogonal shape.

Results and discussion

In control cases, ventricles showed regions of low signal intensity due to a lack of metabolites in CSF in images of NAA, Cr, and Cho. At the level of the third ventricle, marked signal loss in the deep frontal region was observed in all images. This signal loss was considered due to the susceptibility of sphenoidal and ethomoidal air sinuses. Images of Cr and Cho showed area of very high intensity in the cerebellum compared with the cerebrum. This means a high concentration or changes in relaxation time for both Cr and Cho in the cerebellum. In cerebral infarctions at the chronic stage (9 months after stroke), though NAA images showed no signal intensity in the infarcted lesion, Cr and Cho images showed mildly high intensity in the infarction (Fig. 15). In general, glial cells contained no NAA but contained Cr and Cho. Therefore, the tissues in this lesion mainly consisted of glial cells. MRSI was very useful for revealing the metabolic condition of the infarcted lesion, but it was not always adequate for the analysis of the metabolic condition for acute strokes because of the relatively long clinical examination time at present [45]. In the case of brain tumor, though NAA images showed no or hypo- signal intensity in the tumor, Cr and Cho images showed areas of iso or slightly high signal intensity in the tumor (Fig. 16). The Cho signal for MR spectroscopy mainly consisted of phospholylcholine, which is a precursor of membrane phospholipid. Therefore, the increase in Cho signal suggested membrane synthesis and/or degradation [46]. Characteristic findings of ^{1}H-MRS of malignant brain tumor were a high signal intensity of Cho and an increased Lac signal. In this case, however, there was no lactate signal and a mild increase in Cho signal in the legion. Therefore, although these findings suggested neuronal loss and tumor growth in the lesion, they were not indicative of a pure malignant tumor. The pathological diagnosis of this tumor was glioma grade II and was not inconsistent with the results of MRSI.

In conclusion, MRSI has excellent potential for evaluating metabolism in the brain and cerebral disorders.

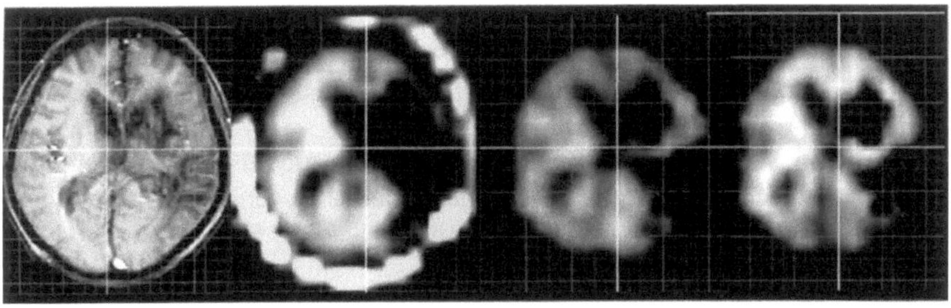

MRI **NAA** **Cr** **Cho**

Fig. 15. MR spectroscopic images of chronic cerebral infarction (9 months after onset). NAA image: N-acetyl aspartate, Cho image:Choline, Cr/Pr image:creatine/phosphocreatine. The NAA iamge shows an area of very low signal intensity in the left MCA territory, resulting in loss of neuronal cells. In this infarcted area, both Cho and Cr images show an area of norm signal intensity, which was suspected to be gilial tissue without neurons.

T1w-MRI **NAA** **Cho**

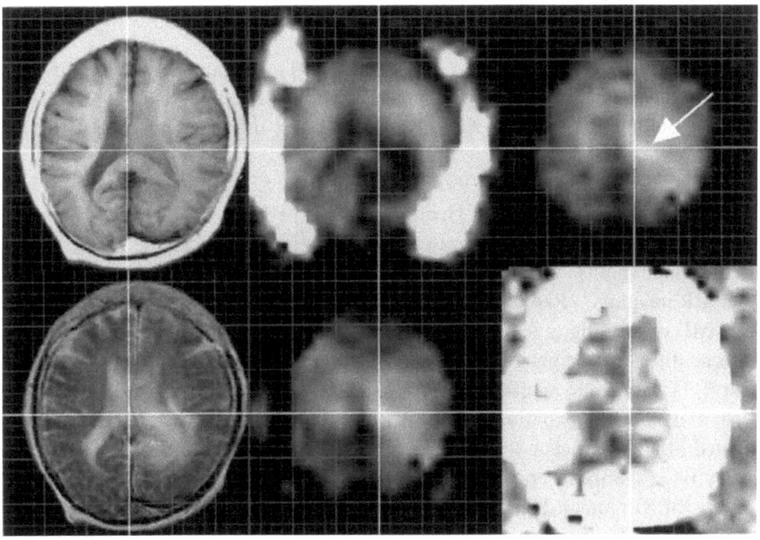

T2w-MRI **Cr/PCr** **Lac/Lipid**

Fig. 16. MR spectroscopic images of a low grade astrocytoma. NAA: N-acetyl asparatate, Cho:choline, Cr/Pcr:ceatine/phosphocreatine, Lac/Lipid: lactate/lipid. The NAA images shows an area of low signal intensity in the habenula of the corpus callosum and surrounding tissue, resulting in a loss of neuronal cells. In this area, both Cho and Cr images showed a region of norm or high signal intensity (arrow), which was considered to reflect increased membrane synthesis creating tumor cells. There was no lactate signal in the tumor. Lactate signal was seen in the malignant tumor or prefifocal edema surrounding the meningioma, therefore this tumor was considered to be a low grade glioma based on this preoperative MR spectroscopic image.

Acknowledgement

We thank Mr. Kiyotaka Katsuta and Mr. Akihiko Fujikawa for their technical advice on this experimental procedures.

This work was supported by Special Coordimation Funds for Promoting Science and Technology of the STA of the Japanese Government and also partly supported by Japan Society for the Promotion of Science; Research for the Future Program (No. 97L00204).

References

1. Moseley ME, Cohen Y, Mintorovitch J, et al (1990) Early detection of regional cerebral ischemia in cats: Comparison of diffusion- and T2- weighted MRI and spectroscopy. Magn Reson Med14: 330-346
2. Moseley ME, Kucharczyk J, Mintorovitch J, et al (1990) Diffusion-weighted MR imaging of acute stroke: correlation with T2-weighted and magnetic susceptibility-enhanced MR imaging in cats. AJNR 11: 423-429
3. Knight RA, Ordidge RJ, Helpern JA, et al (1991) Temporal evolution of ischemic damage in rat brain measured by proton NMR. Stroke 22: 802-808
4. Chien D, Buxton RB, Kwong KK, et al (1990) MR diffusion imaging of the human brain. J Comput Assist Tomogr 14: 514-520
5. Warach S, Chien D, Li W, et al (1992) Fast magnetic resonance diffusion-weighted imaging of acute human stroke. Neurology 42: 1717-1723
6. Sorensen AG, Buonanno FS, Gonzalez RG, et al (1996) Hyperacute stroke: evaluation with combined multisection diffusion-weighted and hemodynamically weighted echo-planar MR imaging. Radiology 199: 391-401
7. Marks MP, de Crespigny A, Lentz D, et al (1996) Acute and chronic stroke: navigated spin-echo diffusion-weighted MR imaging. Radiology 199: 403-408
8. Ebisu T, Katsuda K, Fujikawa A, et al (2001) Early and delayed neuroprotective effects of FK506 on experimental focal ischemia quantitatively assessed by diffusion-weighted MRI. Mag Reson Imaging, 19: 153-160
9. Bradley WG (1993) MR appearance of hemorrhage in the brain. Radiology189:15-26
10. .Gomori JM, Grossman RI, Goldberg HI, et al (1985) Intracranial hematomas: imaging by high field MR. Radiology 157: 87-92
11. Clark RA, Watanabe AT, Bradley WG, et al (1990) Acute hematomas: effect of deoxyhemoglobin, hematocrit, and fibrin-clot formation and retraction on T2 shortening. Radiology 174: 201-206
12. Hayman LA, McArdle C, Taber KH, et al (1989) MR imaging of hyperacute intracranial hemorrhage in the cat. AJNR 10: 681-686
13. Kaibara M. (1996) Rheology of blood coagulation. Biorheology 33:101-117
14. Rapoport S, Sostman HD, Pope C, et al (1987) Venous clots: evaluation with MR imaging. Radiology 162: 527-530
15. Edelman RR, Wielopoloski P, Schmitt F (1994) Echo-planar MR imaging. Radiology 192: 600-612
16. Thulborn KR, McKee A, Kowall NW, et al (1990) Role of ferritin and hemosiderin in the MR appearance of cerebral hemosiderin in the MR appearance of cerebral

hemorrhage: a histopathologic biochemical study in rats. AJNR 11: 291-297
17. Ebisu T, Tanaka C, Umeda M, et al (1996) Discrimination of brain abscess from necrotic or cystic tumors by diffusion-weighted echo planar imaging. Magn Reson Imaging 14: 1113-1116
18. Ebisu T, Tanaka C, Umeda M, et al (1997) Hemorrhagic and nonhemorrhagic stroke: Diagnosis with diffusion-weighted and T2-weighted echo-planar MR imaging. Radiology 203:823-82
19. Kim SG (1995) Quantification of relative cerebral blood flow change by flow-sensitive alternation inversion recovery (FAIR) technique: application to functional mapping. Magn. Reson. Med. 34:293-301
20. Edelman RR, Siewert B, Darby DG, et al (1994) Quantitative mapping of cerebral blood flow and functional localization with echo-planar MR imaging and signal targeting with alternating radio frequency. Radiology 192:513-520
21. Zhang W, Williams DS, Koretsky AP (1993) Meausurement of rat brain perfusion by NMR using spin labeling of arterial water: In vivo determination of the degree of spin labeling. Magn. Reson. Med. 29:416-421
22. Kwong KK, Chesler DA, Weisskoff RM, et al (1995) MR perfusion studies with T1-weighted echo planar imaging. Magn. Reson. Med. 34:878-887
23. Rosen BR, Belliveau JW, Chien D (1989) Perfusion imaging by nuclear magnetic resonance. Magn Reson Med 5:263-281
24. Weisskoff RM, Chesler D, Boxerman JL, et al (1993) Pitfalls in MR measurement of tissue blood flow with intravenous tracers;which mean transient time? Magn. Reson. Med. 29:553-559
25. Belliveau JW, Kennedy DNJr, Mckinstry RC, et al (1991) Functional mapping of the humanvisual cortex by magnetic resonance imaging. Science 254: 716-719
26. Ogawa S, Tank DW, Menon R, et al (1992) Intrinsic signal changes accompanying sensory stimulation: functional brain mapping with magnetic resonance imaging. Proc Natl Acad Sci USA 89: 5951-5955
27. Ogawa S, Lee TM, Nayak AS et al (1990) Oxygen sensitive contrast in MRI in rodent brain at high magnetic fields. Magn Reson Med 14: 68-78
28. Fox P, Raichle ME, Focal (1986) physiological uncoupling of cerebral blood flow and oxidative metabolism during somatosensory stimulation in human subjects. Proc Natl Acad USA 83:1140-1144
29. Fox PT, Raichle ME, Mintun MA et al (1988) Nonoxidative glucose consumption during focal physiologic neural activity. Science 241: 462-464
30. Hammeke TA, Yetkin FZ, Mueller WM, et al (1994) Functional magnetic resonance imaging of somatosensory stimulation. Neurosurgery 35: 677-681
31. Mueller WM, Zetkin FY, Hammeke TA, et al (1996) Functional MRI mapping of the motor cortex in patients with cerebral tumors. Neurosurgery 39: 515-520
32. Yetkin FZ, Mueller WM, Morris GL, et al (1997) Functional MR activation correlated with intraoperative cortical mapping. AJNR 18: 1311-1315
33. Binder JR, Swanson S, Hammecke T, et al (1996) Determination of language dominance using functional MRI: a comparison with the Wada test. Neurology 46: 978-984
34. Sobel DF, Gallen CC, Schwartz BJ, et al (1993) Locating the central sulcus: comparison of MR anatomic and MEG functional methods. AJNR 14: 915-926
35. Maldjian J, Atlas SW, Howard RS, et al (1996) Functional magnetic resonance imaging of regional brain activity in patients with intraverebral arteriovenous malformations

before surgical or endovascular therapy. J Neurosurg 84: 477-483

36. Tanaka C, Fukunaga M, Ebisu T, et al (1999) Clinical application of functional MRI. In: Yoshimoto T, Kotani M, SKuriki S, Karibe H, and Nakasato N (Eds.): Recent advances in biomagnetism, Tohoku University Press, Sendai, pp. 868-871
37. Lin YJ, Koretsky AP (1997) Manganese ion enhances T1-weighted MRI during brain activation: an approach to direct imaging of brain function. Magn Reson Med 38:378-88
38. Hunter DR, Komai H, Haworth RA et al (1980) Comparison of Ca2+, Sr2+, and Mn2+ fluxes in mitochondria of the perfused rat heart. Circ Res 47:721-217
39. Shibuya I, Douglas WW (1993) Indications from Mn-quenching of Fura-2 fluorescence in melanotrophs that dopamine and baclofen close Ca channels that are spontaneously open but not those opened by high [K+]O; and that Cd preferentially blocks the latter. Cell Calcium 14:33-44
40. Drapeau P, Nachshen DA (1984) Manganese fluxes and manganese-dependent neurotransmitter release in presynaptic nerve endings isolated from rat brain. J Physiol 348:493-510
41. Narita K, Kawasaki F, Kita H (1990) Mn and Mg influxes through Ca channels of motor nerve terminals are prevented by verapamil in frogs. BrainRes 510:289-295
42. Luyten PR, Marien AJH, Heindel W, et al (1990) Metabolic imaging of patients with intracranial tumors; ^{1}H-MR spectroscopic imaging and PET. Radiology 176:791-799
43. Naruse S, Furuya S, Tanaka C (1996) Functional MRI and magnetic resonance spectroscopy with clinical MRI scanners. In I. Hashimoto, Y.C..Okada & S. Ogawa (Eds): Visualization of Information Processing in the Human Brain; Recent advances in MEG and Functional MRI, Elsevier Science B.V., Amsterdam, pp. 317-330
44. Duyn JH, Gillen J, Sobering G, et al (1993) Multisection proton spectroscopic imaging of the brain. Radiology 188:277-282
45. Takegami T, Ebisu T, Bito Y, et al (2001) Mismatch between lactate and the apparent diffusion coeficient of water in progressive focal ischemia. NMR Biomed. 14: 5-11
46. Bruhn H, Frahm J, Gyngell ML, et al (1989) Noninvasive differentiation of tumors with use of localized H-1 MR spectroscopy in vivo: initial experience in patients with cerebral tumors. Radiology 172:541-548

Key Word Index

MIX
Papier aus verantwortungsvollen Quellen
Paper from responsible sources
FSC® C105338

If you have any concerns about our products,
you can contact us on
ProductSafety@springernature.com

In case Publisher is established outside the EU,
the EU authorized representative is:
Springer Nature Customer Service Center GmbH
Europaplatz 3, 69115 Heidelberg, Germany

Printed by Libri Plureos GmbH
in Hamburg, Germany